Introduction to Sectional Anatomy

Introduction to Sectional Anatomy

Michael E. Madden, PhD, RT(R), (CT), (MR)

Professor

Department of Allied Health

Fort Hays State University

LIPPINCOTT WILLIAMS & WILKINS

A **Wolters Kluwer** Company

Editor: Lawrence McGrew
Associate Managing Editor: Angela Heubeck
Marketing Manager: Debby Hartman
Production Editor: Jennifer D. Weir

530 Walnut Street
Philadelphia, Pennsylvania 19106

351 West Camden Street
Baltimore, Maryland 21201-2436 USA

The publisher is not responsible (as a matter of product liability, negligence, or otherwise) for any injury resulting from any material contained herein. This publication contains information relating to general principles of medical care which should not be construed as specific instructions for individual patients. Manufacturers' product information and package inserts should be reviewed for current information, including contraindications, dosages and precautions.

Printed in the United States of America

Library of Congress Cataloging-in-Publication Data

Madden, Michael E.
  Introduction to sectional anatomy / Michael E. Madden.
    p. cm.
  Includes bibliographical references and index.
  ISBN 0-7817-2105-9
    1. Human anatomy. 2. Magnetic resonance imaging. 3. Tomography. I. Madden,
Michael E. II. Title.

QM23.2 .M325 2000
611--dc21   00-061820

The publishers have made every effort to trace the copyright holders for borrowed material. If they have inadvertently overlooked any, they will be pleased to make the necessary arrangements at the first opportunity.

To purchase additional copies of this book, call our customer service department at **(800) 638-3030** or fax orders to **(301) 824-7390.** For other book services, including chapter reprints and large quantity sales, ask for the Special Sales department.

For all other calls originating outside of the United States, please call **(301)714-2324.**

Visit Lippincott Williams & Wilkins on the Internet: **http://www.lww.com.** Lippincott Williams & Wilkins customer service representatives are available from 8:30 am to 6:00 pm, EST, Monday through Friday, for telephone access.

00 01 02 03 04
1 2 3 4 5 6 7 8 9 10

This book is dedicated to my parents,
Lee and Eddie,
who taught me the value of education
and whose love and support will shape my life forever.

Pronunciation Key

VOWELS

ā	day, care, gauge
a	mat, damage
ă	about, para
ah	father
aw	fall, cause, raw
ē	be, equal, ear
ě	taken, genesis
e	term, learn
ī	pie
ĭ	pit, sieve, build
ō	note, for, so
o	not, oncology, ought
oo	food
ow	cow, out
oy	troy, void
ū	unit, curable
ŭ	cut

Reprinted from *Stedman's Medical Dictionary, 27th Edition/Stedman's Electronic Medical Dictionary, Version 5.0.* Baltimore: Lippincott Williams & Wilkins, 2001 (www.stedmans.com).

CONSONANTS

b	bad
ch	child
d	dog
dh	this, smooth
f	fit
g	got
h	hit
j	jade
k	kept
ks	tax
kw	quit
l	law
m	me
n	no
ng	ring
p	pan
r	rot
s	so, miss
sh	should
t	ten
th	thin, with
v	very
w	we
y	yes
z	zero
zh	azure, measure

Preface

This manuscript was developed from my teaching materials to provide a learning aid for radiologic science practitioners to better understand anatomy in sectional images. Since about 1990, the number of sectional images generated by computerized modalities for diagnostic interpretation has continued to rise dramatically. Recent statistics estimate that approximately one out of every three diagnostic images taken in the clinical setting is a sectional image. Consequently, individuals practicing in medical diagnostic imaging today are required to identify structures in computer-generated slices of the body.

Although the text is at the introductory level, students are expected to have completed one to two semesters of study in anatomy and physiology before attempting to discern sectional images of anatomy. Except for the Introduction, all chapters include an anatomical overview of the structures within the region. The reviews focus on the relationship between structures, because this is critical to understanding anatomy in sectional images. To provide more emphasis on the most clinically relevant information, structures that are not visualized well on diagnostic images or those of little clinical significance are not described.

To provide the reader with the most widely accepted anatomical terminology, the terms used to describe structures are from the accepted standards in the *Nomina Anatomica* adopted by the 12th International Congress of Anatomists, London, England, 1985. Some useful terms not included in the 6th edition of the *Nomina Anatomica* will be found in the text. Also, to help the reader learn the correct pronunciation of unfamiliar terms, phonetic spelling is found in parenthesis immediately following the name of the anatomical structure. A key for pronunciation is found on the page facing this one.

After the "Anatomical Overview," sectional anatomy is described by labeled CT and MR images. CT and MR images of patient scans are included so the reader can focus on the clinical application of this knowledge.

To provide a highly regimented learning tool, all of the chapters except Chapter 1 begin with a series of objectives and conclude with a series of review exercises to evaluate the reader's understanding of the chapter's material. An accompanying review book is also available and corresponds closely with the textbook. Using most of the sectional images from the textbook, the review book asks the reader multiple choice questions in the format used on CT and MR registry examinations. In lieu of traditional slides, the images from the textbook and review book are available in CD-ROM format for use in the classroom by the instructor, along with a test generator for the instructor's use as well.

Although countless hours have gone into researching, writing, and reviewing the text, constructive comments from readers identifying errors or recommending content changes are certainly welcome and appreciated, because they would improve a subsequent edition of the book.

Acknowledgments

This book would not have been possible without the contributions of many individuals and I would like to express my sincere gratitude to the following:

To Janie Meder and Shelly Flax who spent countless hours developing the sectional anatomy drawings.

To Ron Neseth, Jennifer Wagner, and the other faculty at FHSU for providing their support and encouragement.

To all the students that critically reviewed the manuscript and gave me their ideas for improvement.

To Jennifer Smith, the illustrator of the anatomy drawings, for contributing her talent.

All the staff at Lipincott Williams & Wilkins, especially Jennifer Weir, Production Editor, for their expertise and considerable efforts in developing this project for publication.

Most importantly, I wish to thank Theresa, my wife, for providing more love and support than I deserve, and to Levi and Luke, who are my constant source of inspiration.

Contents

Chapter 1

Introduction

Traditional anatomy courses tend to focus primarily on the names and shapes of anatomical structures. By comparison, sectional anatomy places much more emphasis on the physical relationship among structures. To identify anatomical structures on sectional images, a complete understanding of the basic anatomical information is a requisite from which a three-dimensional understanding develops. This textbook follows this organization beginning with an anatomical overview of structures in the region followed by the labeled CT images and MR images. To demonstrate the application of this knowledge, selected pathology is included as supplemental information in the following chapters.

Compared to conventional radiographs, computer-generated sectional images are especially useful when evaluating soft tissue structures and those not clearly displayed owing to adjacent structures. For example, although proper positioning will show much of the bony anatomy in the lateral skull, it provides little diagnostic information of soft tissue structures and demonstrates the right and left sides of the skull superimposed over each other (Fig. 1-1). By comparison, the CT or MR computer-generated sectional images (Fig. 1-2) eliminate overlapping structures, allowing many structures to be more clearly visualized in a nearly endless variety of planes. Although CT and MR will likely never replace conventional radiography because of affordability and diagnostic value in certain situations, these forms of computerized imaging are found in most clinical facilities.

Similar to conventional radiography, CT and MR images are extremely valuable diagnostic tools. However, for these images to be useful clinically, they must accurately depict the region of the patient's anatomy being studied. Because the image is generated by a computer, technical factors can significantly change or alter the resulting image. If the operator has an introductory knowledge of sectional anatomy,

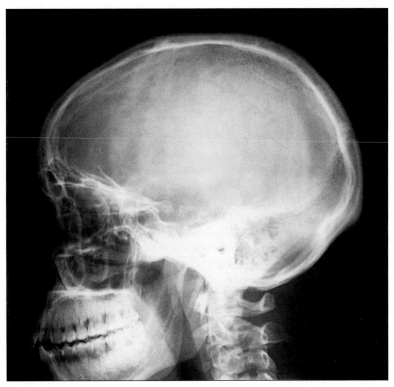

Figure 1-1 Lateral skull radiograph.

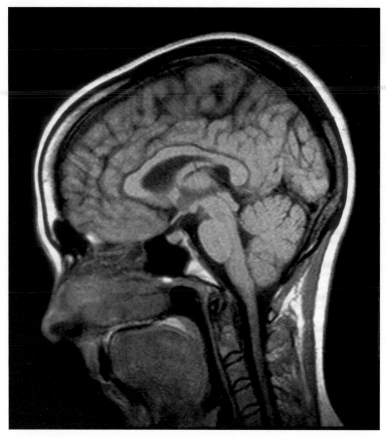

Figure 1-2 Sagittal MR image of head in median plane.

the diagnostic information in the specific region(s) of interest can be altered to best show the patient's condition.

When viewing sectional images, it is important to remember that the image depicts a volume of the body, or what is commonly called a slice of the body (Fig. 1-3). The thickness of the section depends on the technical settings used in generating the sectional images, and usually varies from several millimeters to 1 cm. To visualize all of the structures within a given region of the body, the sections are typically taken in sequence, and the locations are annotated on the scanogram or scout image to provide a regional location. Similar to conventional radiographs, your right side should correspond to the patient's left side. For orientation, when viewing axial images you should picture yourself standing at the patient's feet looking up into the body of the patient with your right always on the left side of the patient. Although *right* and *left* are simple concepts, keeping the proper orientation on sectional images is critical for correct identification of anatomical structures. Initially, the viewer should emphasize whether the structure is on the left or right side of the body.

When viewing sectional images, the initial impulse is to start in the center of the image identifying eye-catching structures without first discerning the location of the scan within the body. Attempting to identify anatomy without first determining the location of the slice will often result in

confusion and errors. Besides the scanogram or scout image that provides general placement, additional information in the image itself can help in more specifically locating the sectioned anatomy. The bones can often provide much of the information necessary to gain a more thoroughly defined perspective. Once this perspective is obtained, identification of structures progresses relatively rapidly and accurately, because the appearance of anatomical structures will vary at different levels (Fig. 1-4).

Unlike learning general anatomy, memorization of vertebral levels or sectional images will lead to mistakes, because no two images will ever be the same. Even if the same patient were scanned at the same level, differences in breathing or involuntary movements would result in a slightly different slice of anatomy. If another patient were used and scanned at the same level, the differences would be even more evident, because their anatomical arrangement would be somewhat different. For example, when we look at people's faces, we see that everyone has two eyes, one nose, and one mouth; but we don't expect the specific arrangement of these structures to be exactly the same for everyone. Just like on the outside, although most people have two kidneys, one superior vena cava, and one aorta, the specific arrangement of these structures will vary from person to person.

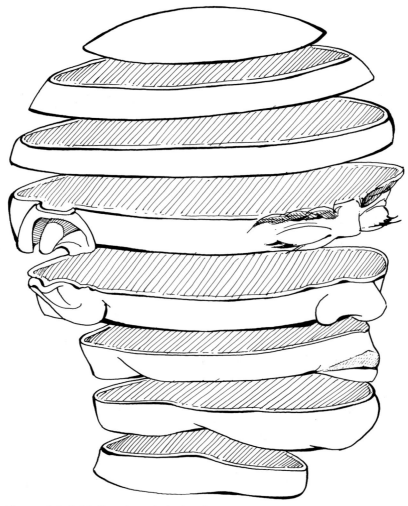

Figure 1-3 Axial slices through the head.

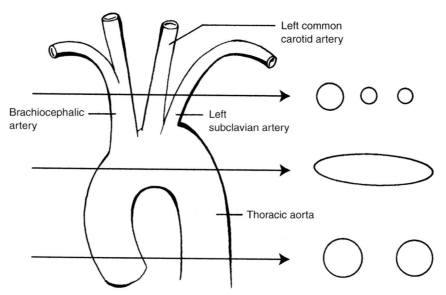

Figure 1-4 The aortic arch demonstrating differences in axial sections taken at several levels.

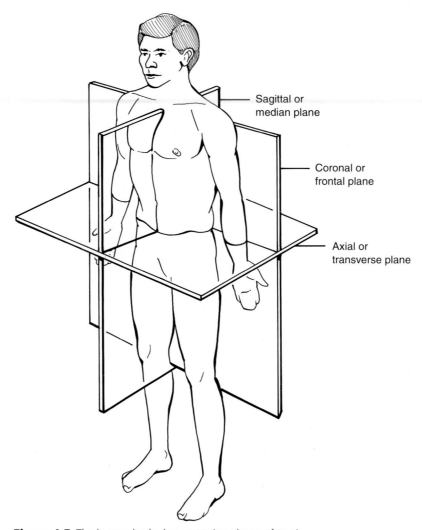

Figure 1-5 The human body demonstrating planes of section.

PLANES OF THE BODY (FIG. 1-5)

Sagittal (*SAJ-i-tăl*). A plane extending along the long axis of the body dividing it into right and left sides.

   Median or midsagittal. A sagittal plane through the body dividing it into equal right and left halves.

Coronal (*KŌR-ŏ-năl*) or **frontal.** A plane extending through the body dividing it into anterior and posterior parts.

Axial (*AK-sĕ-ăl*) or **transverse.** A plane extending across or through the axis of the body, extending from side to side, dividing the body into upper and lower portions.

CLASSIFICATION OF JOINTS

Synarthrosis (*SIN-ar-THRŌ-sis*). An immovable joint with no joint cavity. Examples include the sutures of the cranium and the sternocostal joints.

Amphiarthrosis (*AM-fi-ar-THRŌ-sis*). Slightly movable joints between two bones.

Symphysis (*SIM-fi-sis*). The opposed surfaces of bone are connected through fibrocartilage. Examples include the symphysis pubis and the intervertebral disks.

Syndesmosis (*SIN-dez-MŌ-sis*). The fibrocartilage forms an interosseous ligament between the bones. Examples include the inferior tibiofibular articulation and the bones of the infant skull.

Diarthrosis (*dī-ar-THRŌ-sis*). A freely movable joint that is lubricated by synovial fluid within the joint space. The joints are surrounded by a fibrous capsule lined with synovial membrane, the articular capsule, which is reinforced by ligaments and muscles extending over the joint.

Arthrodia (*ar-THRŌ-dē-ă*). A gliding joint where bones slide face to face and movement is limited by restraining ligaments. Examples include the intercarpal and intertarsal joints.

Ginglymus (*JING-gli-mŭs*). A hinge joint that allows movement in only one plane. Examples include the elbow and the knee joints.

Saddle joint. The opposing bones fit the contour of the other and increase the extent of the hinge movement to include other planes of movement. An example is the first carpometacarpal joint.

Ellipsoid ($\overline{e}$-*LIP-soyd*). A modified ball-and-socket joint in which the opposing surfaces are shaped like a spindle or are ellipsoidal instead of being spherical. An example is the wrist joint.

Trochoid ($TR\overline{O}$-*koyd*). A pivot joint that resembles a pulley and allows movement in a partial ring. Examples include the radioulnar joints.

Enarthrosis (*en-ar-THR$\overline{O}$-sis*). A ball-and-socket joint in which the spherical head fits into a cup-like cavity and provides free movement. Examples include the hip and shoulder joints.

THE HOUNSFIELD SCALE

In CT, x-rays are used to generate the diagnostic information much like conventional radiography. However, the principle of tomography is used to better visualize overlapping structures. Based on a series of complex mathematical processes, the computer reconstructs the image from a series of digital numbers. The numbers generated are registered on the Hounsfield scale by which bone is +1000, water is 0, and air is −1000 (Fig. 1-6). Because CT uses x-rays to generate the image, radiodensity and radiolucency are used to distinguish various tissues within the patient. To enhance the visualization of structures with similar densities, the window level and width can be adjusted to demonstrate only part of the Hounsfield scale.

T1- AND T2-WEIGHTED IMAGES

In MR, the magnetic properties of the hydrogen atoms that constitute 80% of the human body are used to generate data. When the patient is positioned within a strong external magnetic field, the single protons in the hydrogen nuclei align within the field. Radiowaves are then directed at the patient from another angle, causing the nuclei absorbing the energy to flip from their previous positions. Depending on the chemical environment, the hydrogen atoms require different amounts of energy to flip out of the magnetic field. After the termination of the external radio signals, the nuclei within the patient gradually release radio signals as they return to their original state within the magnetic field. Depending on their chemical environment, the hydrogen atoms require different times to return to their original position. The energy released is gathered and used to generate the image; a series of complex mathematical processes produce the digital image. If the technical factors are varied, the signal intensity for a given tissue will change (Fig. 1-7). Similar to CT, adjusting the technical factors can optimize the diagnostic value of the image.

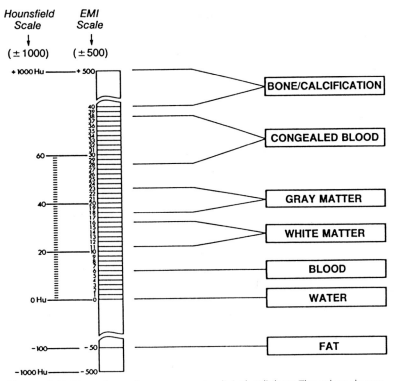

Figure 1-6 Absorption values common to clinical radiology. The values shown are for the EMI and Hounsfield scales.

The optimal technical factors depend on the specific MR scanner, and recommended protocols are provided by the manufacturer. To weight an image, the following relaxation times (T_R) and echo times (T_E) are generally used:

T1-weighted images are generated with a short T_R (250–1100 ms) and a short T_E (10–25 ms).

T2-weighted images are generated with a long T_R (2000+ ms) and a long T_E (60+ ms); this setting often better demonstrates pathologies.

T1-weighted	*T2-weighted*
Bright, high-signal intensity	**Bright, high-signal intensity**
1 Fat	CSF, water 1
2 Marrow	2
3	3
4	Intervertebral disk 4
5 Brain, white matter	Brain, gray matter 5
6	6
7 Liver, pancreas	Spleen 7
8 Brain, gray matter	8
9 Kidney	9
10 Spleen	10
11	11
12	Brain, white matter 12
13	Liver 13
14 Cerebrospinal fluid	Fat 14
15 Water, lung	Iron in basal ganglia 15
16 Cortical bone, flowing blood, air	Bone, flowing blood, air 16
Dark, low-signal intensity	**Dark, low-signal intensity**

Figure 1-7 Comparison of signal intensities in data generated by T1 versus T2 weighting.

Chapter 2

Chest

OBJECTIVES

Upon completion of this chapter, the student should be able to:

1. Describe the superior and inferior boundaries of the chest.
2. Describe the level of the three parts of the sternum as compared to the viscera or thoracic vertebrae.
3. List the number of floating, false, and true pairs of ribs in the chest.
4. Describe the structures separating the mediastinum and the pleural cavities.
5. Correctly identify the chambers of the heart on sectional images.
6. Identify and describe the airway structures within the chest.
7. Follow the course of blood as it passes through the pulmonary circulation system.
8. Describe the major arteries and veins located within the chest and upper arm.
9. Explain the relationships between structures within the mediastinum.
10. Correctly identify anatomical structures on patient CT and MR images of the chest.

ANATOMICAL OVERVIEW

The chest or thorax is the region of the bony thoracic cage located between the neck and the abdomen. The upper boundary of the chest, the thoracic inlet, is formed by the first thoracic vertebra, the first ribs, and the upper margin of the manubrium. Inferiorly, the chest extends to the level of the thoracic outlet, marked by the diaphragm, which extends between the inferior margin of the sternum and the upper lumbar vertebrae.

Skeletal

Thoracic (*thō-RAS-ik*) **vertebra.** In the chest, 12 thoracic vertebrae are found in the vertebral column and form the posterior border of the thoracic cage (Fig. 2-1). Compared to other vertebrae, they are average in size and are distinguishable by costal facets for articulation with the ribs. As with other vertebrae, each can be divided into two parts: a body and a vertebral arch.

Vertebral (*VER-tĕ-brăl*) **body.** The largest and heaviest portion of the vertebra, located anterior to the vertebral arch, forming the anterior margin of the vertebral foramen. When viewed from either the lateral or superior aspect, it is seen anterior to the vertebral foramen. The shape, however, is significantly different in the two views: In the lateral view, the body is wedge shaped, but when viewed from above, it has an oval shape.

Vertebral arch. All the vertebral structures except the body are considered part of the vertebral arch. More specifically, it consists of two pedicles, two laminae, and seven processes (two transverse, four articular, and one spinous).

Pedicles (*PED-ĭ-kls*). The bony projections forming the lateral walls of the vertebral foramen; they connect the vertebral body to the transverse processes.

Laminae (*LAM-i-nē*). The remainder of the vertebral arch is formed by the laminae, which form the posterolateral walls of vertebral foramen, connecting the transverse processes with the spinous process.

Clavicles (*KLAV-i-kls*). Commonly called the collar bones. The clavicle forms part of the shoulder girdle, connecting the acromion process of the scapula with the manubrium of the sternum (Figs. 2-2 and 2-3). Owing to the horizontal course of this long bone, axial sections through the upper chest demonstrate the clavicle in longitudinal section.

Humeri (*HYŪ-mer-ī*). The bones within the upper arms; the longest and largest bones of the upper limbs. On the proximal end of the humerus, the shoulder joint is formed by the head of the humerus and the glenoid process of the scapula.

Scapulae (*SKAP-yū-lē*). Frequently called the shoulder blades. They are located bilaterally along the posterolateral margin of the thoracic cage. Considered part of the shoulder girdle, the scapula articulates with the humerus to form the shoulder joint. The broad, flat bone is roughly triangular in shape and contains the following features.

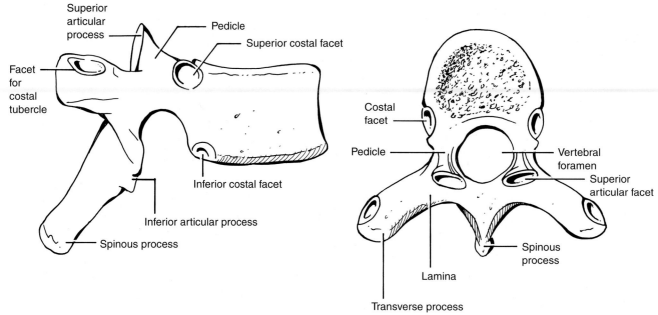

Figure 2-1 Lateral and superior views of a thoracic vertebra.

Acromion (ă-KRŌ-mē-on) process. The part of the bone that projects over the top of the shoulder joint and articulates with the lateral end of the clavicle.

Coracoid (KOR-ă-koyd) process. The bony projection on the anterior surface of the scapula found just inferior to the lateral clavicle. Its primary function is to provide a site of attachment for the pectoralis minor muscle.

Glenoid (GLĒ-noyd) process. The bony projection from the lateral margin of the scapula that forms the socket for the head of the humerus.

Sternum. The elongated, flat bone forming the anterior wall of the thoracic cage (Fig. 2-2). The sternum is divided into three parts.

Manubrium (mŭ-NU-brē-ŭm). The roughly quadrangular-shaped bone forming the superior division of the sternum. The superior margin, the jugular notch, can be easily palpated along with the distal ends of the clavicles where they articulate with the superolateral margins of the manubrium. It is generally located at the level of the 3rd and 4th thoracic vertebrae.

Body. The middle division of the sternum is long and slender and is generally at a level of the 5th to 9th thoracic vertebrae. The juncture of the body with the inferior margin of the manubrium, called the sternal angle, is often palpable and corresponds to the intervertebral disk between the 4th and 5th thoracic vertebrae.

Xiphoid (ZIF-oyd) process. The most inferior portion of the sternum is small and often bifid in shape. The process is easily located as the lower margin of the bony thoracic cage

in the median plane and corresponds to approximately the 9th thoracic vertebrae.

Ribs. There are 12 pairs of ribs in the chest: 7 true and 5 false, 2 of which are floating. In general, the long slender bones all articulate with the respective thoracic vertebra and are curvilinear in shape (Figs. 2-2 and 2-3). As the ribs extend from the vertebrae, they slope downward toward their anterior ends. This downward slope of the ribs causes them to be obliquely sectioned in axial images.

True ribs. The upper (1st to 7th pairs) ribs are classified as true ribs, because they articulate with thoracic vertebrae posteriorly and, through cartilage, with the sternum anteriorly.

False ribs. The 8th to 12th pairs of ribs are not considered true ribs because they do not articulate with the sternum. The 8th and 10th ribs articulate with the costal cartilage of the ribs above. The 11th and 12th pairs of ribs also are considered floating because they articulate only posteriorly with the vertebrae. Similar to all the other ribs, the floating ribs generally move downward toward their lateral ends and will be obliquely sectioned in axial images.

Enclosing Structures

Mediastinal *(MĒ-dē-as-TĪ-năl)* **pleura.** The thick connective tissue membrane that surrounds the region between the lungs, encompassing the heart, the great vessels, and the major divisions of the bronchial tree (Figs. 2-4 and 2-5).

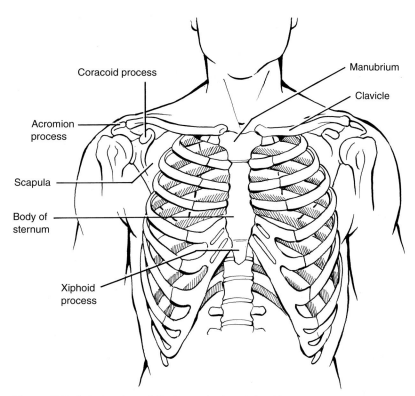

Figure 2-2 Anterior view of the bony chest and shoulder.

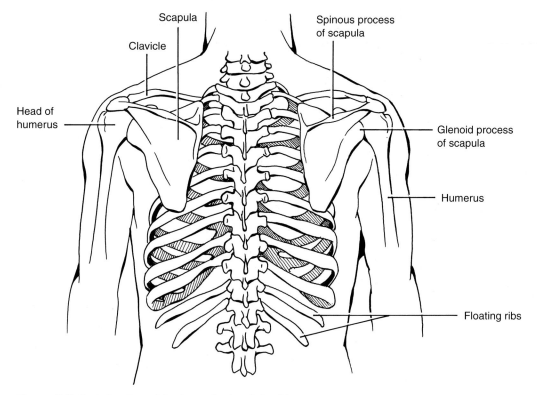

Figure 2-3 Posterior view of the bony chest and shoulder.

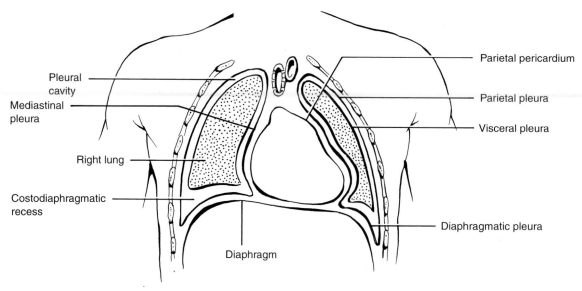

Figure 2-4 Coronal section through the chest demonstrating the enclosing structures.

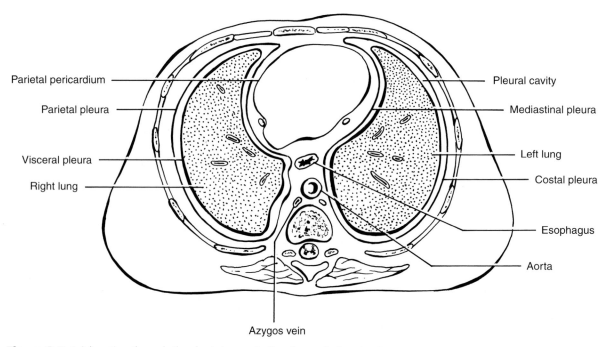

Figure 2-5 Axial section through the chest demonstrating the enclosing structures.

Pericardium (*per-i-KAR-dē-ŭm*). Within the mediastinum, the pericardium is a tough fibrous sac surrounding the heart and separating it from the other mediastinal structures. It has two layers: the parietal pericardium, or the tougher outer layer, and the visceral pericardium, which lines the entire surface of the heart and extends several centimeters along the base of the great vessels until they pass through the parietal pericardium. Regarding function, both the visceral and parietal layers have facing serous membranes that provide a smooth, lubricated surface between the two constantly moving structures.

Diaphragm (*DĪ-ă-fram*). This dome-shaped muscular sheet forms a convex floor for the chest and serves as a septum between the thoracic and abdominal cavities. Its periphery has broad, flat muscle fibers that converge on a central region of dense connective tissue, the central tendon.

Pleura (*PLŪR-ă*). There are two separable pleural membranes in the chest: the parietal (*pă-RĪ-ĕ-tăl*) pleura lines the inside of the thoracic musculoskeletal wall and the visceral pleura surrounds the surface of the lungs. Together, the pleural membranes reduce friction between the constantly moving lungs and thoracic musculoskeletal structures. The following spaces are between the pleural membranes.

Pleural cavity. The space filled with small amounts of serous fluid situated between the pleural membranes. In some pathologic conditions, fluid or blood outside the lungs accumulates in this space and limits respiration (e.g., pleurisy).

Costodiaphragmatic (kos-tō-DĪ-ă-frag-MAT-ik) recesses. The most inferior regions of the pleural cavity at the juncture of the ribs with the posterolateral margins of the diaphragm. In the erect position, fluid within the pleural cavity will be concentrated within the recesses.

Airway Structures

Right lung. The lung on the right side has three lobes: upper, middle, and lower (Fig. 2-6). Although this nomenclature describes the position of the lobes with respect to one another, as shown in a lateral view (Fig. 2-7), it would be incorrect to assume that the middle lobe separates the upper and lower lobes. In an axial section through the upper lung, both the upper and lower lobes are often demonstrated, with the lower lobe being more posterior.

Oblique (*ob-LĒK*) **fissure.** The space separating the upper and middle lobes from the lower lobe of the right lung.

Horizontal fissure. The space separating the upper and middle lobes of the right lung.

Left lung. The lung on the left side has two lobes: upper and lower (Figs. 2-6 and 2-8). Similar to the right lung, this nomenclature generally describes the position of the lobes within the lung. However, in axial sections through the middle of the lung, both lobes will be seen. Because of the course of the oblique fissure, the upper lobe will be more anterior than the lower lobe.

Oblique fissure (left lung). As the name implies, the fissure divides the upper and lower lobes of the left lung in an oblique fashion.

Hilum (*HĪ-lŭm*). A region near the center on the medial aspect of both the right and left lungs where the bronchi, veins, and arteries enter and exit the lungs next to the heart.

Trachea (*TRĀ-kē-ă*). The most superior airway structure in the chest, the trachea extends inferiorly from the larynx, located within the neck, until it bifurcates in the right and

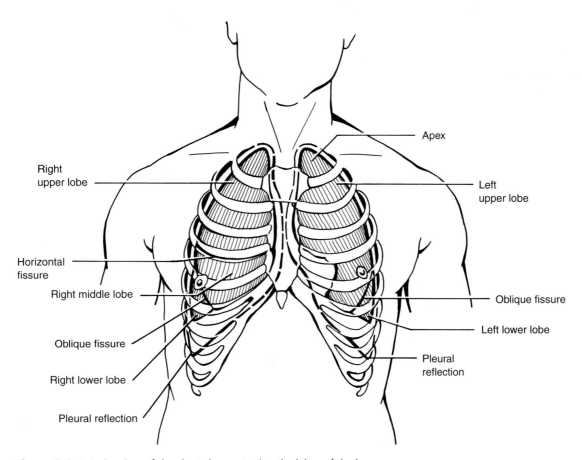

Figure 2-6 Anterior view of the chest demonstrating the lobes of the lungs.

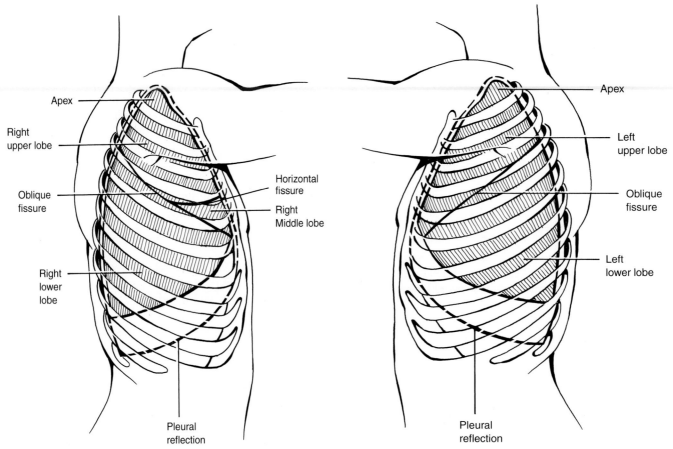

Figure 2-7 Lateral view of the right lung demonstrating the location of the superior, middle, and inferior lobes.

Figure 2-8 Lateral view of the left lung demonstrating the superior and inferior lobes.

left main bronchi (Fig. 2-9). Although the exact level may vary, the trachea terminates at the level of the 5th or 6th thoracic vertebra. Compared to other structures within the region, the trachea is posterior to the great vessels and anterior to the esophagus.

Carina (kă-RĪ-nă). At the terminal end of the trachea, a ridge extends superiorly, originating the bifurcation of the trachea into the right and left main bronchi. Although the level may vary among individuals, the carina is seen near the level of the pulmonary artery. In an axial section through the terminal trachea, the carina can often be seen within the center of the opening dividing the right and left bronchi.

Main bronchi (BRONG-kī). The principal divisions of the trachea, dividing the airway into right and left halves. Note that the right main bronchus is the larger and more vertical of the two. Both main bronchi are just posterior to the pulmonary arteries at a level of the 6th or 7th thoracic vertebra.

Upper lobe bronchi. The first division of the main bronchi on both the right and left sides, the upper lobe bronchi transport air to and from the superior lobes of the lungs.

The right upper lobe bronchus originates more superiorly than the left.

Bronchus intermedius. The other major branch of the right main bronchus that divides to give rise to both the middle and lower bronchi.

Middle lobe bronchus. This airway structure is found on the right side as it branches from the bronchus intermedius to transport air to and from the middle lobe of the lung.

Lower lobe bronchi. Air is transported to and from the inferior lobes of the lungs via the lower lobe bronchi on both the right and left sides.

Other Viscera (VIS-er-a)

Heart. The heart contains four chambers: the right atrium, the right ventricle, the left atrium, and the left ventricle (Fig. 2-10). Although this nomenclature implies the chambers are located on either the right side or left side, the in vivo chambers of the heart are not truly arranged in this simple fashion (Fig. 2-11). Because the heart rests on the diaphragm, the apex of the heart is shifted toward the right

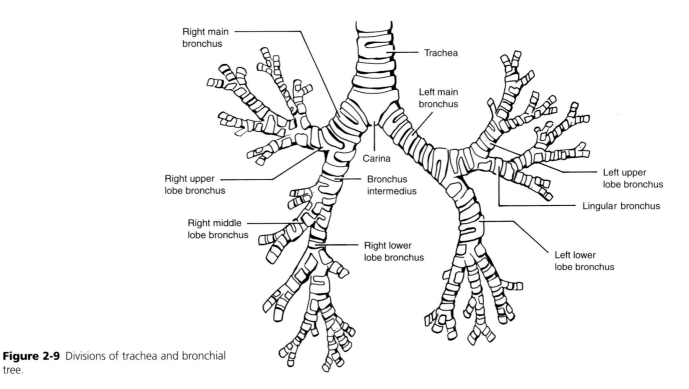

Figure 2-9 Divisions of trachea and bronchial tree.

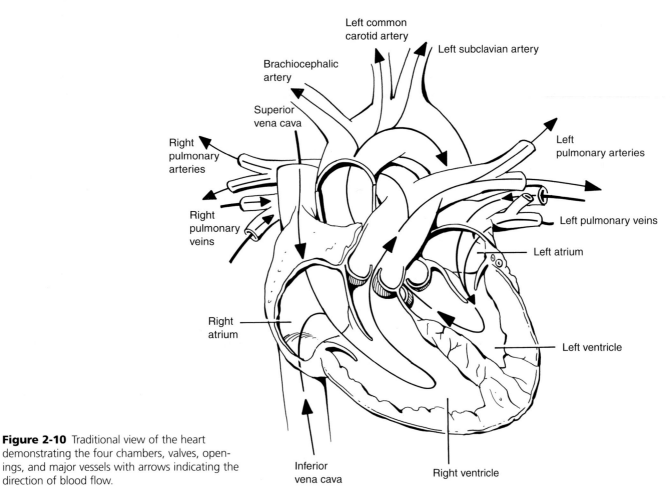

Figure 2-10 Traditional view of the heart demonstrating the four chambers, valves, openings, and major vessels with arrows indicating the direction of blood flow.

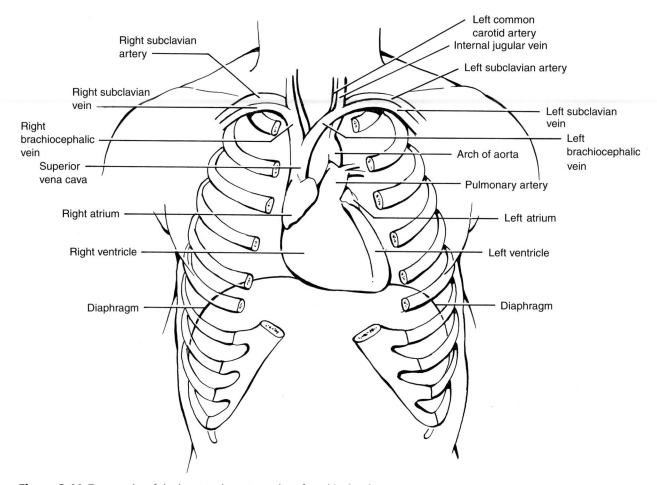

Figure 2-11 Topography of the heart and great vessels as found in the chest.

side, placing the right ventricle of the heart in front of the left. In sectional images, the chambers appear skewed off-center, with the right ventricle being the most anterior chamber of the heart and the left atrium being most posterior.

Right atrium ($\overline{A}$-$tr\overline{e}$-$\breve{u}m$). The drainage point of the superior and inferior vena cavae, it pumps venous blood into the right ventricle through the tricuspid valve (Fig. 2-10). Within the mediastinum, the right atrium is on the right side of the heart slightly above the ventricles.

Right ventricle. This chamber receives venous blood from the right atrium during relaxation. During contraction, the chamber pumps blood into the pulmonary trunk through the pulmonary semilunar valve. In the chest, this chamber of the heart is the most anterior and forms most of the anterior surface of the heart inferior to the right atrium (Fig. 2-11).

Left atrium. This chamber receives blood from the four pulmonary veins and pumps it into the left ventricle through the mitral or bicuspid valve. Within the chest, the left atrium is the most posterior chamber at approximately the level of the right atrium.

Left ventricle. This chamber receives blood from the left atrium and pumps it into the aorta through the aortic semilunar valve. In the body, this chamber is farthest to the left side of the heart and lies posterior to much of the right ventricle.

Esophagus ($\overline{e}$-SOF-$\breve{a}$-$g\breve{u}s$). This gastrointestinal tube extends from the pharynx to the stomach. In the upper mediastinum, the esophagus lies in the midline between the trachea and vertebral column. Below the level of the trachea, the esophagus occupies a position between the heart and vertebral column.

Arteries

The major arterial structures within the body are within the mediastinum and are adjacent to corresponding venous structures (Fig. 2-12). In the upper mediastinum, the adjacent veins are more superficially located than the corresponding arteries.

Aorta ($\overline{a}$-$\overline{O}R$-$t\breve{a}$). This major artery is the largest in the body and originates from the left ventricle. The thoracic aorta is divided into three parts.

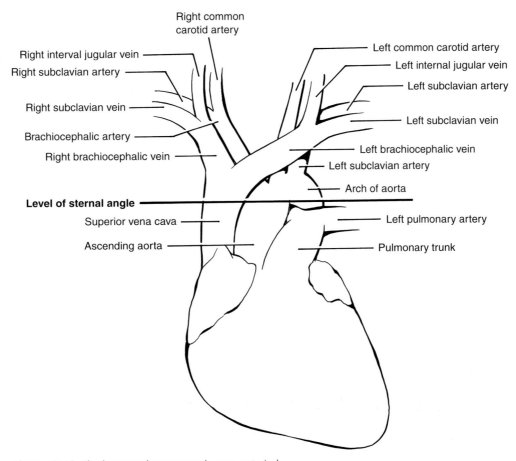

Right common carotid artery

Right interval jugular vein

Right subclavian artery

Right subclavian vein

Brachiocephalic artery

Right brachiocephalic vein

Level of sternal angle

Superior vena cava

Ascending aorta

Left common carotid artery

Left internal jugular vein

Left subclavian artery

Left subclavian vein

Left brachiocephalic vein

Left subclavian artery

Arch of aorta

Left pulmonary artery

Pulmonary trunk

Figure 2-12 The heart and great vessels seen anteriorly.

Ascending aorta. The first portion of the artery ascending from the heart. Although originating from the left ventricle, the ascending aorta in an axial image is superior to the right ventricle and next to the superior vena cava.

Aortic arch. The second arch-shaped portion of the artery that curves over the pulmonary trunk. This segment originates from the ascending aorta on the right side of the heart and arches toward the left side to form the descending thoracic aorta. The arch of the aorta passes over both the pulmonary trunk and left main bronchus.

Descending aorta. The last segment of the thoracic aorta between the aortic arch and the abdominal aorta. This major artery descends along the left side of the thoracic vertebrae in the posterior mediastinum.

Brachiocephalic ($BR\bar{A}$-$k\bar{e}$-$\bar{o}$-se-FAL-ik) **artery.** The first major branch off the aortic arch; it extends to the right and divides into the right subclavian and the right common carotid arteries. Note that there is no left brachiocephalic artery, because the aorta arches to the left side of the body and gives rise to the branches that would have been derived from the left brachiocephalic artery.

Common carotid (ka-ROT-id) **arteries.** The arteries on either side of the trachea that supply arterial blood to much of the head and neck. Although both arteries have the same structure and location, their origins differ, because the right artery originates from the brachiocephalic artery and the left artery is the second major branch off the aortic arch.

Subclavian ($s\breve{u}b$-$KL\bar{A}$-$v\bar{e}$-an) **arteries.** Similar to the common carotid arteries, these arteries are bilateral with the same structure and function but have different origins. On the right side, the subclavian artery arises from the brachiocephalic artery. On the left side, the subclavian artery is the third major branch off the aortic arch. Compared to the common carotid arteries, the subclavian arteries are more laterally located and ascend through the upper thorax to exit through the thoracic inlet to form the axillary arteries (Fig. 2-13).

Axillary (AK-sil-$\bar{r}$-$\bar{e}$) **arteries.** The bilateral arterial structures that supply blood to the pectoral girdle and arm. As just described, the axillary arteries originate from the subclavian arteries at the level of the first rib. In axial images through the upper chest, the axial vessels are seen

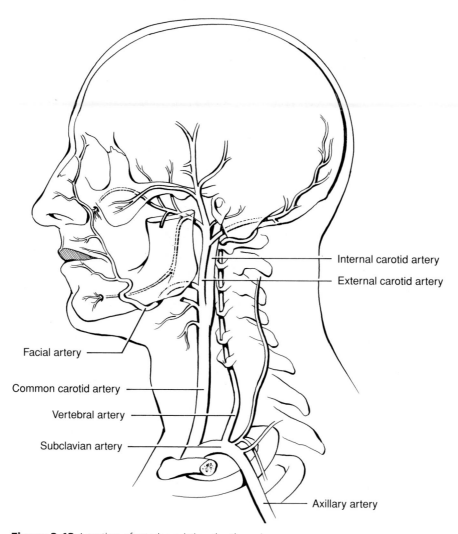

Figure 2-13 Location of arteries existing the thoracic cage.

longitudinally sectioned outside the ribs, extending toward the region of the shoulder.

Vertebral arteries. From the subclavian arteries, the arteries are found bilaterally and run superiorly through the foramen transversarium of the cervical vertebrae. At the level of the skull, they enter the cranium through the foramen magnum to supply the posterior part of the brain with arterial blood.

Main pulmonary (*PŬL-mō-nār-ē*) **artery or trunk.** This major artery from the right ventricle moves posteriorly as it ascends to form the right and left pulmonary arteries (Fig. 2-14). Together, the pulmonary trunk and the pulmonary arteries form the characteristic T-shape of the pulmonary arteries. The pulmonary trunk lies below the aortic arch and in front of the esophagus.

Pulmonary arteries. Arteries located bilaterally and arising from the pulmonary trunk; they carry deoxygenated blood to the lungs. The pulmonary arteries are the only arteries in the body that carry deoxygenated blood.

Veins

Superior vena cava (*VĒ-nă KĀ-vă*). The major vein located on the superior aspect of the right side of the heart adjacent and slightly posterior to the ascending aorta (Fig. 2-15). It is above the right atrium and lies anterior to the right pulmonary artery and the right main bronchus. Regarding function, this major vein drains blood from the upper trunk into the right atrium.

Brachiocephalic veins. Bilateral veins that originate at the juncture of the internal jugular veins and the subclavian veins; they drain into the superior vena cava. Compared to the adjacent arteries, the veins are more superficial and are found at or above the level of the aortic arch. Although the veins are markedly similar, the course of the right vein is much more

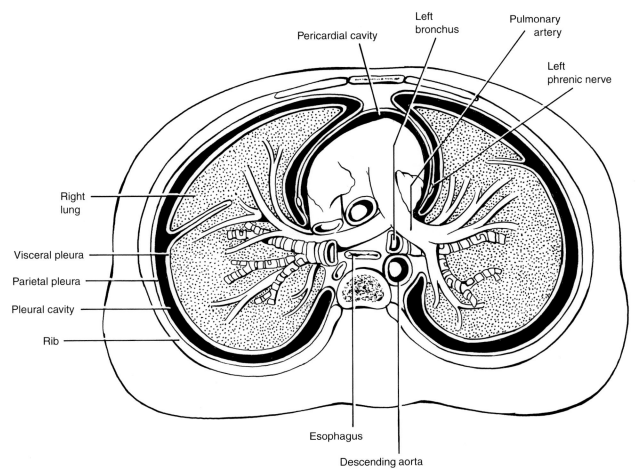

Figure 2-14 Transverse section through the thorax.

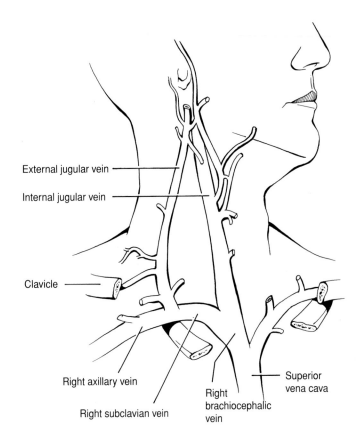

Figure 2-15 Location of veins exiting the thoracic cage.

vertical than the left vein. In an axial section, the oblique course of the left vein will often result in an oblique section, whereas the right vein will be shown as a transverse section.

Subclavian veins. Bilateral veins that are continuations of the axillary veins originating from the upper limb and shoulder girdle. The veins begin at the thoracic inlet as they cross over the first rib and drain into the brachiocephalic veins. Found within the lateral parts of the upper mediastinum, the veins lie just anterior to the adjacent subclavian arteries.

Axillary veins. Serve to drain venous blood from the upper extremity and shoulder girdle on both sides of the body. The veins terminate as they cross over the first ribs to join the subclavian veins. Similar to the subclavian vessels, the course of the veins are superficial to the adjacent axillary arteries.

Internal jugular (*JŬG-yū-lar*) **veins.** The bilateral veins originate from the sigmoid sinuses inside the skull and drain most of the venous blood from the brain. The veins descend deep in the neck, superficial to the common carotid arteries, and drain into the brachiocephalic veins.

Azygos (*AZ-ī-gos*). A vein in the right posterior thoracic cage adjacent to the right side of the vertebral bodies (Fig. 2-16). The vessel drains much of the venous blood from the posterior thorax and upper abdomen into the superior vena cava.

Hemiazygos (*HEM-ē-AZ-ī-gos*). The major vein located on the left side of the vertebral bodies below the accessory hemiazygos or approximately the level of T6. The hemiazy-

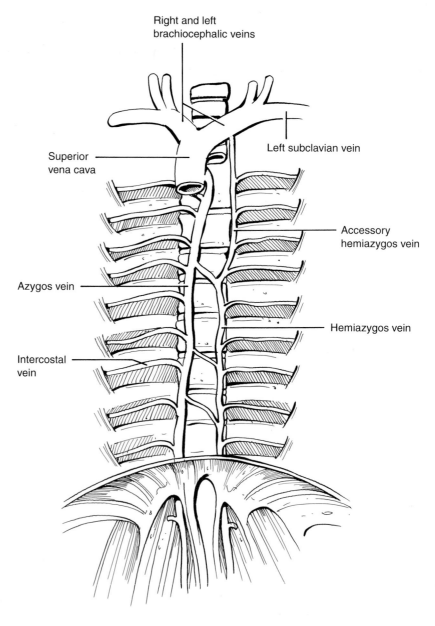

Right and left brachiocephalic veins

Superior vena cava

Left subclavian vein

Accessory hemiazygos vein

Azygos vein

Hemiazygos vein

Intercostal vein

Figure 2-16 Veins of the posterior thoracic cage.

gos vein drains the inferior half of the left posterior thoracic cage into the azygos vein.

Accessory hemiazygos vein. The vein located inside the posterior thoracic cage next to the vertebral column on the left side above the level of T6. At the level of T6, the vessel drains blood from the superior half of the left posterior thoracic cage into the hemiazygos vein.

Inferior vena cava. A large vein draining most of the lower half of the body into the right atrium (Fig. 2-10). The vessel extends upward through the diaphragm to the right side of the heart and joins to the lower part of the right atrium. At the level of the diaphragm, the inferior vena cava is anterior to the esophagus and the descending aorta.

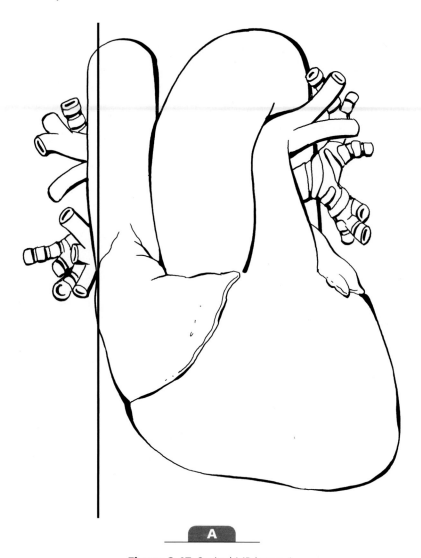

Figure 2-17 Sagittal MR image 1.

SAGITTAL MR IMAGES

Because of the relatively long acquisition time and the constant move-ment of the heart and lungs, MR images of the chest provide very limited visualization of moving structures. This section examines eight sequential images taken at 5.0 mm intervals through the middle of the chest from right to left. The images were generated at the following technical factors: TR = 500, TE = 20, RF = 90°, FOV = 45 cm. Abbreviations: TR = repetition time, TE = echo-time, RF = radiofrequency, FOV = field of view.

Figure 2-17 (A,B,C). Review of the bony anatomy in the MR image reveals that the ver-tebral bodies are not yet included within the section, and the anterior musculoskeletal wall demonstrates ribs in cross-section. Regarding soft tissue structures, the right lung forms a background for the mediastinal structures located centrally within the chest. Anteriorly, the upper lobe of the right lung is seen adjacent to the superior vena cava, demonstrated in lon-gitudinal section. Just posterior to the superior vena cava, the hilum is seen, demonstrating vessels and airways in cross-section extending between the right lung and the mediastinum. Posteriorly in the chest cavity, the lower lobe of the right lung can be seen extending inferior to the hilum.

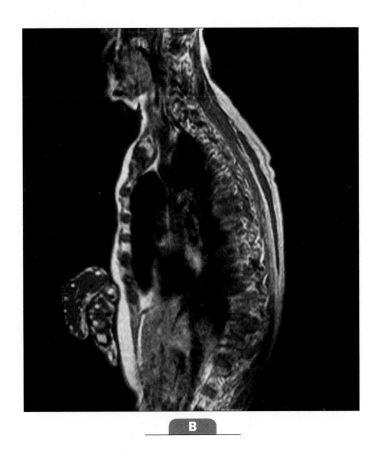

B

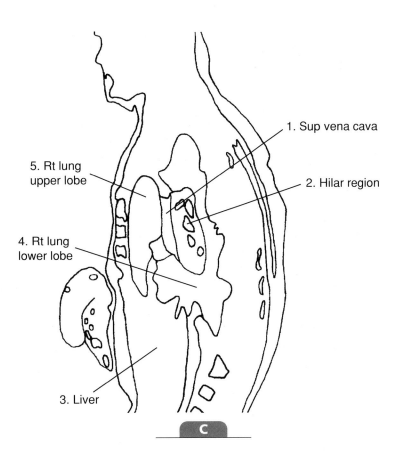

5. Rt lung
upper lobe

1. Sup vena cava

2. Hilar region

4. Rt lung
lower lobe

3. Liver

C

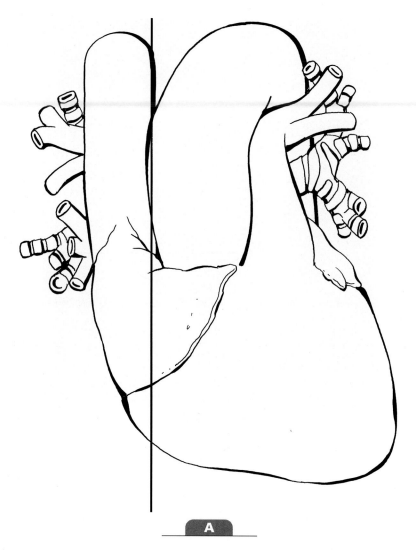

Figure 2-18 Sagittal MR image 2.

Figure 2-18 (A,B,C). This second MR scan demonstrates structures 5 mm to the left of the first MR image and is slightly closer to the center of the chest. Consequently, less of the right lung is seen and more of the mediastinal structures are visualized. In addition to the superior vena cava just described, the wall of the aortic arch is between the superior vena cava and the upper lobe of the right lung. Posterior to the superior vena cava, the structures within the hilum are more discernible and, based on their positions, can be labeled as the right pulmonary artery and the right pulmonary vein, respectively. Inferior to the pulmonary vessels, the right atrium appears to be resting on the liver, and the inferior vena cava is seen in longitudinal section within the upper abdomen.

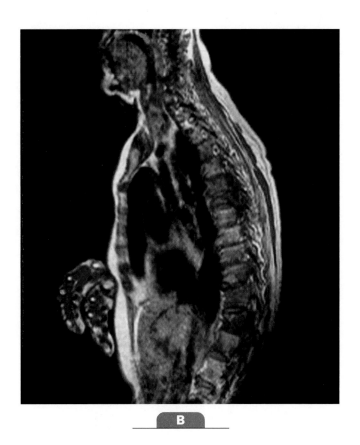

B

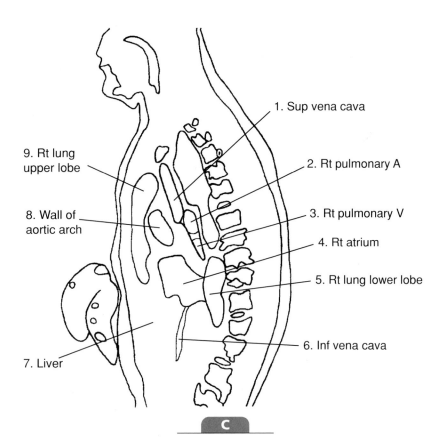

C

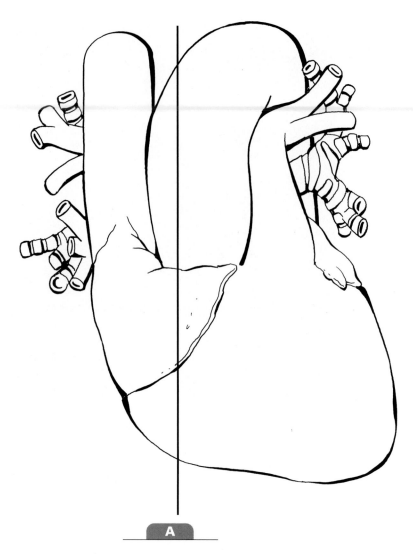

Figure 2-19 Sagittal MR image 3.

Figure 2-19 (A,B,C). Many of the structures just described are also seen in the section shown in this figure, including the aortic arch, pulmonary artery, right atrium, and liver. However, the superior vena cava is no longer present and two vessels are demonstrated above the aortic arch. Based on their location, the vessels are labeled as the left brachiocephalic vein and the brachiocephalic artery. As described earlier in this chapter, the veins of the chest are generally located superficial to the corresponding arteries. Immediately posterior to the vessels, two openings are seen extending upward into the region of the neck. Given the large size and its location adjacent to the vessels, the more anterior opening is the trachea; the smaller opening, adjacent to the vertebrae, is within the esophagus. Inferior to the trachea and esophagus, the pulmonary artery is seen above a structure larger than the pulmonary veins. The pulmonary veins empty into the left atrium, and a small section of the left atrium is seen posterior to the right atrium.

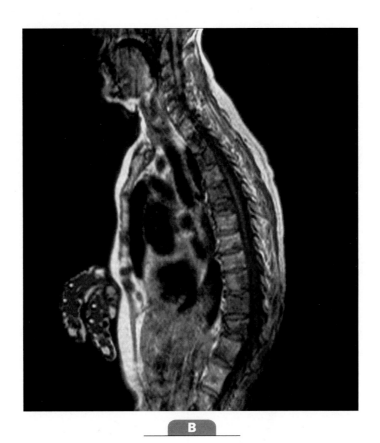

B

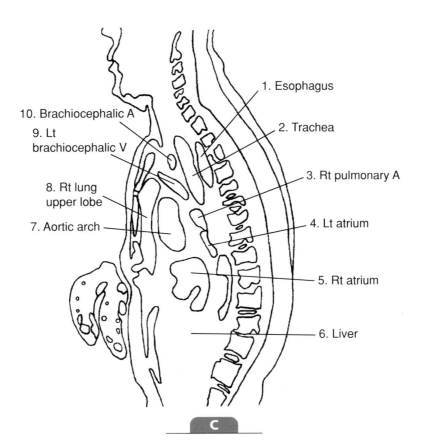

1. Esophagus

10. Brachiocephalic A

9. Lt brachiocephalic V

2. Trachea

8. Rt lung upper lobe

3. Rt pulmonary A

7. Aortic arch

4. Lt atrium

5. Rt atrium

6. Liver

C

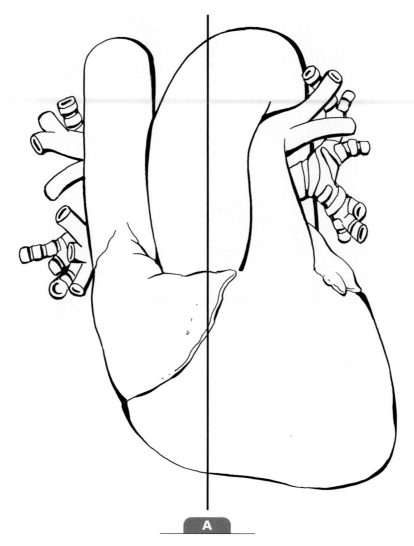

Figure 2-20 Sagittal MR image 4.

Figure 2-20 (A,B,C). The vertebral bodies are demonstrated in cross-section in front of the spinal cord, indicating the section is nearing the median plane. The large and most noticeable opening near the center of the chest represents the arch of the aorta. The brachiocephalic artery is originating from the arch, and the left brachiocephalic vein (seen in cross-section) is demonstrated anteriorly. Similar to the previous image, the right pulmonary artery is found just posterior to the aortic arch and superior to the left atrium. Below the great vessels, the right atrium is shown anterior to the left atrium within the heart.

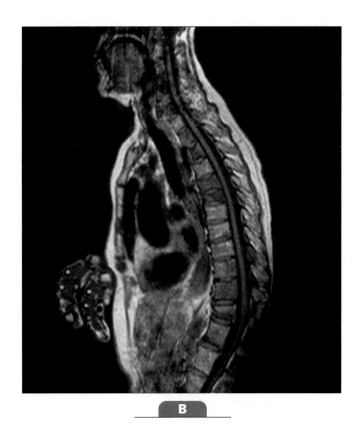

B

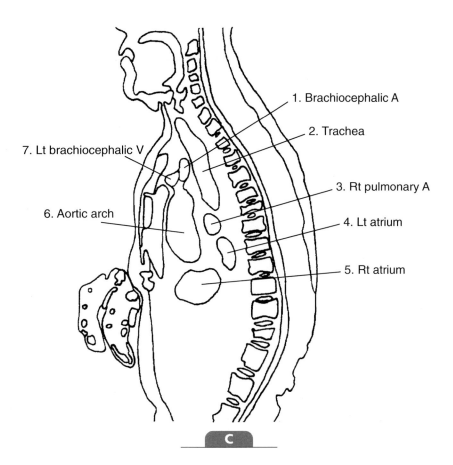

1. Brachiocephalic A

2. Trachea

7. Lt brachiocephalic V

3. Rt pulmonary A

6. Aortic arch

4. Lt atrium

5. Rt atrium

C

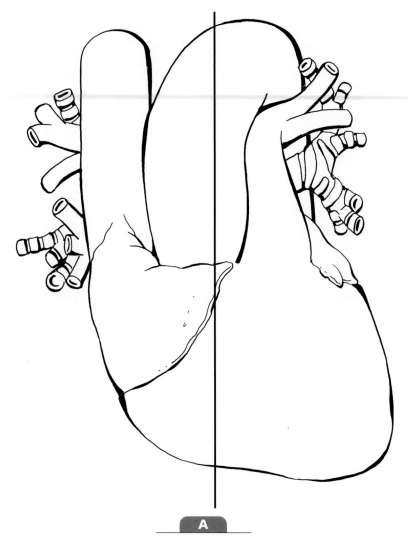

A

Figure 2-21 Sagittal MR image 5.

Figure 2-21 (A,B,C). The aortic arch, near the center of the chest, appears larger in this image than in the previous images. The only vessel seen above the aortic arch, the left brachiocephalic vein, is situated anterior to the opening of the trachea, shown extending up through the neck to the head. As described previously, the right pulmonary artery is sectioned just posterior to the aorta and just superior to the left atrium. Although the specific division is not demonstrated, the right atrium has been replaced by the right ventricle within the heart.

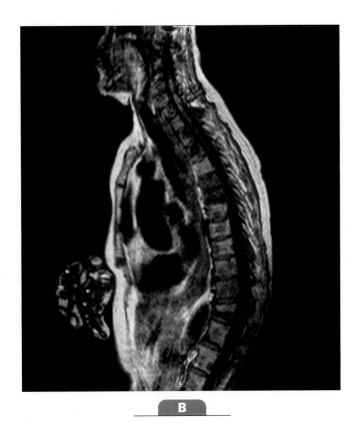

B

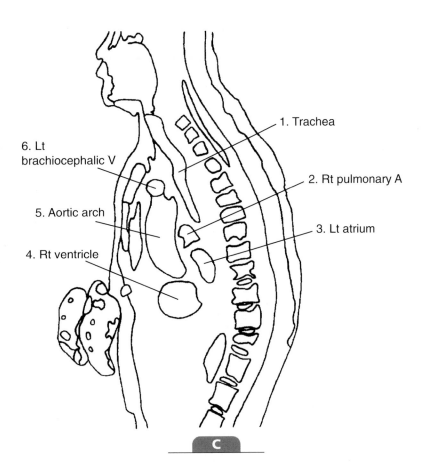

6. Lt
brachiocephalic V

5. Aortic arch

4. Rt ventricle

1. Trachea

2. Rt pulmonary A

3. Lt atrium

C

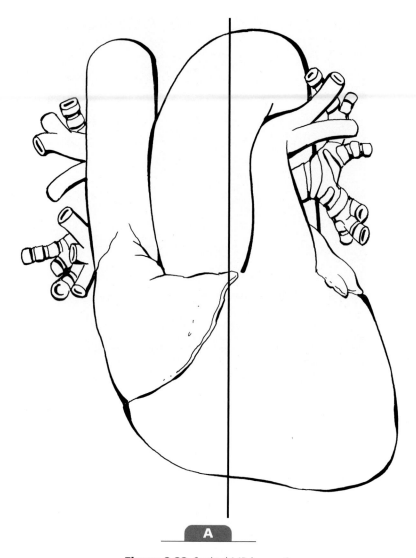

Figure 2-22 Sagittal MR image 6.

Figure 2-22 (A,B,C). Many of the structures just described are seen in the next section, including the aortic arch, the left brachio-cephalic vein, the right pulmonary artery, the left atrium, and the right ventricle. In contrast to the previous image, the trachea is no longer seen and the left bronchus is shown in cross-section extending into the left lung. Also, the pleural cavity is larger than in the previous section, signifying the beginning of the left lung.

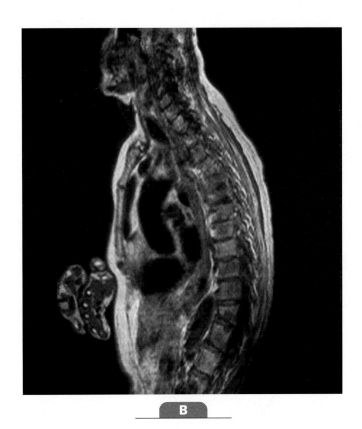

B

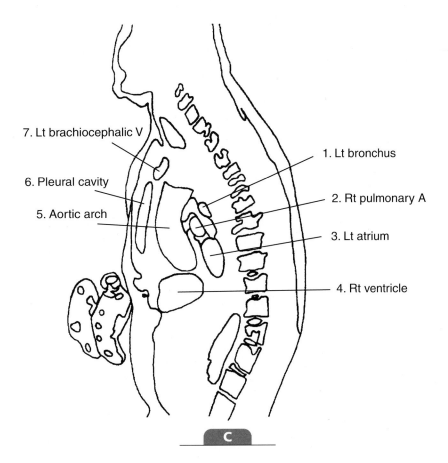

7. Lt brachiocephalic V

6. Pleural cavity

5. Aortic arch

1. Lt bronchus

2. Rt pulmonary A

3. Lt atrium

4. Rt ventricle

C

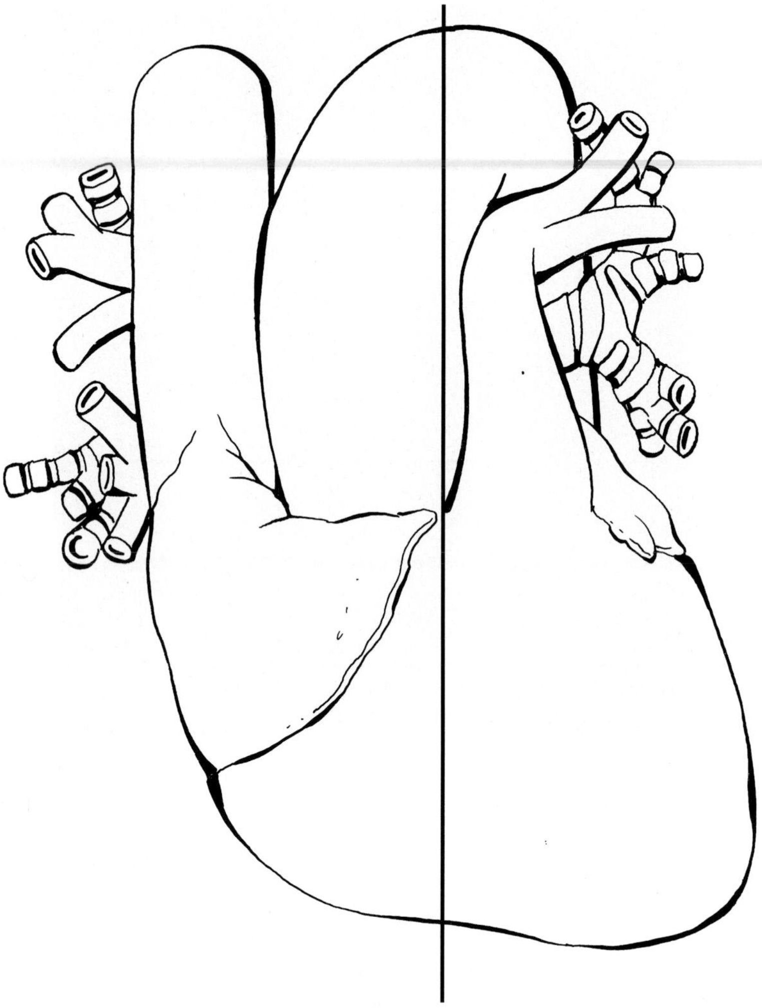

Figure 2-23 Sagittal MR image 7.

Figure 2-23 (A,B,C). Near the center of the chest, all three parts of the thoracic aorta are clearly visualized in this figure; the ascending aorta originating from the left ventricle, the arch moving posteriorly, and the descending aorta on the left side of the posterior thoracic cage. As described earlier, the aorta is arching over the left bronchus and the right pulmonary artery. Below the aorta, three chambers of the heart are included within this section. The right ventricle is the most anterior chamber and lies in front of the left ventricle. Behind the left ventricle, the left atrium is shown to be the most posterior chamber of the heart.

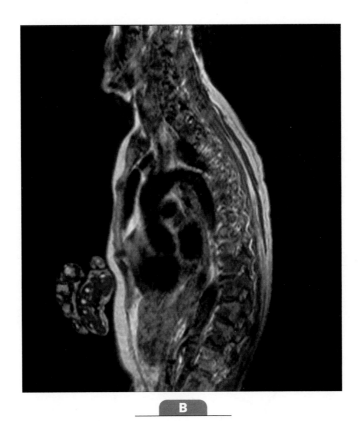

B

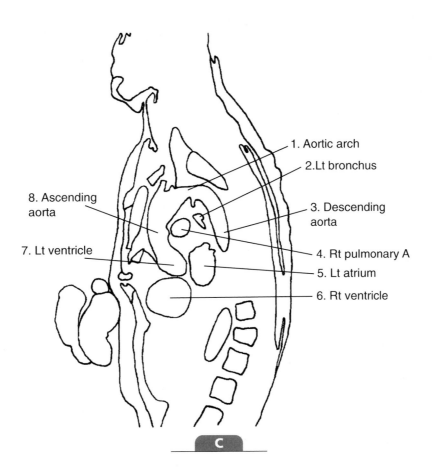

8. Ascending aorta

7. Lt ventricle

1. Aortic arch

2. Lt bronchus

3. Descending aorta

4. Rt pulmonary A

5. Lt atrium

6. Rt ventricle

C

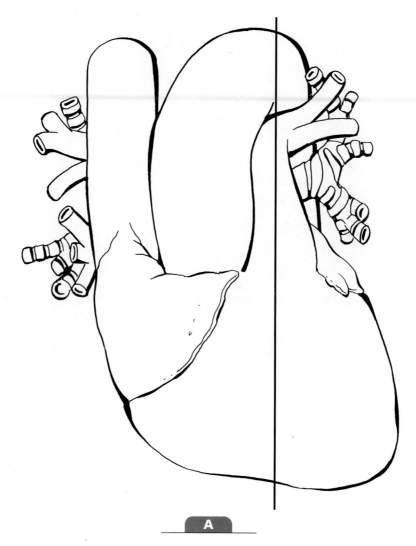

Figure 2-24 Sagittal MR image 8.

Figure 2-24 (A,B,C). The aortic arch and descending aorta are easily identified adjacent to the heart, but the ascending portion is no longer demonstrated adjoining the left ventricle. Instead, the pulmonary trunk is seen in longitudinal section as a large vessel extending between the upper right ventricle and the arch of the aorta. Adjacent to the arch, the pulmonary trunk divides into the right and left pulmonary arteries, which extend laterally to the right and left lungs along with the bronchi and pulmonary veins. Within the heart, the right ventricle is located most anteriorly and the left atrium is most posterior. If additional sagittal sections were described moving toward the left side of the chest, the left ventricle would enlarge, becoming slightly larger than the right ventricle.

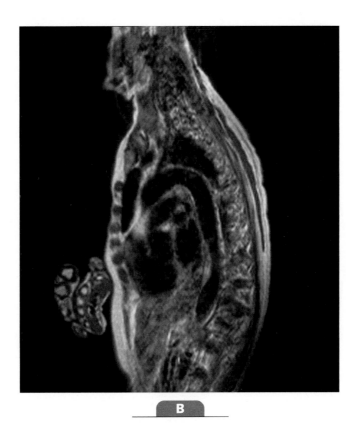

B

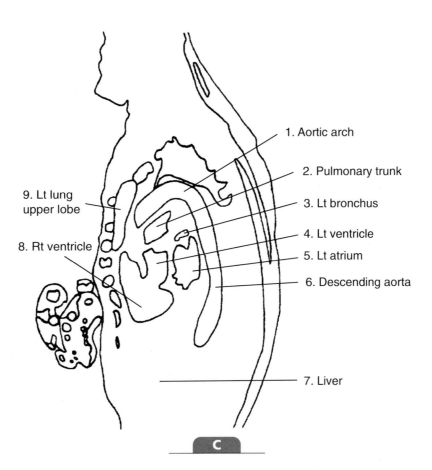

1. Aortic arch

2. Pulmonary trunk

9. Lt lung
upper lobe

3. Lt bronchus

4. Lt ventricle

8. Rt ventricle

5. Lt atrium

6. Descending aorta

7. Liver

C

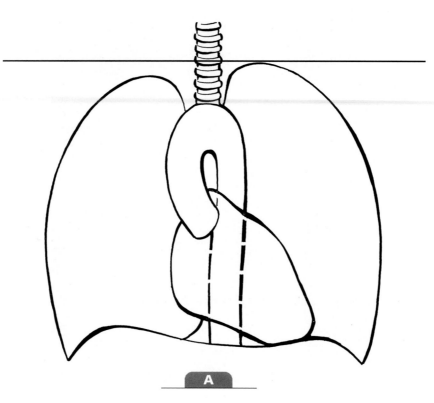

Figure 2-25 Axial CT image 1.

AXIAL CT IMAGES

This section examines 26 axial CT images of the chest taken at 10.0 mm intervals through the chest from superior to inferior. In a typical scan of the chest, images are generated throughout the region of the bony thoracic cage. The images were generated immediately after the administration of 100 ml venous contrast media at the following technical factors: 120 kVp and 150 mA-s. Abbreviations: kVp = kilovolt peak, mA-s = milliampere-second.

Figure 2-25 (A,B,C). In this first CT image at the top of the chest, the vertebra can clearly be labeled as the first thoracic vertebra by the absence of any ribs except the small sections shown articulating with costal facets on the transverse processes bilaterally. Although one might expect to find the first rib articulating with the vertebral body in this same section, it is demonstrated on the next image, because the transverse processes angle superiorly above the vertebral body. In addition to the other vertebral structures identified, the clavicle is obliquely sectioned on the left side, and the upper head of the humerus is demonstrated anterior to the acromion process of the scapula. Looking at the soft tissues of the upper chest, the trachea is easily identified and serves as a landmark for identification of adjacent structures. The esophagus, located directly posterior to the trachea, appears flattened with little or no lumen evident. On the left side, the contrast has enhanced the left vertebral artery lateral to the esophagus and vertebral body. On either side of the trachea, the deep vessels of the neck are shown with the slightly larger internal jugular veins superficial to the common carotid arteries.

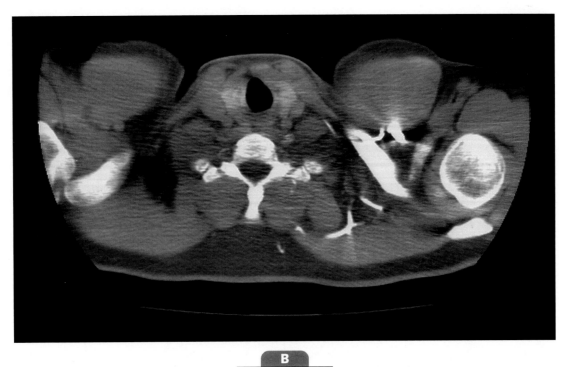

B

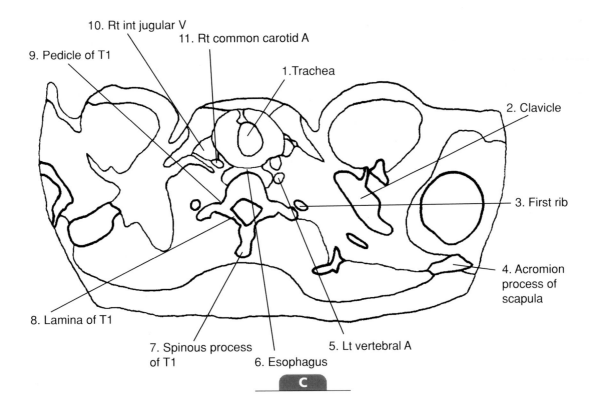

10. Rt int jugular V

11. Rt common carotid A

9. Pedicle of T1

1.Trachea

2. Clavicle

3. First rib

4. Acromion process of scapula

8. Lamina of T1

7. Spinous process of T1

6. Esophagus

5. Lt vertebral A

C

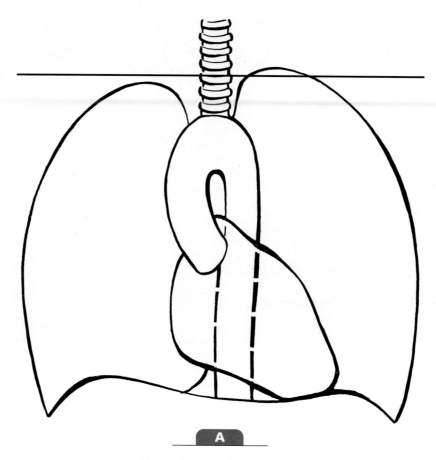

Figure 2-26 Axial CT image 2.

Figure 2-26 (A,B,C). Following the anatomy from the previous image, most of the structures just described are also found within this lower section. However, the first rib is articulating with the costal facet on the vertebral body, and the second rib is sectioned at the costal facet of the transverse process of the second thoracic vertebra. The head of the humerus (shown in full on the left side) is articulating with the glenoid process of the scapula, and the acromion process is no longer seen. When the attention is shifted to soft tissue structures, the center of the thyroid gland is apparent wrapping around the anterior trachea. Lying behind the lobes of the thyroid gland, the internal jugular vein and common carotid artery are on either side. On the left side, the left vertebral artery is shown in cross-section near the first rib, and the vessel highlighted with contrast lateral to the internal jugular vein is the left subclavian vein. Outside of the bony thoracic cage (over the first rib), the left axillary vein is sectioned as it extends from the region of the shoulder.

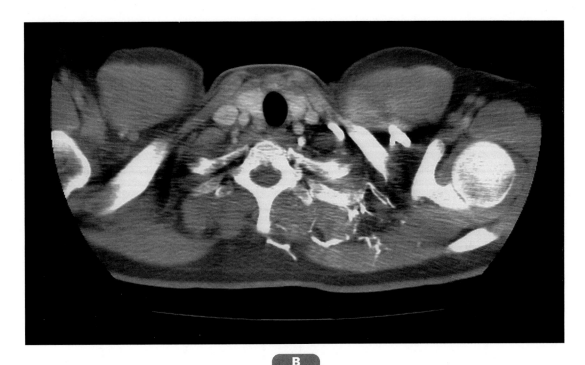

B

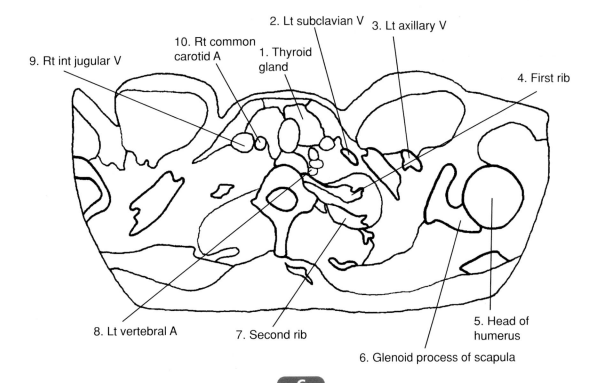

9. Rt int jugular V

10. Rt common carotid A

2. Lt subclavian V

3. Lt axillary V

1. Thyroid gland

4. First rib

8. Lt vertebral A

7. Second rib

5. Head of humerus

6. Glenoid process of scapula

C

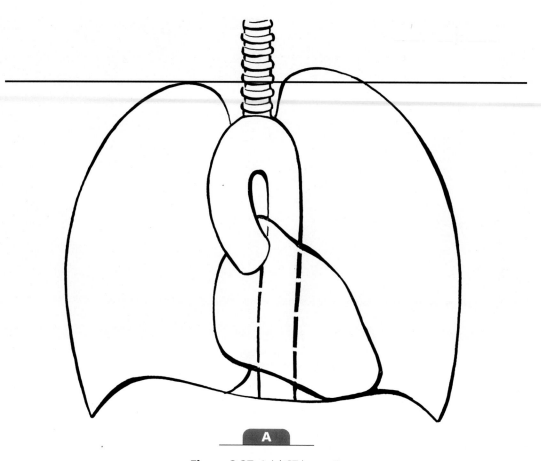

Figure 2-27 Axial CT image 3.

Figure 2-27 (A,B,C). The ribs are shown obliquely sectioned encasing the upper lobes of the right and left lungs. The "hook," or coracoid process of the scapula, is shown bilaterally extending toward the anterior chest wall. Within the mediastinum, the trachea is again shown centrally between the common carotid arteries and internal jugular veins. On the left side, the vertebral artery is cross-sectioned behind the common carotid artery, and the subclavian vein is sectioned lateral to the internal jugular vein.

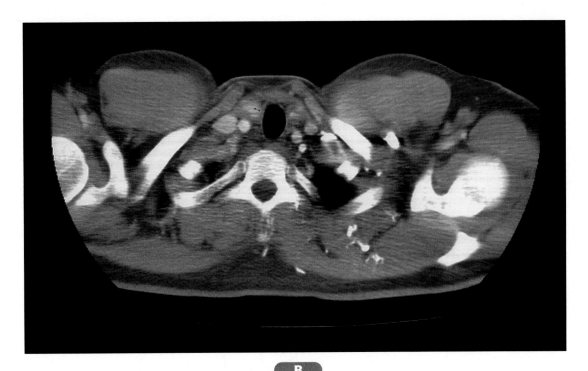

B

10. Rt int jugular V

2. Lt common carotid A

3. Lt int jugular V

4. Lt subclavian V

1. Trachea

5. Ribs

6. Coracoid process of scapula

9. Upper lobe of rt lung

8. Lt vertebral A

7. Upper lobe lt lung

C

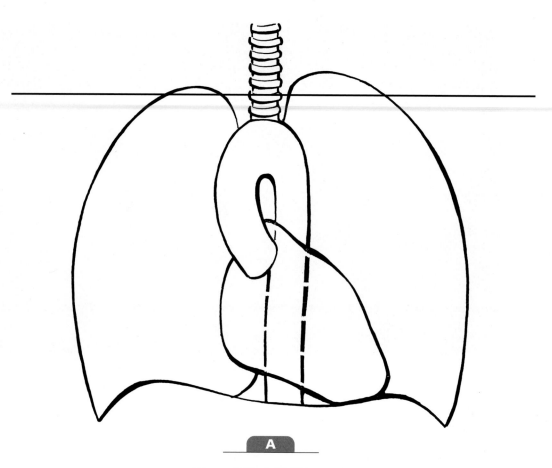

Figure 2-28 Axial CT image 4.

Figure 2-28 (A,B,C). The humerus is no longer seen on the left side, but the head is still demonstrated on the right, indicating the patient's shoulders are asymmetrical. Within the midline, the trachea is sectioned in front of the esophagus and separates the common carotid arteries. In distinction to the earlier images in the series, the left internal jugular vein and left subclavian vein are not distinctly separable, indicating the level of bifurcation of the left brachiocephalic vein. At this lower level, the left subclavian artery lies adjacent to the vertebral artery. Outside of the thoracic cage, the axillary artery is demonstrated in longitudinal section.

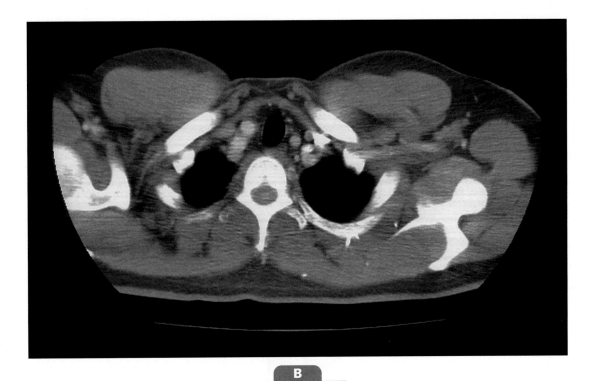

B

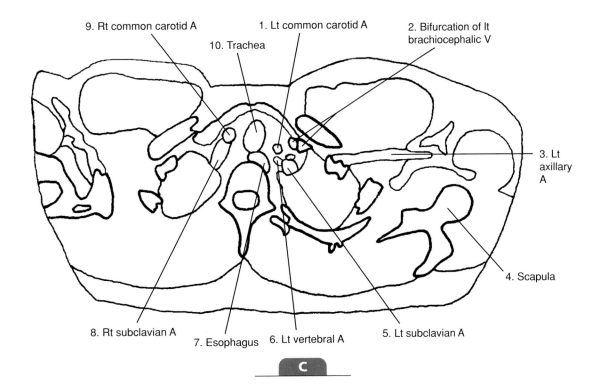

9. Rt common carotid A

1. Lt common carotid A

2. Bifurcation of lt brachiocephalic V

10. Trachea

3. Lt axillary A

4. Scapula

8. Rt subclavian A

7. Esophagus

6. Lt vertebral A

5. Lt subclavian A

C

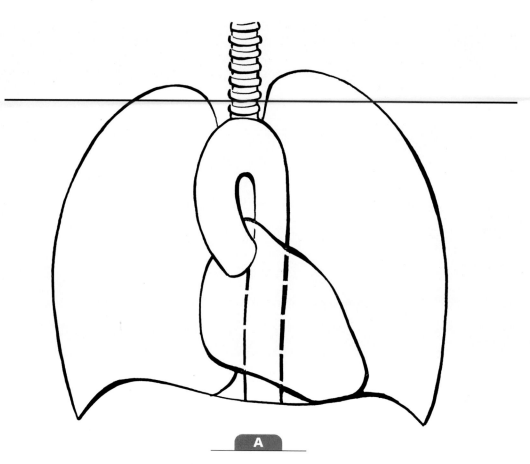

Figure 2-29 Axial CT image 5.

Figure 2-29 (A,B,C). This bony anatomy depicts the inferior parts of the scapulae, and the clavicles are obliquely sectioned in front of the thoracic cage. The right common carotid and subclavian arteries are no longer distinctly separate and are shown at their origin from the brachiocephalic artery. Adjacent to the clavicles, the brachiocephalic veins are superficial to the adjacent arterial structures. On the left side of the patient, the subclavian and common carotid arteries are shown just above their origin, the aortic arch. The left common carotid artery lies near the trachea, and the subclavian artery is found in cross-section near the upper lobe of the left lung.

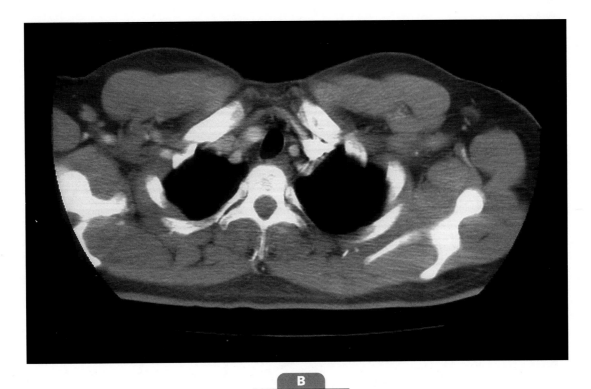

B

7. Rt brachiocephalic V

1. Lt clavicle

2. Lt brachiocephalic V

6. Origin of rt
subclavian A

5. Origin of rt
common carotid A

4. Lt common
carotid A

3. Lt subclavian A

C

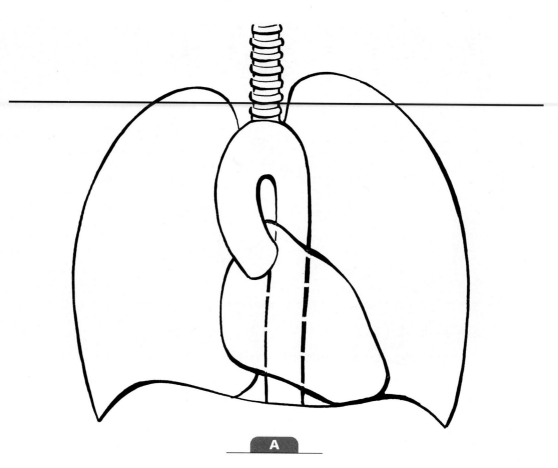

Figure 2-30 Axial CT image 6.

Figure 2-30 (A,B,C). All three of the brachiocephalic vessels can be identified. The right and left brachiocephalic veins are located immediately posterior to the clavicles. Owing to the more horizontal course of the left brachiocephalic vein, an oblique section is highlighted with contrast, whereas the right brachiocephalic vein is in cross-section with little contrast enhancement. Between the veins, the brachiocephalic artery (not labeled right or left because there is only one located on the right side) is just anterior to the trachea. Because the three major arteries within this image all originate from the aortic arch, they can be identified as the brachiocephalic artery, left common carotid artery, and the left subclavian artery. Centrally, the esophagus is found between the opening within the trachea and the vertebral body.

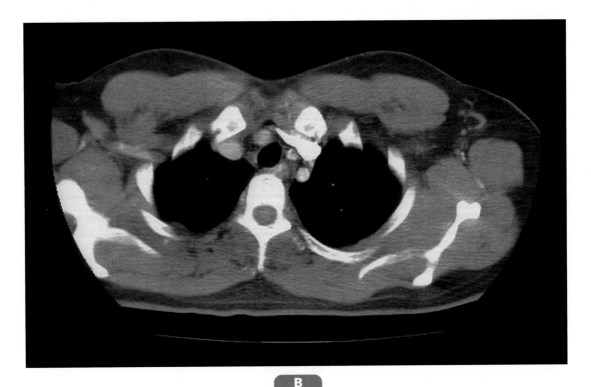

B

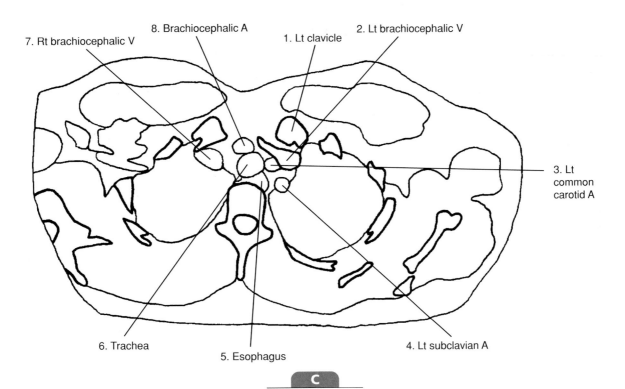

7. Rt brachiocephalic V

8. Brachiocephalic A

1. Lt clavicle

2. Lt brachiocephalic V

3. Lt common carotid A

4. Lt subclavian A

5. Esophagus

6. Trachea

C

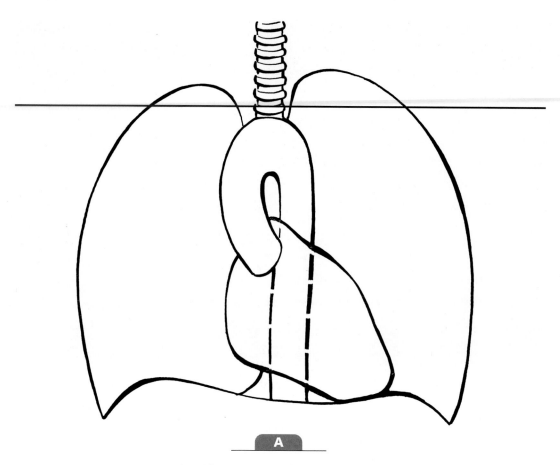

Figure 2-31 Axial CT image 7.

Figure 2-31 (A,B,C). On the anterior aspect of the chest wall, the manubrium of the sternum is shown articulating with the ends of the clavicles. Within the mediastinum, the anatomy is markedly similar to the previous section. The right and left brachiocephalic veins are just behind the clavicles, and the left vein is obliquely sectioned owing to its more horizontal projection within the mediastinum. Behind the veins, the three branches off the aortic arch are shown in order from right to left as the brachiocephalic artery, the left common carotid artery, and the left subclavian artery. The opening within the trachea is shown between the brachiocephalic artery and the vertebral body. Compared to the previous figure, the esophagus has moved to the left of the trachea at this lower level.

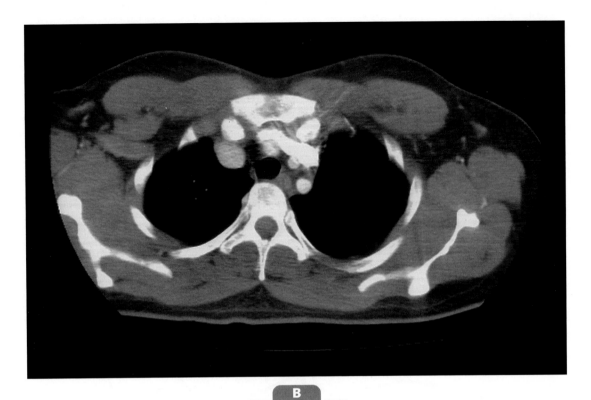

B

9. Rt brachiocephalic V

1. Manubrium

2. Lt clavicle

3. Lt brachiocephalic V

4. Lt common carotid A

8. Brachiocephalic A

7. Trachea

6. Esophagus

5. Lt subclavian A

C

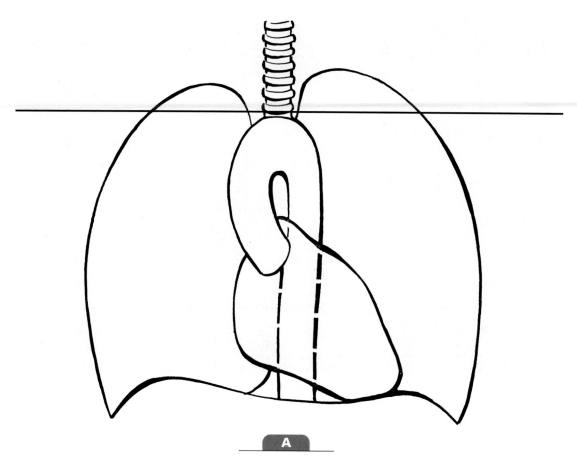

Figure 2-32 Axial CT image 8.

Figure 2-32 (A,B,C). The clavicles are no longer present, and the great vessels are tightly arranged within the mediastinum behind the manubrium. Similar to previous images, the right brachiocephalic vein is found in cross-section, and the left brachiocephalic vein is obliquely sectioned. The left brachiocephalic vein lies just anterior to the three arterial vessels originating from the aortic arch: the brachiocephalic artery, the left common carotid artery, and the left subclavian artery. Within the posterior mediastinum, the esophagus is again shown slightly to the left of the trachea.

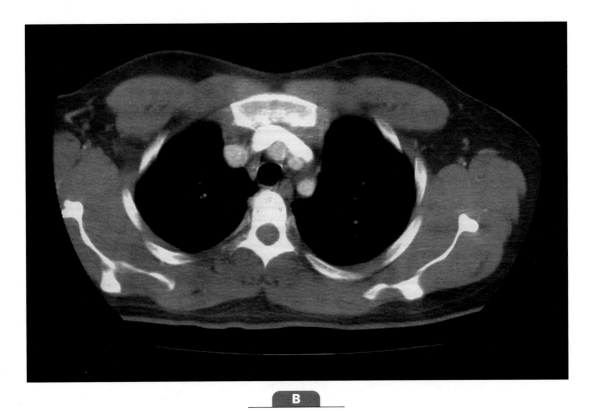

B

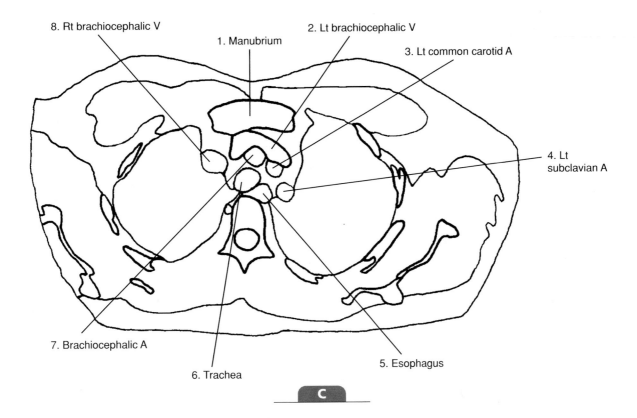

8. Rt brachiocephalic V

1. Manubrium

2. Lt brachiocephalic V

3. Lt common carotid A

4. Lt subclavian A

7. Brachiocephalic A

5. Esophagus

6. Trachea

C

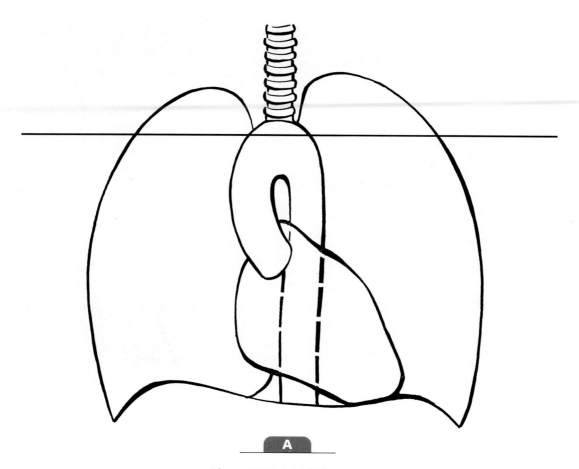

Figure 2-33 Axial CT image 9.

Figure 2-33 (A,B,C). The manubrium, the large, flat bone forming the anterior boundary of the mediastinum. The most distinctive difference between this image and the previous one is the absence of the three arteries, which have merged together to form one large arterial structure, the aortic arch. Also, the brachiocephalic veins are not as distinctly separable as in the previous section and will later be shown to join to form the superior vena cava. Within the posterior mediastinum, the trachea is still centrally located in front of the esophagus.

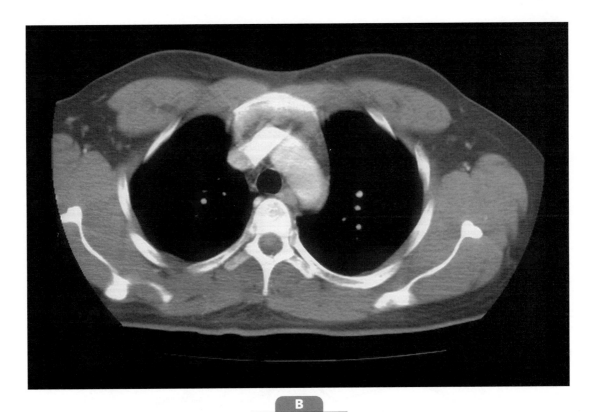

B

5. Lt brachiocephalic V

6. Manubrium

4. Rt brachiocephalic V

1. Aortic arch

2. Esophagus

3. Trachea

C

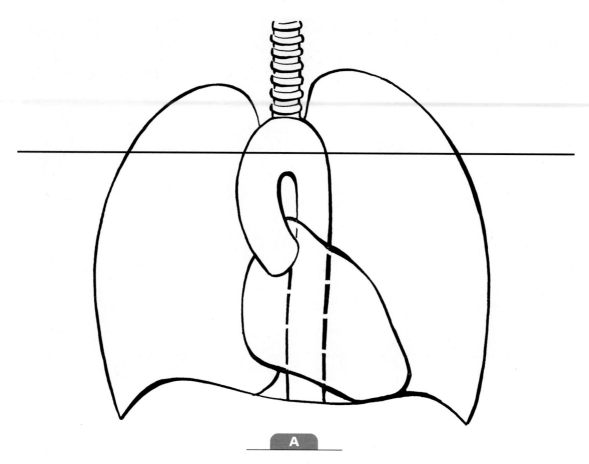

Figure 2-34 Axial CT image 10.

Figure 2-34 (A,B,C). Behind the manubrium, only two large vessels are seen anterior to the trachea. The aortic arch can easily be followed as it extends toward the left side of the posterior thoracic cage. The other major vessel, the superior vena cava, occupies a position adjacent to the right side of the aortic arch. In addition, a portion of a smaller vessel, the azygos arch, is shown on the right side of the trachea, extending from the right posterior thoracic cage toward the superior vena cava.

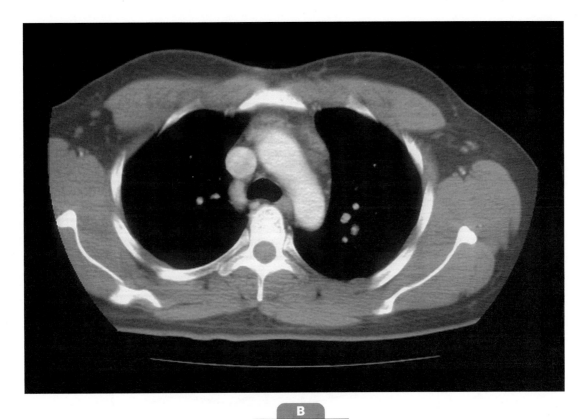

B

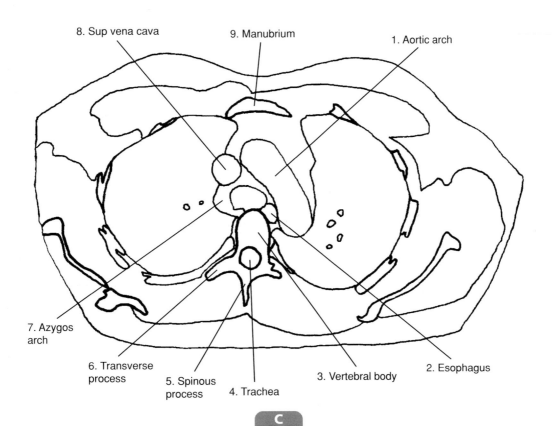

8. Sup vena cava   9. Manubrium   1. Aortic arch

7. Azygos arch

6. Transverse process   5. Spinous process   4. Trachea   3. Vertebral body   2. Esophagus

C

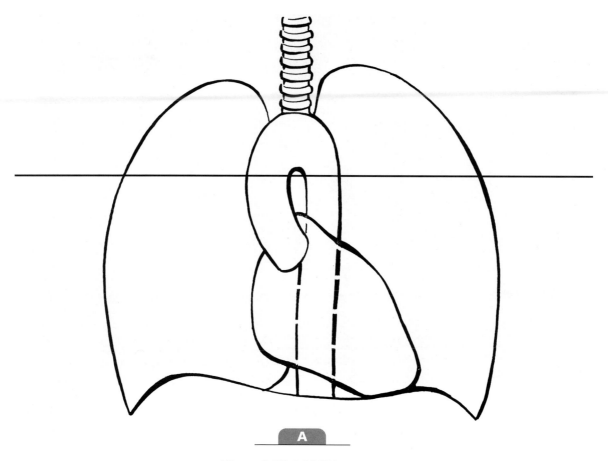

Figure 2-35 Axial CT image 11.

Figure 2-35 (A,B,C). At this level, the aorta can be separated into three parts: ascending (originating from the left ventricle), arch (extending over the pulmonary trunk and left bronchus), and descending (located on the left side of the thoracic vertebral bodies). Near the aorta, the location of the mediastinal pleura marks the boundary between the mediastinum and the pleural space, containing the lungs on either side. Posterior to the superior vena cava, the trachea appears "flattened out," indicating the section is nearing the point of bifurcation into the right and left main bronchi.

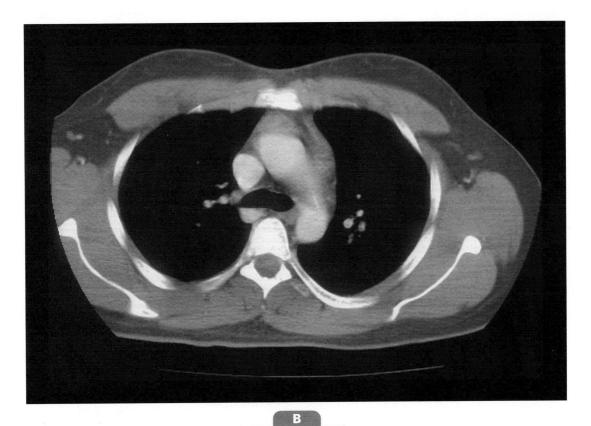

B

6. Sup vena cava   1. Ascending aorta   2. Mediastinal pleura

3. Bottom of aortic arch

5. Tracheal bifurcation   4. Descending aorta

C

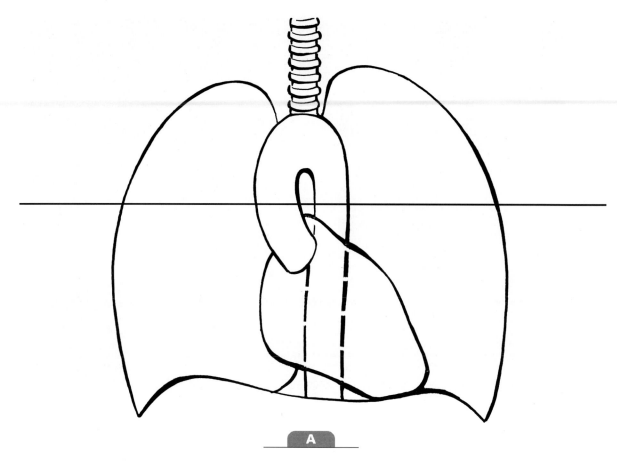

Figure 2-36 Axial CT image 12.

Figure 2-36 (A,B,C). Compared to the previous images, the most notable distinction in this figure is the absence of the arch between the ascending and descending parts of the aorta. Because this section is below the level of the arch, the left pulmonary artery is demonstrated extending into the left lung. At this level, a thin ridge representing the carina is separating the trachea into the right and left main bronchi. In addition, the right upper lobe bronchus is extending anteriorly from the main bronchus within the hilum of the right lung.

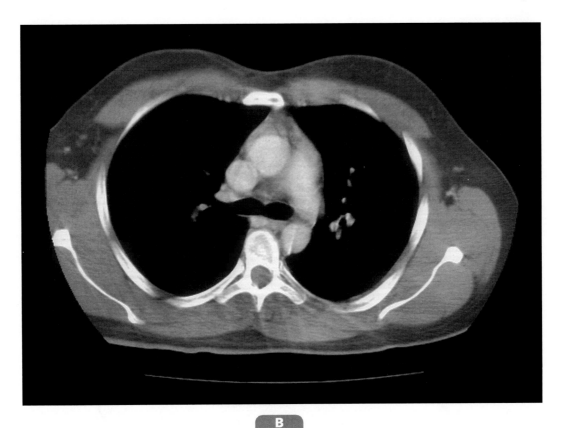

B

1. Ascending aorta

8. Sup vena cava

2. Lt pulmonary A

7. Rt
upper lobe
bronchus

6. Rt main bronchus

5. Carina

4. Lt main
bronchus

3. Descending aorta

C

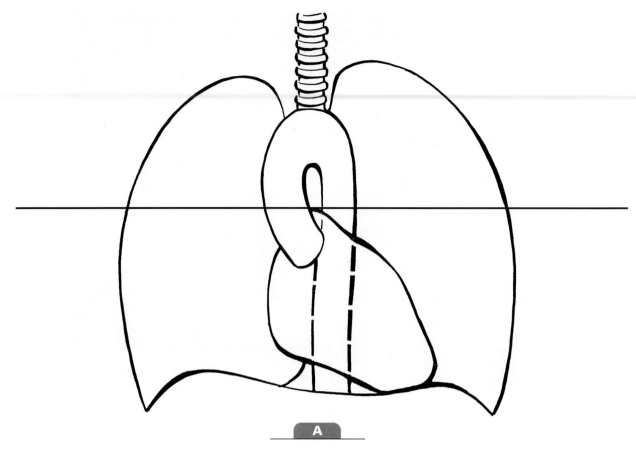

Figure 2-37 Axial CT image 13.

Figure 2-37 (A,B,C). The T-shape of the pulmonary trunk and arteries is demonstrated as obliquely sectioned in this figure, because the left pulmonary artery was demonstrated in the previous section. The pulmonary trunk (originating from the right ventricle) is longitudinally sectioned, originating from the anterior mediastinum and extending posteriorly. At the terminal end, the pulmonary trunk bifurcates forming the right and left pulmonary arteries. Together, these three arterial structures form a T, which can be described as "laying down on the top of the heart" to "go under" the arch of the aorta. Adjacent to the pulmonary trunk, the left superior pulmonary vein is demonstrated inferior to the left pulmonary artery included within the previous section. On the right side of the pulmonary trunk, the ascending aorta and the superior vena cava are shown in cross-section above the heart. Similar to previous images, the descending aorta and esophagus are found within the posterior mediastinum.

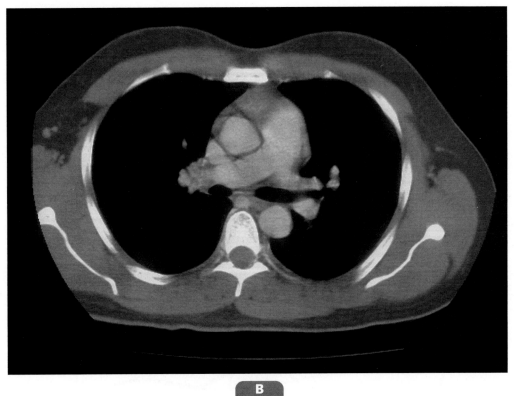

B

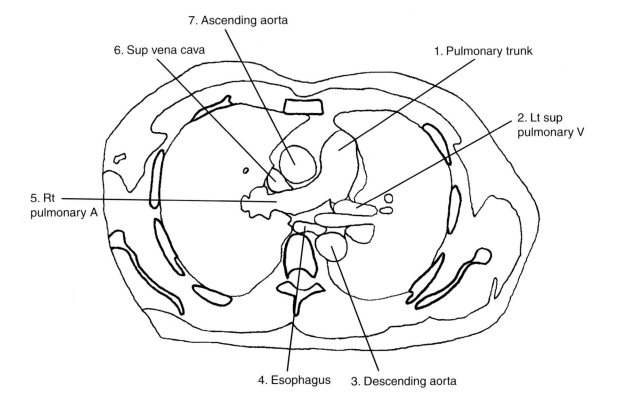

7. Ascending aorta

6. Sup vena cava

1. Pulmonary trunk

2. Lt sup
pulmonary V

5. Rt
pulmonary A

4. Esophagus　　3. Descending aorta

C

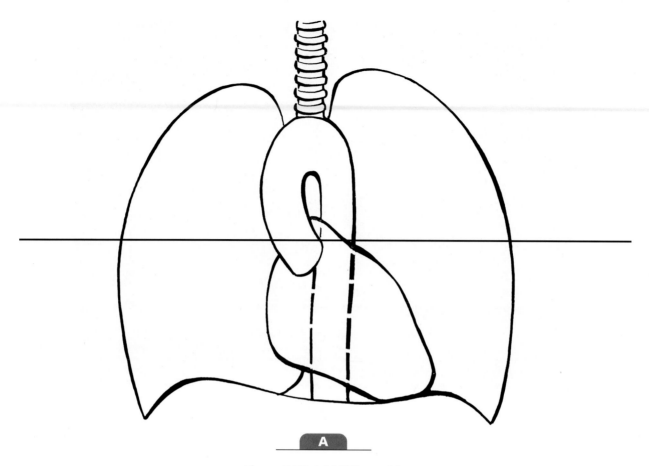

Figure 2-38 Axial CT image 14.

Figure 2-38 (A,B,C). The major vessels closely associated with the heart are not clearly demonstrated because of the movement caused by the beating of the heart during the scan. However, several major vessels can be identified by location on the anterior aspect of the heart: the superior vena cava, the ascending aorta, and the pulmonary trunk. Posterior to the three major vessels, the superior pulmonary veins from the right and left lungs are shown draining into the left atrium. Posterior to the atrium, the left main bronchus is giving rise to the left upper lobe bronchus, which lies just anterior to the descending branch of the left pulmonary artery. On the right side, the bronchus intermedius (continuation of right main bronchus after the origin of the upper lobe bronchus) is directly behind the superior pulmonary vein.

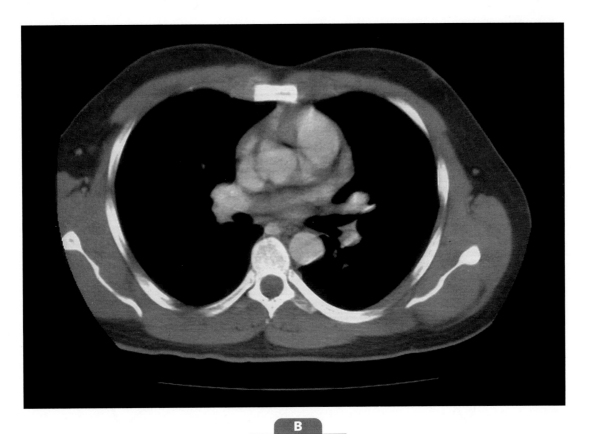

B

9. Sup vena cava

1. Origin of
pulmonary trunk

10. Ascending aorta

8. Rt sup pulmonary V

2. Lt atrium

3. Lt superior
pulmonary V

4. Lt upper
lobe bronchus

5. Desc branch
of lt pulmonary A

7. Bronchus intermedius

6. Lt main bronchus

C

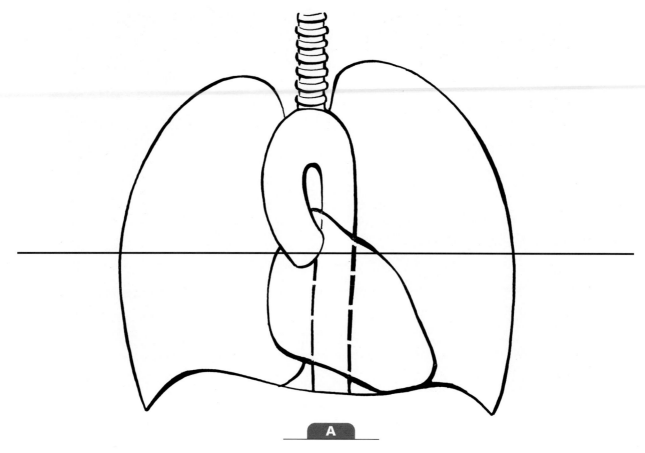

Figure 2-39 Axial CT image 15.

Figure 2-39 (A,B,C). Within the heart, the chambers are labeled as follows: the left atrium is most posterior, the right atrium is farthest to the right, the right ventricle is most anterior. Near the center of the heart, the ascending aorta is sectioned as it originates from the left ventricle. Outside of the heart, the upper and lower lobe bronchi are seen on the left side. Because the upper lobe lies more anterior to the lower lobe as a result of the course of the oblique fissure, the upper lobe bronchus is more anterior. On the right side of the mediastinum, the superior pulmonary vein is labeled near its termination at the left atrium. Behind the left atrium, the esophagus continues to be shown in cross-section in front of the vertebral column.

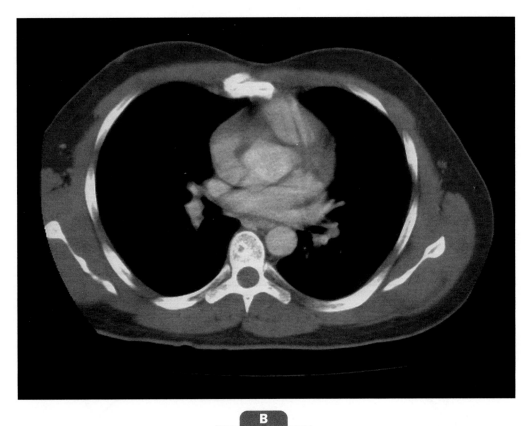

B

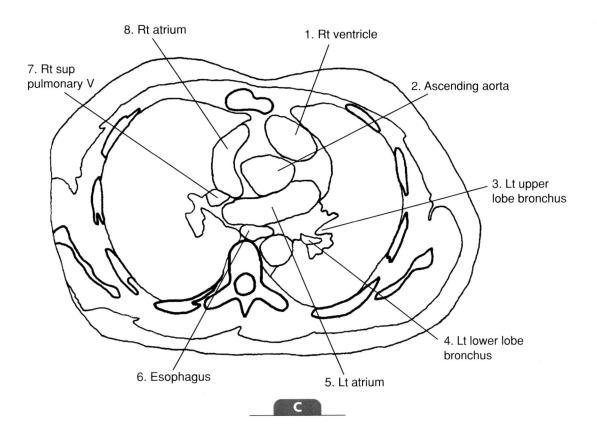

8. Rt atrium

1. Rt ventricle

7. Rt sup
pulmonary V

2. Ascending aorta

3. Lt upper
lobe bronchus

4. Lt lower lobe
bronchus

6. Esophagus

5. Lt atrium

C

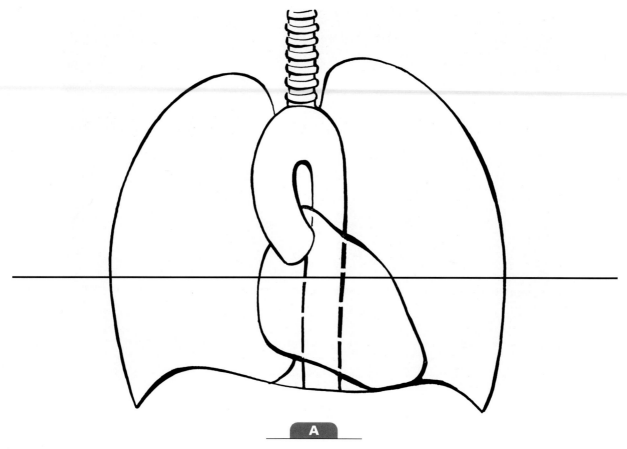

Figure 2-40 Axial CT image 16.

Figure 2-40 (A,B,C). All four chambers can be identified within the heart. The left atrium is most posterior and the right atrium is farthest to the right. As described earlier, the right ventricle is most anterior and the left ventricle is farthest to the left. Outside of the heart, the middle and lower lobe bronchi are seen on the right side near the position previously occupied by the bronchus intermedius.

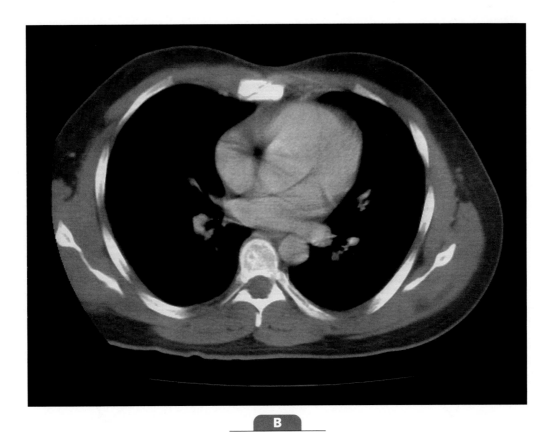

B

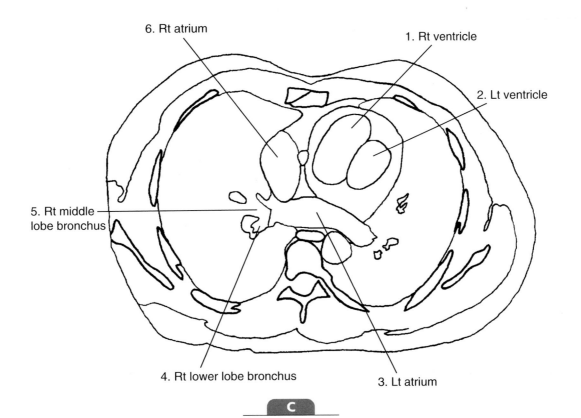

6. Rt atrium

1. Rt ventricle

2. Lt ventricle

5. Rt middle lobe bronchus

4. Rt lower lobe bronchus

3. Lt atrium

C

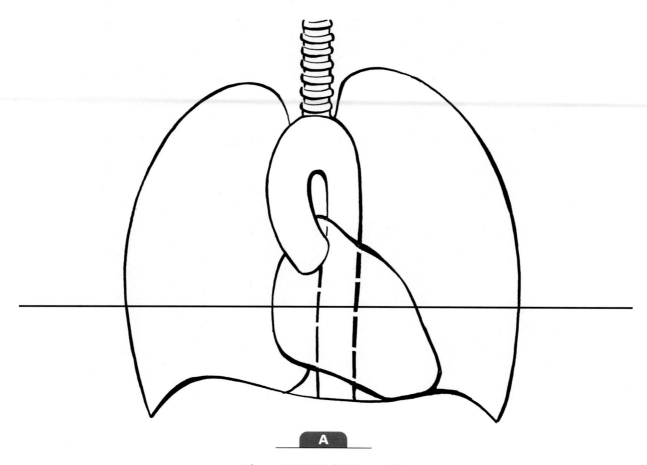

Figure 2-41 Axial CT image 17.

Figure 2-41 (A,B,C). Although the margin of the heart appears "shadowed" as an artifact of movement, all four chambers are seen in this figure. At this level, the left atrium is shown continuous with the left inferior pulmonary vein. As described in the previous image, the right atrium is farthest to the right, the right ventricle is most anterior, and the left ventricle is farthest to the left. Posterior to the heart, the esophagus and descending aorta are found beside the thoracic vertebral body. Within the vertebra, a pedicle and lamina, forming the vertebral arch, are labeled.

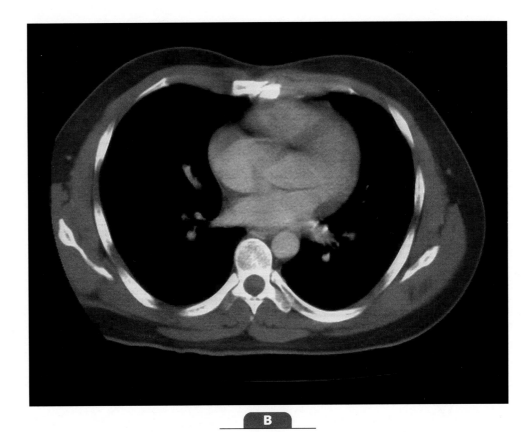

B

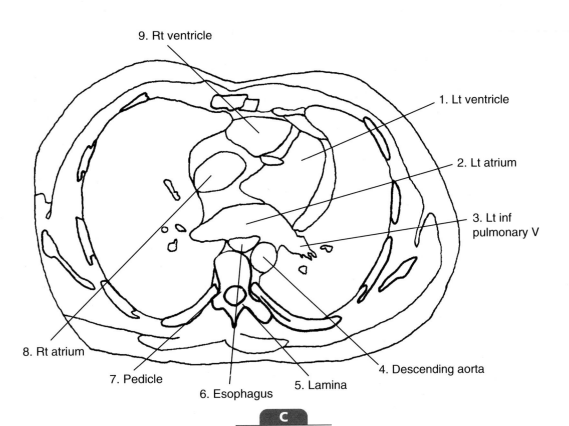

9. Rt ventricle

1. Lt ventricle

2. Lt atrium

3. Lt inf
pulmonary V

4. Descending aorta

5. Lamina

6. Esophagus

7. Pedicle

8. Rt atrium

C

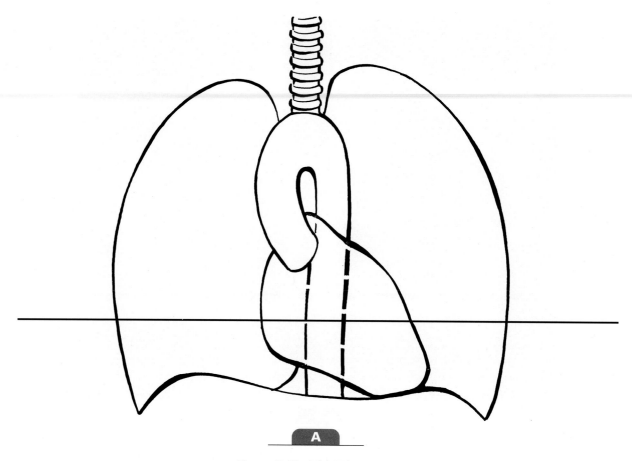

Figure 2-42 Axial CT image 18.

Figure 2-42 (A,B,C). The most remarkable difference in this section compared to the previous two images is the demonstration of the ventricular walls. Despite the shadowing caused by heart movement, the interventricular septum and the outer ventricular wall are shown encasing the ventricular chambers (filled with blood). Because the septum extends toward the left side of the anterior thorax, the right ventricle and atrium are generally found in front of the left ventricle and atrium. Behind the heart, the esophagus and descending aorta are beside the thoracic vertebra.

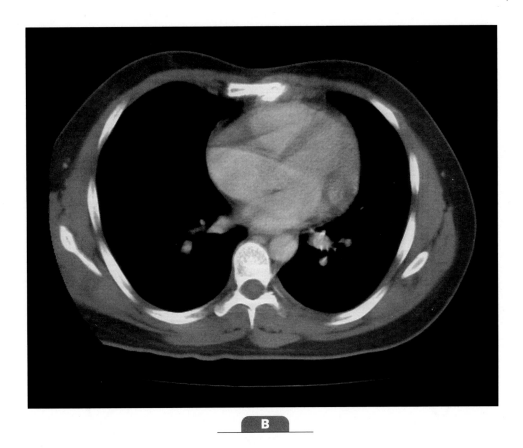

B

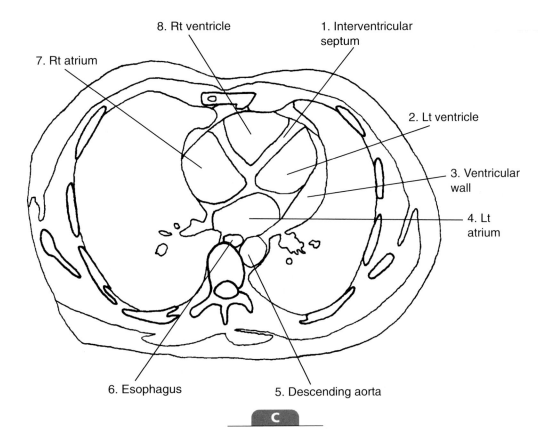

8. Rt ventricle

1. Interventricular septum

7. Rt atrium

2. Lt ventricle

3. Ventricular wall

4. Lt atrium

6. Esophagus

5. Descending aorta

C

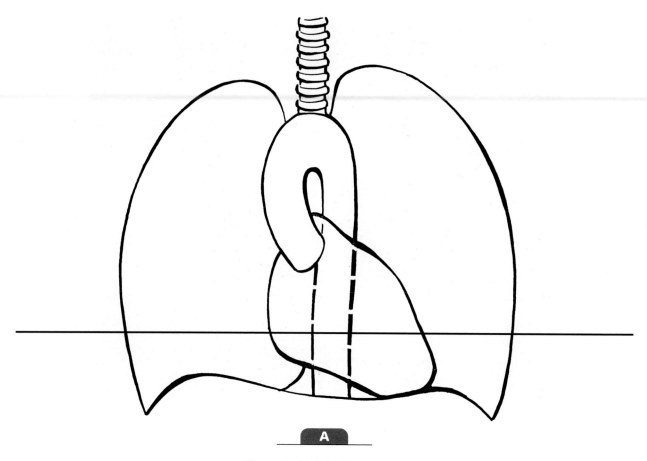

Figure 2-43 Axial CT image 19.

Figure 2-43 (A,B,C). The left atrium is no longer found on the posterior aspect of the heart, and the chambers of the ventricles are larger at this lower level. Similar to previous views, the right atrium is farthest to the right, the right ventricle is most anterior, and the left ventricle is farthest to the left. Although the esophagus and descending aorta are again shown behind the heart, the azygos vein is clearly discernible between the esophagus and the vertebral body.

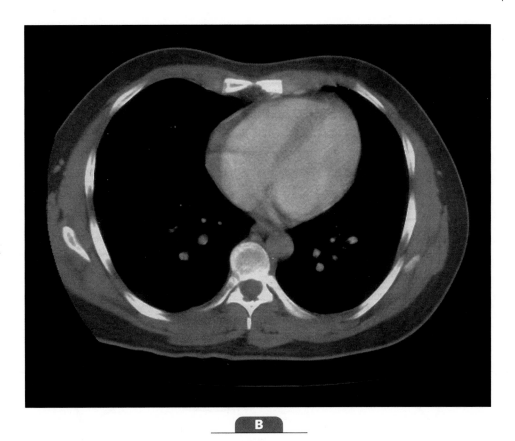

B

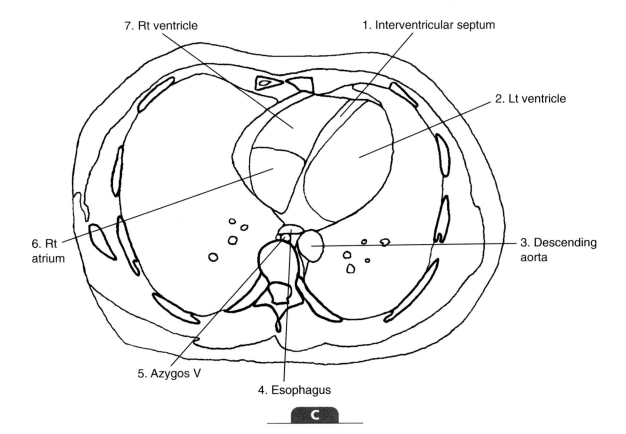

7. Rt ventricle

1. Interventricular septum

2. Lt ventricle

6. Rt atrium

3. Descending aorta

5. Azygos V

4. Esophagus

C

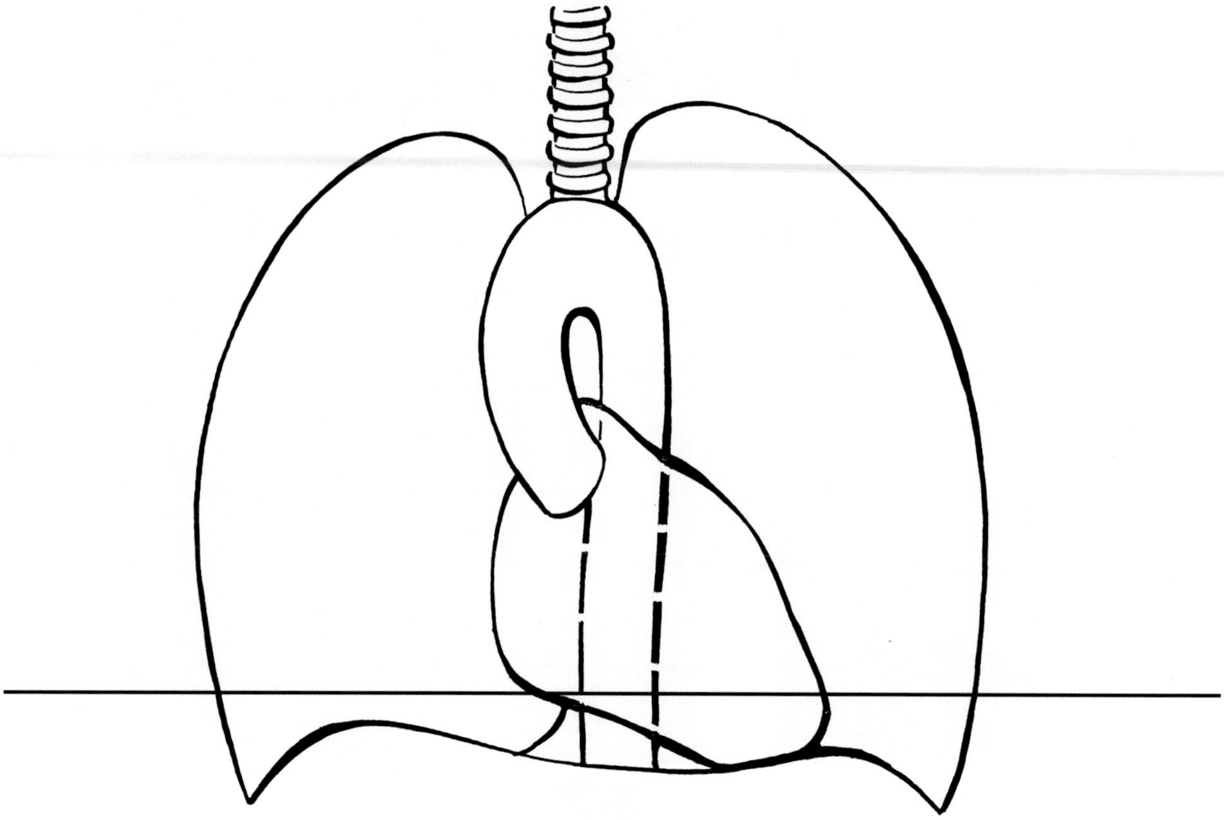

Figure 2-44 Axial CT image 20.

Figure 2-44 (A,B,C). This image shows a section through the middle region of the heart and includes the bottom of the right atrium. The larger chambers, the right and left ventricles, are separated by the interventricular septum and are larger than in previous views. Behind the heart, the esophagus and descending aorta are labeled within the posterior mediastinum.

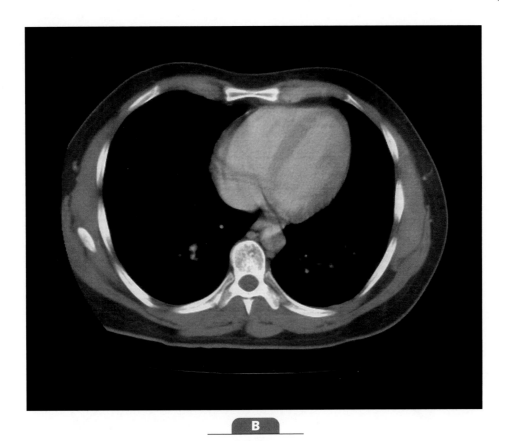

B

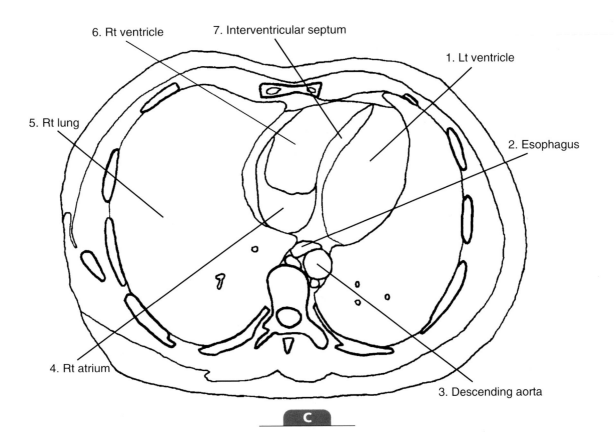

6. Rt ventricle   7. Interventricular septum

1. Lt ventricle

5. Rt lung

2. Esophagus

4. Rt atrium

3. Descending aorta

C

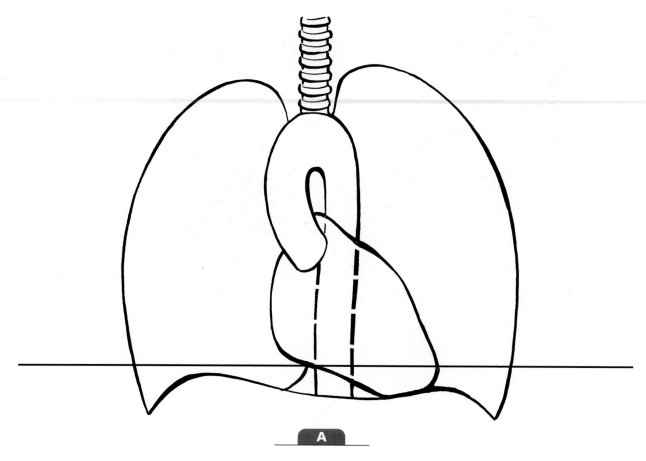

Figure 2-45 Axial CT image 21.

Figure 2-45 (A,B,C). At this level, the right atrium is continuous with the inferior vena cava and can be distinguished by contrast enhancement. As in the previous image, the interventricular septum divides the left and right ventricles. Posterior to the heart, the esophagus and descending aorta are again shown within the posterior mediastinum. On either side of the aorta, the azygos vessels are cross-sectioned adjacent to the vertebral body. Although the azygos vein was previously labeled on the right side of the aorta, this section is the first to clearly show the hemiazygos vein on the left side of the vertebral body. If this section were above the level of T6, a small vein in this position would be the accessory hemiazygos vein.

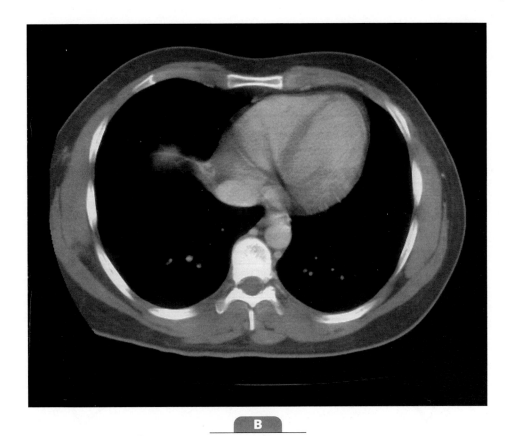

B

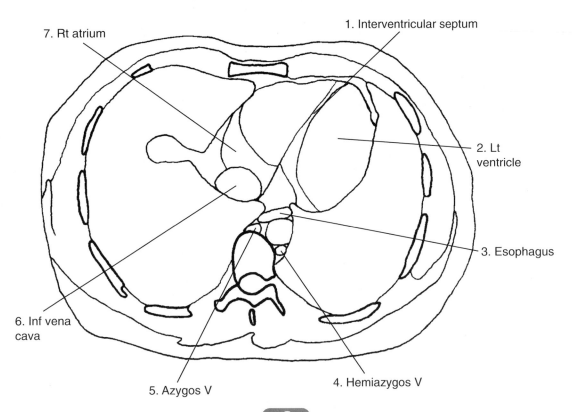

7. Rt atrium

1. Interventricular septum

2. Lt ventricle

3. Esophagus

6. Inf vena cava

5. Azygos V

4. Hemiazygos V

C

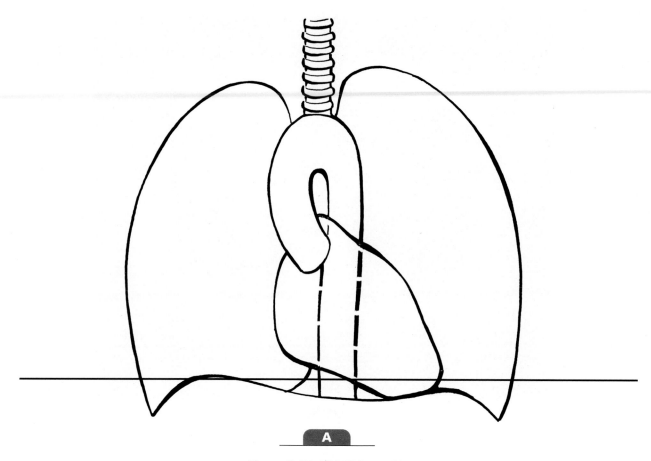

Figure 2-46 Axial CT image 22.

Figure 2-46 (A,B,C). The unique feature of this figure is the appearance of a dense structure, the top of the liver, surrounded by the right lung. The liver appears nearly continuous with the heart, because the central tendon of the diaphragm is obscured by the shadow caused by the beating of the heart during the scan. Between the liver and the heart, the contrast-enhanced inferior vena cava is found in the place previously occupied by the right atrium. Similar to previous views, the interventricular septum separates the right and left ventricles.

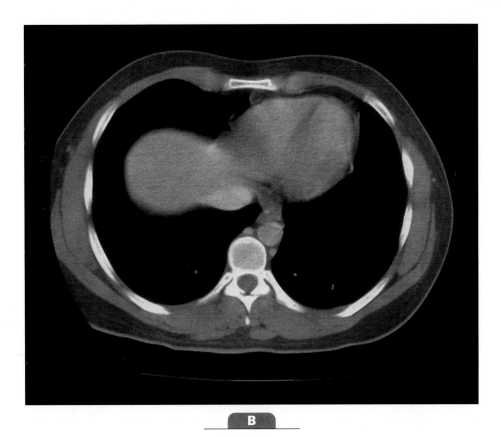

B

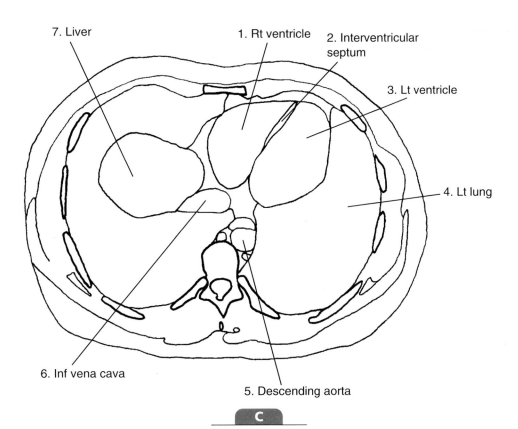

7. Liver

1. Rt ventricle

2. Interventricular septum

3. Lt ventricle

4. Lt lung

6. Inf vena cava

5. Descending aorta

C

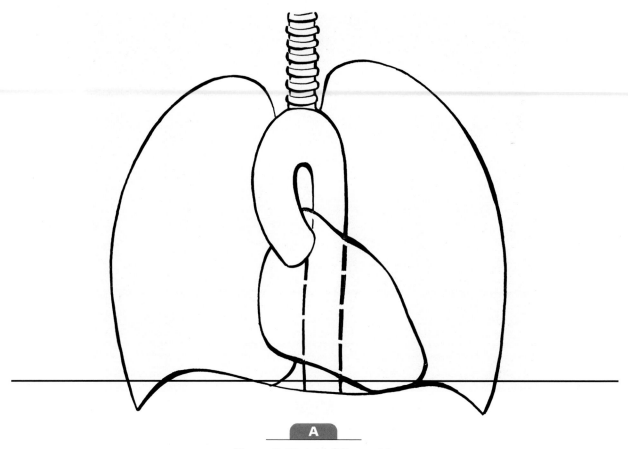

Figure 2-47 Axial CT image 23.

Figure 2-47 (A,B,C). The liver is readily identified on the right side surrounded by the right lung. Within the mediastinum, the section passes through the lower heart, demonstrating the bottom right and left ventricles. As described previously, the right ventricle is more anterior and lies next to the chest wall. The small part of the left ventricle is more posteriorly situated on the left side. Posterior to the heart, the esophagus is near the midline, and the fundus of the stomach is surrounded by the left lung. Because of the shape of the stomach, the fundus is superior to the gastroesophageal junction. Within the posterior mediastinum, the azygos and hemi-azygos veins are shown in cross-section beside the descending aorta.

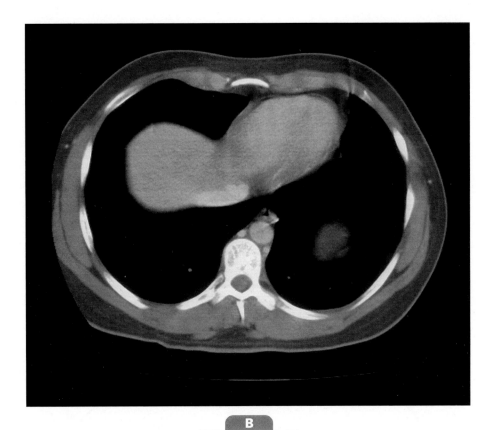

B

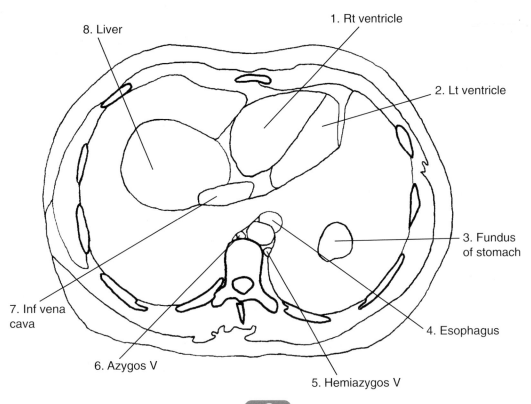

8. Liver

1. Rt ventricle

2. Lt ventricle

3. Fundus of stomach

4. Esophagus

7. Inf vena cava

6. Azygos V

5. Hemiazygos V

C

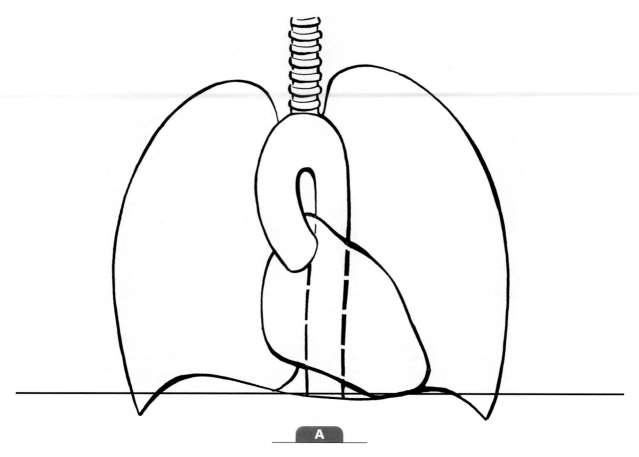

Figure 2-48 Axial CT image 24.

Figure 2-48 (A,B,C). At this level, the heart is no longer seen, and most of the structures demonstrated are contents of the abdominal cavity. The liver occupies much of the section and extends across the midline to the left side. Within the posterior edge of the liver, the contrast-enhanced inferior vena cava is embedded within the liver. On the left, the fundus of the stomach is slightly closer to the esophagus and the base of the left lung is seen only adjacent to the chest wall. Posterior to the stomach, the crescent-shaped spleen is demonstrated as a dense structure bordering the base of the left lung. Anterior to the stomach, the splenic flexure of the colon is shown inferior to the left lung as an irregular-shaped structure containing pockets of air.

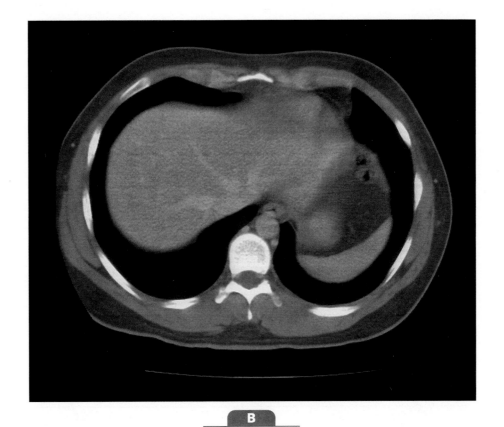

B

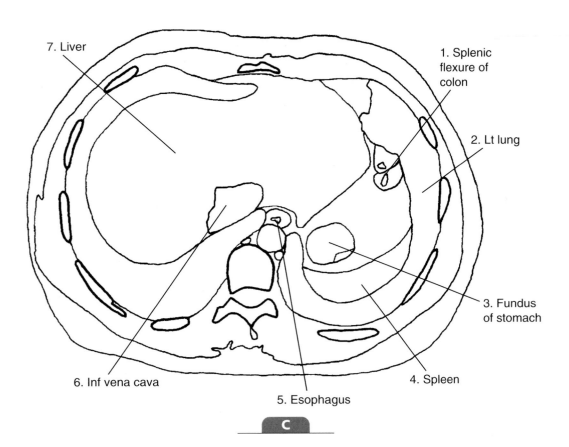

7. Liver

1. Splenic
flexure of
colon

2. Lt lung

3. Fundus
of stomach

6. Inf vena cava

4. Spleen

5. Esophagus

C

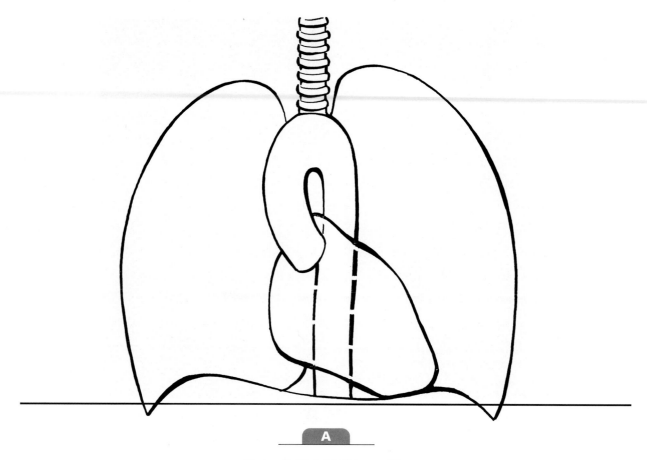

Figure 2-49 Axial CT image 25.

Figure 2-49 (A,B,C). The right lung forms a thin margin around the liver next to the chest wall. Near the midline, the contrast-enhanced inferior vena cava is again found within the posterior margin of the liver. Adjacent to the inferior vena cava, the gastroesophageal junction marks the beginning of the body of the stomach, which is considerably larger than the fundus. On the left side, both the spleen and the splenic flexure of the colon are bordered by the left lung. Although this section is almost below the chest, the descending aorta, azygos vein, and hemiazygos vein are still found within the posterior mediastinum.

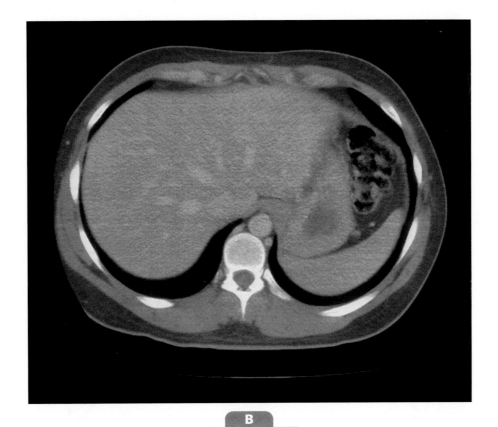

B

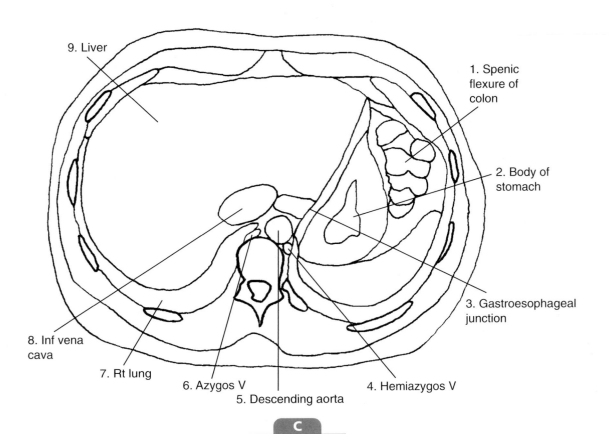

9. Liver

1. Spenic flexure of colon

2. Body of stomach

3. Gastroesophageal junction

8. Inf vena cava

7. Rt lung

6. Azygos V

5. Descending aorta

4. Hemiazygos V

C

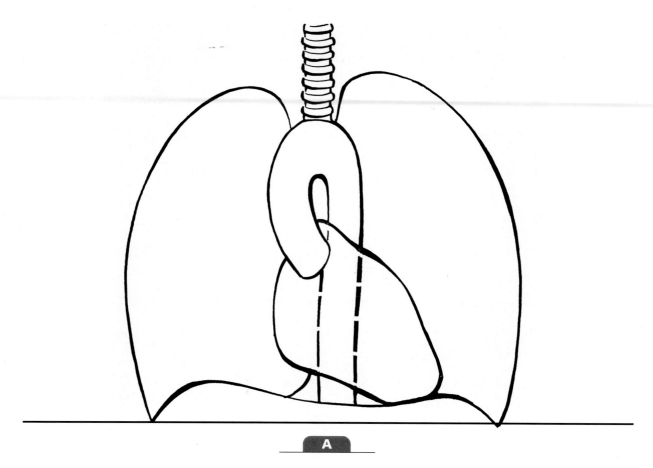

Figure 2-50 Axial CT image 26.

Figure 2-50 (A,B,C). The costophrenic angles of the right and left lungs are just inside the chest wall, indicating this is the last image necessary for an examination of the chest. Within the abdomen, the liver occupies most of the right side and appears to wrap around the inferior vena cava. On the left side, the body of the stomach is sectioned by the splenic flexure of the colon and the spleen. Within the lower mediastinum, the descending aorta lies between the azygos vein on the right and the hemiazygos vein on the left.

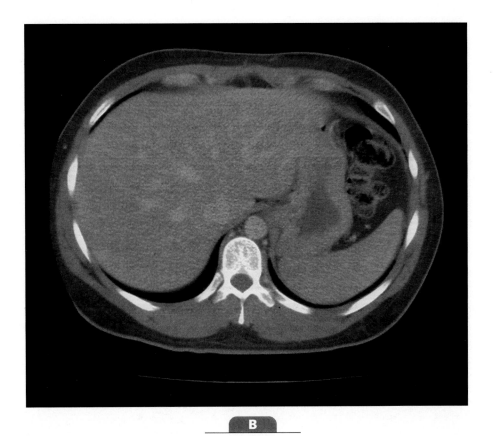

B

9. Liver

1. Splenic flexure of colon

2. Body of stomach

3. Spleen

8. Costophrenic angle

7. Inf vena cava

6. Azygos V

5. Descending aorta

4. Hemiazygos V

C

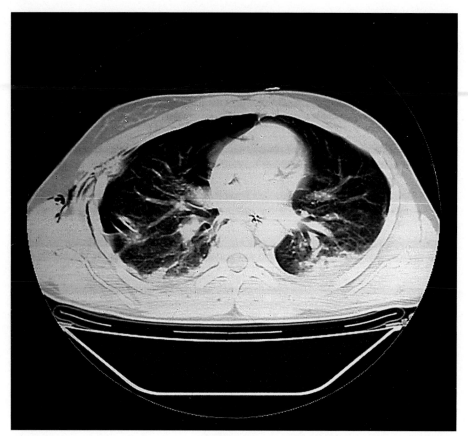

Figure 2-51

Supplement 2-1. *Figure 2-51 shows a 27-year-old man who was injured in a motor vehicle accident. The image was obtained at lung parenchymal window settings after the administration of contrast media. Within the chest wall, multiple rib fractures are found on the right side. Inside the right anterior chest wall, a pneumothorax is shown outside the lung parenchyma as an area of decreased density owing to the absence of bronchial markings. Behind both lungs, there are collections of fluid, representing a bilateral hemothorax. Within the parenchyma of the right lung, a chest tube is obliquely sectioned (in subsequent images, it is seen exiting through the upper anterolateral chest wall).*

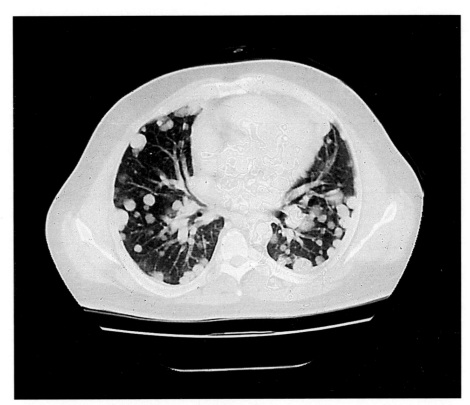

Figure 2-52

Supplement 2-2. *Figure 2-52 shows a 52-year-old male chronic smoker. The patient complained of a persistent cough and a lack of energy. The advanced pulmonary carcinoma is readily apparent in the axial CT image of the chest. Multiple lesions are present in both lungs and appear to be concentrated in the mediastinal and distal parts of the lungs. In addition, the bronchioles are irregular in shape and appear expanded with edema. Shortly after the CT scan, the patient decided to undergo radiation therapy treatment for his disease.*

REVIEW QUESTIONS

1. Describe the azygos vein.
2. Which of the following does not originate from the aorta?
   A. Brachiocephalic artery
   B. Left subclavian artery
   C. Left vertebral artery
   D. Left common carotid artery
3. The spinous process is connected to the transverse process of the vertebra by the_____.
4. The pulmonary arteries carry deoxygenated blood. True or False?
5. The ascending aorta originates from what part of the heart?
   A. Left ventricle
   B. Left atrium
   C. Right ventricle
   D. Right atrium
6. Which chamber of the heart lies most posteriorly?
   A. Left ventricle
   B. Right ventricle
   C. Left atrium
   D. Right atrium
7. Which of the following structures is located anterior to the hilum of the lungs?
   A. Superior vena cava
   B. Esophagus
   C. Descending aorta
   D. Accessory hemiazygos vein
8. Which of the following lobes of the lungs receive air via the bronchus intermedius?
   A. Right middle and lower
   B. Right upper and middle
   C. Left middle and lower
   D. Left upper and middle
9. When you are viewing an axial image of a patient, your right side should always be the patient's_____side.
10. The aorta arches over all of the following structures except the
    A. Pulmonary trunk
    B. Left brachiocephalic vein
    C. Left main bronchus
    D. Left pulmonary veins
11. The hemiazygos vein is located on which side of the body? Right or Left.
12. The_____lines the inside of the chest musculoskeletal wall and the_____lines the surface of the lungs to form a smooth lubricated surface for movement resulting from breathing.
13. In an axial section through the oblique fissure of the left lung, which lobe of the lung would be most anterior?
14. Which of the following structures is most posterior in the chest?
    A. Trachea
    B. Esophagus
    C. Ascending aorta
    D. Pulmonary trunk
15. Describe the left subclavian vein.
16. Which chamber of the heart pumps blood directly into the pulmonary artery?
    A. Right atrium
    B. Right ventricle
    C. Left atrium
    D. Left ventricle
17. The vertebral arteries originate from the
    A. Subclavian arteries
    B. Common carotid arteries
    C. Aorta
    D. Axillary arteries
18. The_____is the region on the medical aspect near the center of both the right and the left lungs, and is the site where the bronchi, venis, and arteries, enter and exit the lungs next to the heart.
19. The vertebral arch consists of_____pedicles,_____laminae, and_____processes (_____transverse,_____articular, and_____spinous).
20. In an MR image of the median sagittal chest, which chamber of the heart would be located most posteriorly?

Chapter 3

Abdomen

OBJECTIVES

Upon completion of this chapter, the student should be able to:

1. Describe the superior and inferior boundaries of the abdomen.
2. Describe the general location of the segments of small and large intestine within the abdomen.
3. Identify and describe the location and lobes of the liver.
4. Describe the enclosing structures separating the abdomen.
5. Explain the location and general function of the gallbladder, pancreas, spleen, adrenal glands, and kidneys.
6. Describe the bile duct system.
7. Follow the course of blood as it passes through portal system.
8. Describe the major arteries and veins located within the lower chest and abdomen.
9. Explain the relationships between structures located within the abdomen.
10. Correctly identify anatomical structures on patient CT images of the abdomen.

ANATOMICAL OVERVIEW

The abdomen is generally considered as the region of the body between the chest and pelvis. Although this seems quite simple, the boundaries of the abdomen are often defined differently by different texts because the abdominal cavity extends well into each of the adjacent regions. The most superior boundary of the abdominal cavity is the dome-shaped diaphragm, which allows a considerable part of the abdomen to lie within the bony thoracic cage. Inferiorly, the abdominal cavity extends into the pelvis and occupies most of the false or greater pelvis, leading some individuals to consider the pelvis as the lower part of the abdomen. Because the abdomen and pelvis are often imaged separately, the pelvis will be further described in the next chapter.

Skeletal

Lumbar (*LŬM-bar*) **vertebrae.** Typically, the vertebral column contains five lumbar vertebrae, which form the posterior border of the abdominal cavity. Owing to the highly variable division of lumbar vertebrae with adjacent thoracic and sacral vertebrae, four and six lumbar vertebrae are common anomalies that may confuse the viewer when determining image location. Compared to the other vertebrae, these can be distinguished by their large size and the absence of costal facets and transverse foramina.

Enclosing Structures

Diaphragm (*DĪ-ă-fram*). The diaphragm is a broad, flat muscle made up of skeletal muscle along the periphery that converges on a broad flat tendon, the central tendon (Fig. 3-1). It is often described as two hemidiaphragms (the right and left), because the right side is usually more superior because of the underlying liver. Its muscular portion originates from several sources: (*a*) the sternal process, (*b*) the costal cartilages and bone of ribs 7 through 12, and (*c*) the upper lumbar vertebrae. Although the diaphragm forms a septum between the thoracic and abdominal cavities, several structures (inferior vena cava, esophagus, and descending aorta) pass through openings within the diaphragm to pass between the chest and abdomen.

Crura (*KRŪ-ră*). The muscular parts of the diaphragm that originate from the lumbar vertebrae and ascend to the central tendon. The right crus arises from the upper three or four lumbar vertebrae, and the left crus originates from the upper two or three. The crura combine with ligaments to form the openings for the aorta and esophagus.

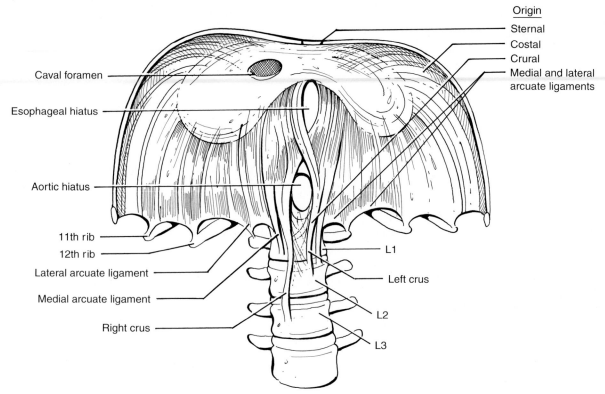

Figure 3-1 Inferior surface of the diaphragm.

Peritoneum (*PER-i- tŏ-NĒ-ŭm*). Its structure and function are similar to those of the pleura, described in Chapter 2 (Fig. 3-2). It is a smooth membrane lining the abdominal cavity (parietal peritoneum) and the abdominal viscera (visceral peritoneum), creating the peritoneal cavity. Because the organs within the abdominal cavity are closely arranged, the peritoneal cavity is normally only a small space containing a thin film of serous fluid produced by the membranes. Much like the pleura, the peritoneum minimizes friction and acts as a barrier to the spread of infection within the abdomen.

Mesentery (*MES-en-ter-ē*). In addition to the parietal and visceral peritoneum, the mesentery is a double layer of peritoneum that encloses the intestine and attaches it to the abdominal wall. Because of constant moving and changes in shape, much of the intestine is described as having no fixed position, being only loosely organized by the mesentery. The mesentery also contains the arteries and veins of the intestines and is a primary site for fat storage within the body.

Retroperitoneal (*RE-trō-PER-i-tō-NĒ-ăl*). Behind the peritoneal cavity, this space is adjacent to the posterior abdominal wall and contains the following abdominal organs: kidneys, pancreas, distal duodenum, and ascending and descending portions of the colon.

Viscera (*VIS-er-ă*)

Stomach. A mobile organ situated in the upper left side of the abdominal cavity just below the left hemidiaphragm. The esophagus descends through the esophageal hiatus in the diaphragm to join the body of the stomach. Above the gastroesophageal junction, the fundus is the part of the stomach found next to the esophagus directly under the diaphragm. Below the body of the stomach, the pyloric part is the narrowing region that is continuous with the duodenum (Fig. 3-3). Although the location and shape of the stomach will vary between individuals and can change over time within a single individual, the relationship of the three segments from superior to inferior will usually remain the same.

Small intestine. The site of the major part of digestion. It extends from the termination of the stomach to the large intestine, ranging from 5 to 8 m in length. It includes the duodenum, jejunum, and ileum.

Duodenum (*dū-ō-DĒ-nŭm*). The first segment of the small intestine, extending from the pyloric part of the stomach to the jejunum. It is approximately 25 cm long. Its C shape wraps around the head of the pancreas and the superior mesenteric vessels (Fig. 3-4). Only the superior part of the duodenum lies within the peritoneum, the

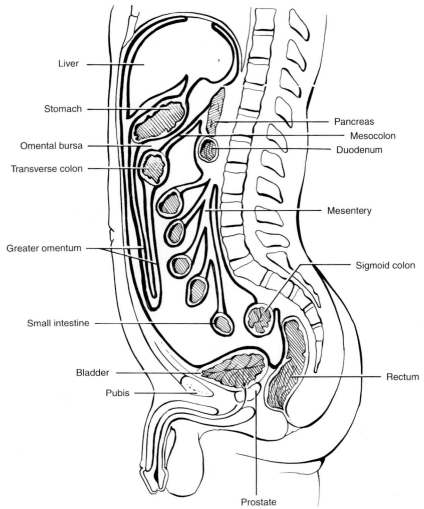

Figure 3-2 Median sagittal view of abdomen demonstrating the peritoneum and mesentery.

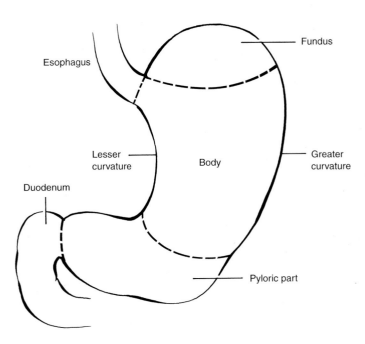

Figure 3-3 Sketch illustrating the three parts of the stomach.

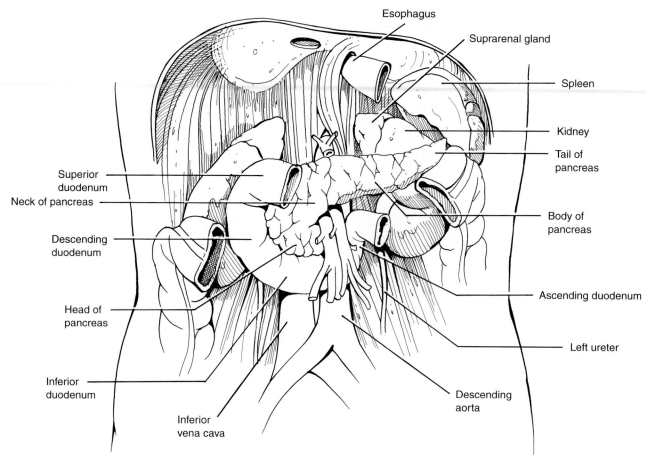

Figure 3-4 Anterior view of the structures within the upper abdominal cavity after removal of the stomach, jejunum, and the transverse colon.

remaining three parts (descending, inferior, and ascending) are all retroperitoneal and are fixed in position.

Jejunum (jĕ-JŪ-nŭm). The second segment of the small intestine is arranged in numerous coils or loops and is approximately 2.4 m long and extends from the duodenum to the ileum (Fig. 3-5). It is difficult to distinguish from the ileum, even though it has a thicker wall, greater diameter, and larger vascular supply. In the average patient, location typically provides a general means for distinguishing between the jejunum and ileum; the jejunum usually lies in the umbilical region, whereas the ileum lies in the lower abdomen and pelvis.

Ileum (IL-ē-ŭm). The third segment is also arranged in numerous coils or loops and is the longest segment of the small intestine, averaging 3.6 m in length. As noted, the ileum is difficult to distinguish from the jejunum, except for its lower position in the abdominal cavity. It terminates in the lower right quadrant of the abdominal cavity at the ileocecal valve and is continuous with the first part of the large intestine. *Helpful hint:* The spelling of the ileum of the intestine is often confused with the ilium of the bony pelvis. If one notes that the shape of the coiled intestine resembles

the letter e, then one should remember the proper spelling for both anatomical structures.

Large intestine. The large intestine is approximately 1.5 m in length and extends from the terminal ileum to the anus (Figs. 3-5 and 3-6). The material passing from the terminal ileum to the large intestine is about 90% water, most of which is absorbed by the large intestine. Many individuals will use the term *colon* synonymously with *large intestine;* however, this is incorrect. The large intestine is made up of two parts: the cecum and the colon.

Cecum (SĒ-kŭm). The first segment of the large intestine located in the lower right side of the abdomen posterior to the peritoneum. It is below the ileocecal valve and forms a blind pouch that is continuous with the ascending colon. At 1 to 2 cm below the opening of the ileocecal valve within the cecum, a smaller opening leads into the appendix. The appendix is a long narrow tube averaging about 8 cm in length with a highly variable position that partially depends on the shape and contents within the cecum.

Ascending colon. The segment originating above the ileocecal valve that is continuous with the cecum and extends

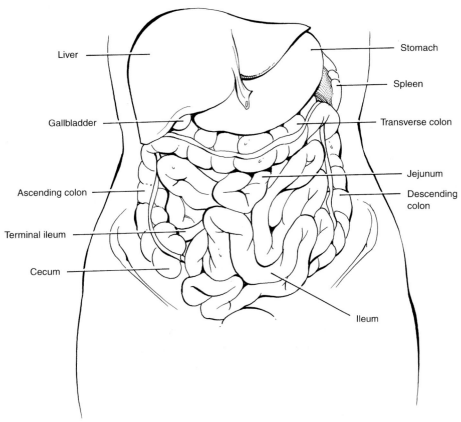

Figure 3-5 Anterior view of the contents within the abdomen following removal and reflection of the anterior abdominal wall.

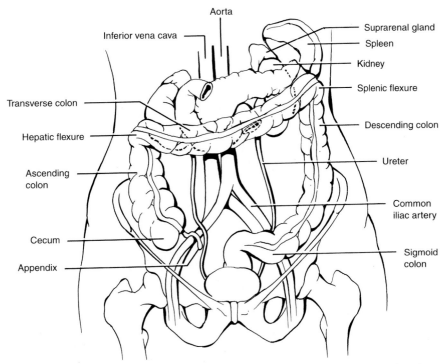

Figure 3-6 Sketch demonstrating the location of the large intestine as compared to the selected structures adjacent to the posterior abdominal wall.

upward to the hepatic flexure next to the liver on the right side of the abdomen. Similar to the cecum, it is retroperitoneal and relatively fixed in position along the posterior wall of the abdomen. In the lower abdomen, it lies adjacent to the musculature forming the posterior abdominal wall; and in the upper abdomen, it lies anterior to the right kidney.

Hepatic (he-PAT-ik) flexure of colon. The bend or right flexure of the colon between the ascending and transverse segments of the colon. As the name implies, the flexure is next to the liver on the upper right side of the abdomen. Owing to the more anterior position of the transverse colon, the hepatic flexure is best demonstrated in an oblique view from the right anterior side.

Transverse colon. The segment of the colon traversing across the abdomen between the hepatic and splenic flexures. In contrast to the ascending colon, it is invested with peritoneum and is suspended from the posterior abdominal wall by mesentery (the transverse mesocolon). Although the ends have a fixed position, the location of the middle region is highly variable and may be found from the upper abdomen to the greater pelvis. Despite the level, the middle region usually lies adjacent to the anterior abdominal wall.

Splenic (SPLEN-ik) flexure of colon. At the terminal end of the transverse colon, the left flexure of the colon redirects the colon downward to become the descending colon. Unlike the hepatic flexure, this flexure is best demonstrated in the oblique view from the left anterior side and is usually more superiorly situated, adjacent to the spleen.

Descending colon. The part of the large intestine originating at the splenic flexure that extends along the left posterior wall to the level of the pelvic brim or inlet. Within the greater pelvis, it travels downward to join the sigmoid colon. Similar to the ascending colon, it is retroperitoneal and is fixed in position by the musculature of the posterior abdominal wall.

Liver. The largest gland in the body, found in the upper abdominal cavity on the right side. For the most part, it lies within the bony thoracic cage, and its superior surface is covered by the diaphragm. The superior liver is dome shaped, following the contour of the diaphragm; and the inferior or visceral surface is somewhat flattened, facing downward toward the other viscera within the abdomen. On the visceral surface, an H-shaped arrangement of fissures and fossae is found dividing the liver into four separate lobes (Fig. 3-7). The transverse part of the H is formed by the porta hepatis,

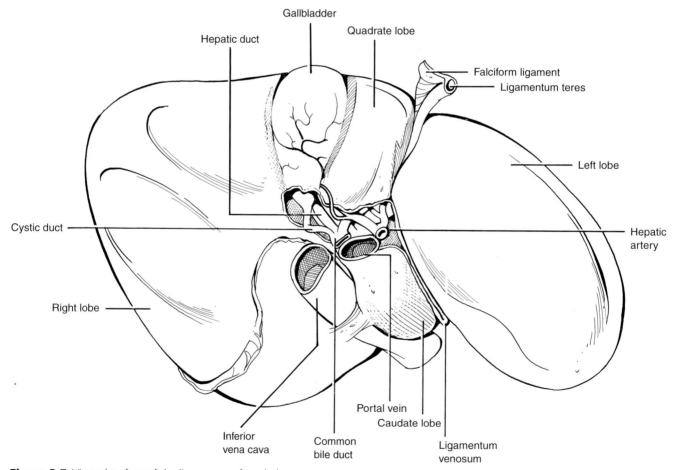

Figure 3-7 Visceral surface of the liver as seen from below.

which includes the hepatic ducts, portal vein, and proper hepatic artery. The sides of the H are formed by the gallbladder and the inferior vena cava on the left side and the ligamentum teres (obliterated remains of the left umbilical vein) and ligamentum venosum (the fibrous remains of the embryologic ductus venosum) on the right side.

Left lobe. The left part of the liver demarcated on the diaphragmatic surface by the falciform ligament. On the visceral side, the ligamentum teres in front and the ligamentum venosum in back form the boundary for the left lobe. In the abdomen, the left lobe of the liver usually lies anterior to body of the stomach.

Right lobe. The largest part of the liver opposite the left lobe. On the visceral surface, the hepatic flexure of the colon lies by the anterior part of the right lobe and lateral to the gallbladder.

Caudate (KAW-dat) lobe. The small, posterior lobe located between the inferior vena cava and the ductus venosus, posterior to the porta hepatis. *Helpful hint:* The "c" in caudate can help you remember that it lies next to the inferior vena cava (also starts with a "c").

Quadrate (KWAH-drăt) lobe. The small, anterior lobe located between the gallbladder and the ligamentum teres.

Helpful hint: The Q of quadrate is shaped much like the G of gallbladder.

Gallbladder. Lies just below the anterior liver within its fossa on the visceral surface and acts as a reservoir for bile produced by the liver.

Common bile duct. Transports bile from the gallbladder (via the cystic duct) and the liver (via the hepatic duct) to the duodenum (Fig. 3-8). In its course, it lies posterior to the superior duodenum and beside the head of the pancreas. It is approximately 7.5 cm in length and ends at the duodenal wall, where it joins with the main pancreatic duct.

Pancreas (*PAN-krē-as*). A collection of glandular tissue with little connective tissue; it has both exocrine and endocrine functions (Figs. 3-8 and 3-9).

Head. The expanded part of the pancreas lying within the curvature of the duodenum. Because the pancreas is covered only on its anterior surface by peritoneum, it is considered retroperitoneal similar to the adjacent parts of the duodenum. The head of the pancreas is divided by the superior mesenteric artery and vein that partially separate the uncinate process, the part of the pancreas located inferior to the mesenteric vessels.

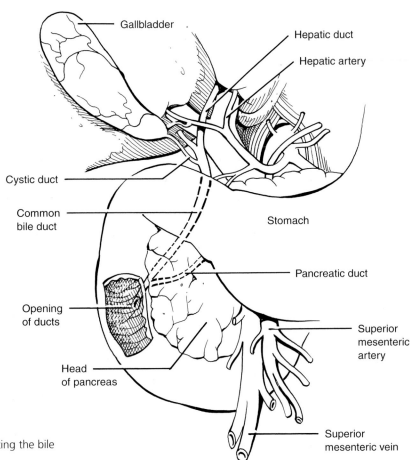

Figure 3-8 Drawing from an anterior view illustrating the bile duct system and adjacent structures.

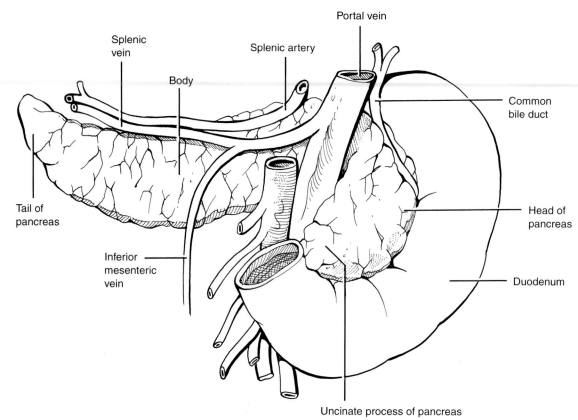

Figure 3-9 Drawing from a posterior view illustrating the pancreas and adjacent structures.

Body. The central region of the pancreas primarily located posterior to the stomach and anterior to the left kidney.

Tail. The narrowed left end of the pancreas extending toward the surface of the spleen.

Spleen (*splēn*). The soft, lymphatic organ that lies against the diaphragm on the upper left side of the abdomen within the thoracic cage (Fig. 3-4). Its size and shape vary considerably, depending somewhat on the adjacent structures. Its anterior surface is next to the stomach, its posterior surface is next to the left kidney, its superior surface is next to the diaphragm, and its inferior surface is next to the left splenic flexure of the colon.

Kidneys. The bean-shaped, retroperitoneal organs on either side of the vertebral column typically centered at the level of the first lumbar vertebra. Anomalies in formation are common during development, resulting in variations in the shape and location of the kidneys. Within the kidney, fluid and waste products are filtered from the blood to form urine, which is collected in the renal pelvis and drains into the ureters (Fig. 3-10).

Ureters (*yū-RĒ-terz*). Retroperitoneal, originating from the renal pelves and extending downward to drain urine into the bladder. Although most people have two ureters (one for each kidney), common congenital anomalies include duplication of part or all of the ureter.

Adrenal (*Ă-DRĒ-năl*) **glands.** Also referred to as the suprarenal glands, these soft, glandular organs are located on the top pole of the kidneys (Fig. 3-11). Roughly triangular in shape, their average dimensions in the adult are approximately 5 cm long, 3 cm wide, and 1 cm thick. Although these endocrine glands are relatively small, they produce hormones with widespread effects, including epinephrine and norepinephrine, which are responsible for the fight-or-flight response. In axial images, the glands are considerably thinner and are less dense than the underlying kidneys (which average 3 cm thick).

Arteries

Abdominal or descending aorta (*ā-OR-tă*). The continuation of the thoracic aorta, it originates at the level of the diaphragm and extends to the pelvis (Fig. 3-6). The retroperitoneal artery lies on the left side of the vertebral column and terminates at the origin of the right and left common iliac arteries.

Celiac (*SĒ-lē-ak*) **trunk.** The first branch off the abdominal aorta, it originates just below the diaphragm between the

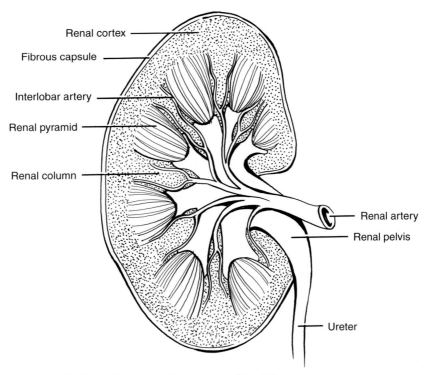

Renal cortex

Fibrous capsule

Interlobar artery

Renal pyramid

Renal column

Renal artery

Renal pelvis

Ureter

Figure 3-10 Sketch illustrating the contents of the kidney.

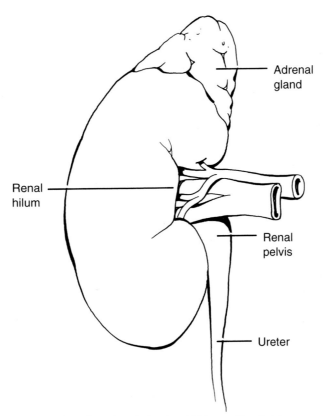

Adrenal gland

Renal hilum

Renal pelvis

Ureter

Figure 3-11 The adrenal gland and kidney with adjoining structures.

lesser curvature of the stomach and the liver (Fig. 3-12). The artery is relatively short (1 to 2 cm long) and originates nearly perpendicular to the aorta. It gives rise to the common hepatic artery, left gastric artery, and splenic artery.

Common hepatic artery. The branch of the celiac trunk that gives rise to the proper hepatic artery (supplies the liver and gallbladder) and the gastroduodenal artery (supplies the stomach, duodenum, and pancreas). Anomalies of the artery are quite common. Approximately 41% of patients have aberrant common hepatic arteries, including instances in which the artery originates directly from the aorta or the superior mesenteric artery.

Splenic artery. The largest branch of the celiac trunk, it travels behind the stomach to end at the spleen. It usually travels a tortuous path, giving it a distinctive appearance and facilitating its identification in sectional images.

Superior mesenteric artery. It originates from the abdominal aorta approximately 1 cm below the celiac trunk. It extends downward to supply blood to the small intestine and the first half of the large intestine, including the cecum, ascending colon, and the right half of the transverse colon (Fig. 3-13). Originating posterior to the pyloric part of the stomach, it extends at an oblique angle from the aorta. Compared to the perpendicular origin of the nearby celiac trunk, its oblique course can be a distinguishing characteristic in sectional images. As the artery descends into the abdomen, it travels through the head of the pancreas within the C loop of the duodenum to enter the mesentery.

Renal ($\overline{RE}$-năl) arteries. Two large trunks arising on either side of the aorta just below the superior mesenteric artery. Each artery forms a nearly right angle with the aorta as it extends to the kidneys (Fig. 3-14). Because the right renal

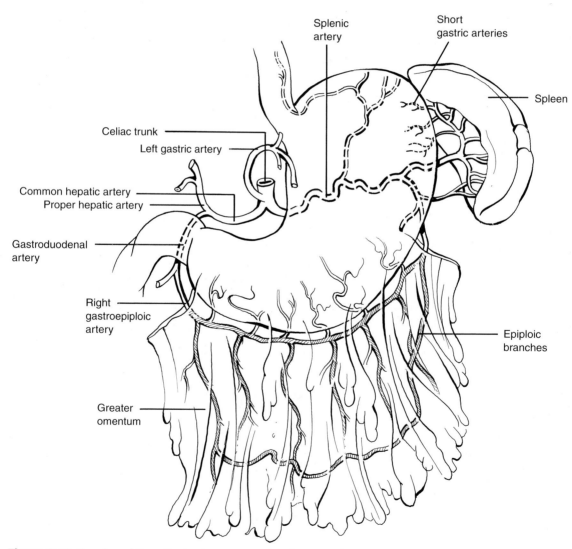

Figure 3-12 Branches of the celiac trunk as compared to the stomach and spleen.

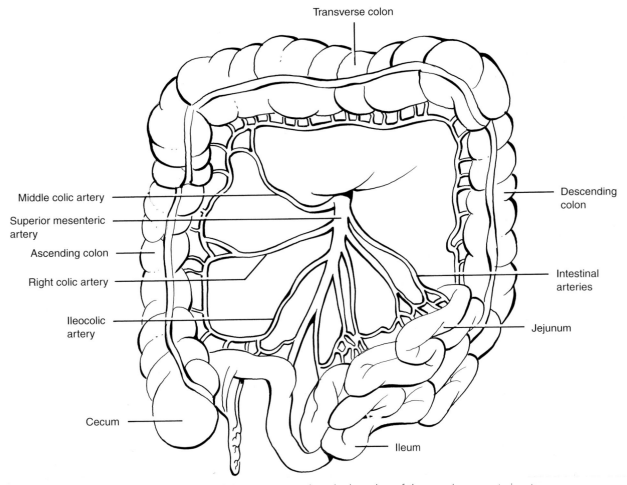

Figure 3-13 Following superior reflection of the transverse colon, the branches of the superior mesenteric artery.

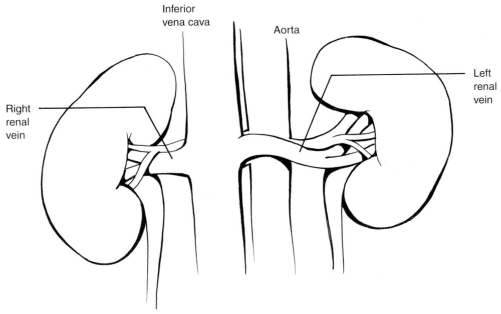

Figure 3-14 Sketch illustrating the renal arteries and veins.

artery passes behind the inferior vena cava and the right renal vein, it is usually slightly longer than the left. In approximately one out of four cases, additional renal arteries are present and are more frequently found on the left side. Instead of entering the kidney at the hilum, additional renal arteries usually join with either the upper or the lower poles of the kidney.

Inferior mesenteric artery. Originating from the aorta in the mid-lumbar region, it enters the mesentery to supply blood to the left half of the transverse colon, descending colon, sigmoid colon, and the upper rectum (Fig. 3-15).

Common iliac arteries. Bilateral arteries arising from the abdominal aorta at the level of the fourth lumbar vertebra; they diverge laterally as they enter the pelvis. Within the greater pelvis, each artery bifurcates to give rise to the internal and external iliac arteries.

Veins

Inferior vena cava ($\overline{VE}$-nă $\overline{KA}$-vă). The major route for drainage of venous blood from the abdomen, pelvis, and lower extremities (Fig. 3-16). It lies parallel to the abdominal aorta, on the right side near the lumbar vertebral bodies.

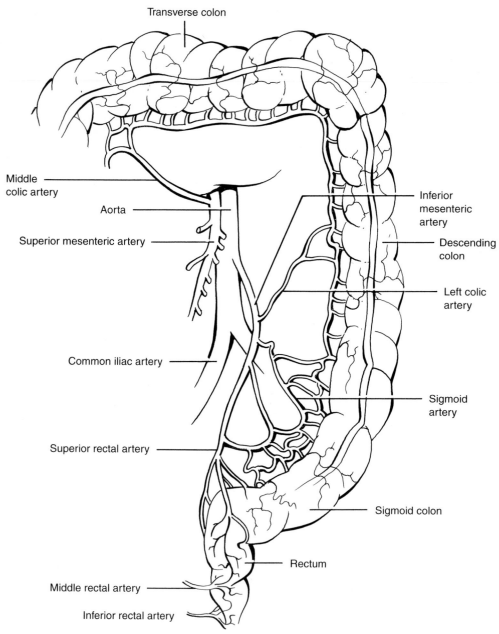

Figure 3-15 The lower abdominal aorta including the branches of the inferior mesenteric artery and the common iliac arteries.

Originating from the joining of the common iliac veins within the upper pelvis, it ascends through the abdomen and thoracic cavity to drain into the right atrium of the heart.

Hepatic veins. The right and left hepatic veins drain the filtered blood from the liver into the inferior vena cava. The vessels are short and are surrounded by liver tissue molded around the inferior vena cava.

Portal (*POR-tăl*) **vein.** Originating from the veins draining most of the gastrointestinal system, it carries nutrient-rich blood to the middle of the visceral surface of the liver. Lying adjacent to the hepatic bile ducts and the hepatic artery proper, it forms part of the porta hepatis, the transverse part of the H on the visceral surface of the liver.

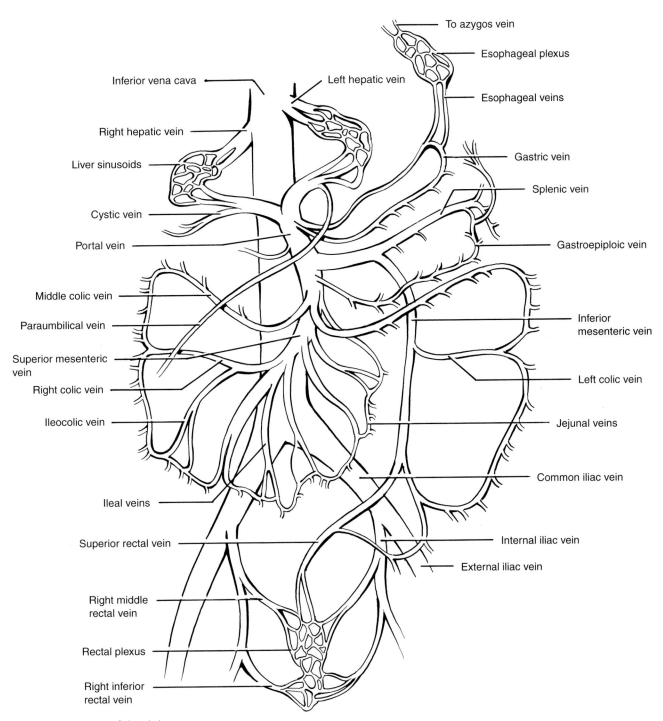

Figure 3-16 Veins of the abdomen.

Splenic vein. Found traversing the abdomen posterior to the stomach and the pancreas, it drains nutrient-rich blood from the spleen and the inferior mesenteric vein into the portal vein. In contrast to the tortuous path of the splenic artery, the course of the vein is nearly linear; this difference can be used to distinguish the two neighboring vessels.

Inferior mesenteric vein. The vessel draining blood from the rectum, sigmoid colon, and ascending colon, to the splenic vein located posterior to the stomach and pancreas. During its course, the vein lies within the mesentery, attaching the intestine to the posterior abdominal wall.

Superior mesenteric vein. Ending at the portal vein immediately posterior to the pancreas, the branches of this vessel drain blood from the stomach, duodenum, jejunum, ileum, cecum, appendix, ascending colon, transverse colon, and pancreas. Like the other mesenteric veins, it lies within the mesentery and carries nutrient-filled venous blood from the intestine to the portal vein.

Renal veins. The right and left renal veins drain venous blood from the kidneys to the inferior vena cava (Fig. 3-17).

Because the abdominal aorta is on the left side of the inferior vena cava, the longer left renal vein crosses in front of the abdominal aorta.

Common iliac veins. These two veins (the right and left) drain venous blood from the lower limbs and pelvis into the inferior vena cava. Arising at the juncture of the internal and external iliac veins, they originate anterior to the L5-S1 joint space and extend only a short distance to join in front of the L4 vertebral body. Unlike most regions of the body, here the veins are more posteriorly and inferiorly situated than the adjacent common iliac arteries.

Muscles

Psoas ($\overline{SO}$-*as*). Originating from the transverse processes of L1-L5 and inserting on the lesser trochanter of the femur on either side, these muscles form part of the posterior abdominal wall. In axial section, the large muscles are round and readily identified lying on either side of the vertebral column and aid in the identification of the adjacent ureters and vessels.

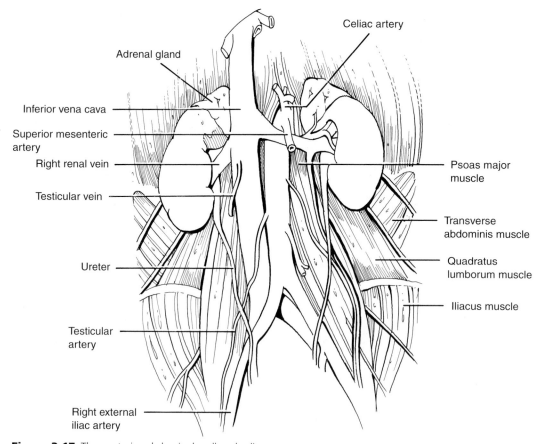

Figure 3-17 The posterior abdominal wall and adjacent structures.

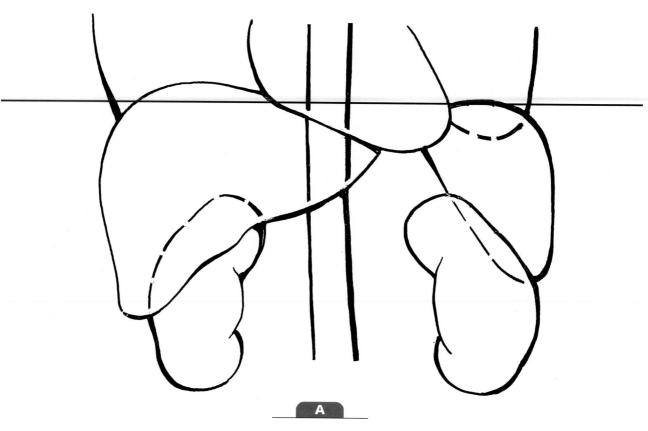

A

Figure 3-18 Axial CT image 1.

AXIAL CT IMAGES

This section describes 24 axial CT images of the abdomen taken at 8.0 mm intervals through the abdomen from superior to inferior. The patient ingested 1000 mL oral contrast media over a 60-min period, and the images were generated immediately after the administration of 100 mL venous contrast media. The following technical factors were used: 120 kVp, 150 mA-s. Abbreviations: kVp = kilovolt peak, mA-s = milliampere-second.

Figure 3-18 (A,B,C). In the first CT image at the top of the abdomen, the liver is shown occupying most of the right side surrounded by the lower lobe of the right lung. On the left side, the lower lobe of the lung is forming a margin around the contents of the upper abdomen. Within the window, the upper pole of the dense spleen and the contrast-filled fundus of the stomach are both demonstrated. Within the mediastinum, the bottom of the heart is sectioned, and the right ventricle is more anterior than the left ventricle. Behind the heart, the esophagus is found extending downward to the stomach in front of the descending aorta and the azygos vein. On the right side of the patient, the inferior vena cava is difficult to discern from the surrounding liver tissue.

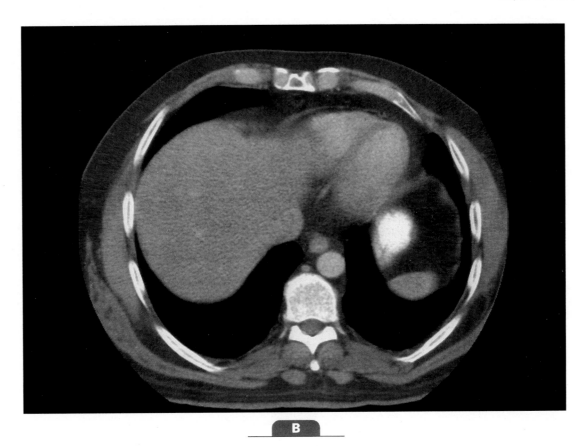

B

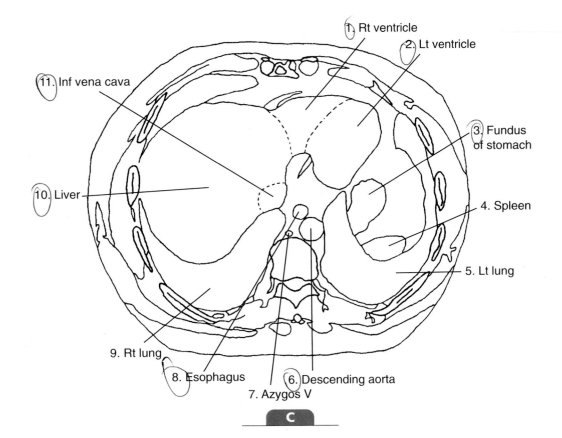

1. Rt ventricle
2. Lt ventricle
11. Inf vena cava
3. Fundus of stomach
10. Liver
4. Spleen
5. Lt lung
9. Rt lung
8. Esophagus
6. Descending aorta
7. Azygos V

C

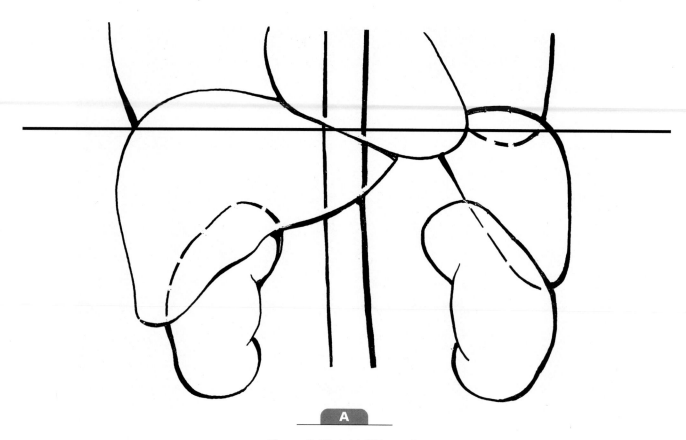

Figure 3-19 Axial CT image 2.

Figure 3-19 (A,B,C). The body of the liver fills most of the right side and is difficult to distinguish from the base of the heart. Even though the diaphragm is not seen between the two organs, the interventricular septum can be seen separating the right and left ventricles of the heart. Next to the heart, the fundus of the stomach, filled with contrast, is shown on the left side. Although the esophagus is still between the descending aorta and inferior vena cava, the stomach is much closer compared to the previous image. Posterior to the stomach, the spleen appears as a dense organ bordered by the lower lobe of the left lung.

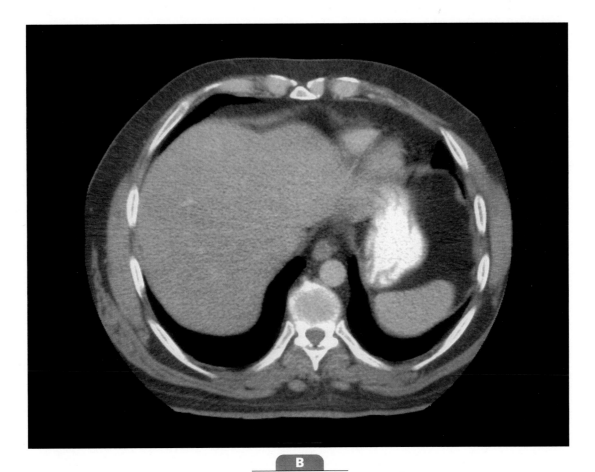

B

1. Rt ventricle

2. Lt ventricle

11. Liver

3. Fundus
of stomach

10. Inf
vena cava

4. Spleen

5. Lt lung

9. Rt lung

8. Azygos V   7. Esophagus   6. Descending aorta

C

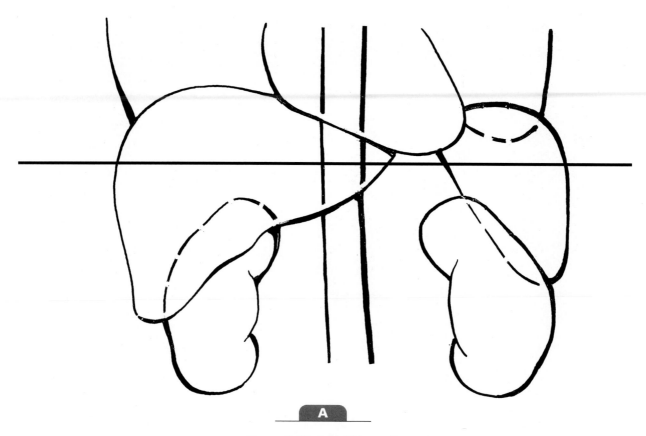

Figure 3-20 Axial CT image 3.

Figure 3-20 (A,B,C). Unlike the previous image, the liver is occupying most of the right side and extending through the midline to lie beside the fundus of the stomach. The esophagus, no longer between the inferior vena cava and descending aorta, is nearing the point where it joins the stomach. On the left side, the costodiaphragmatic recess of the lung is forming a margin around the spleen. Between the lungs, the small azygos and hemiazygos veins are cross-sectioned on either side of the descending aorta.

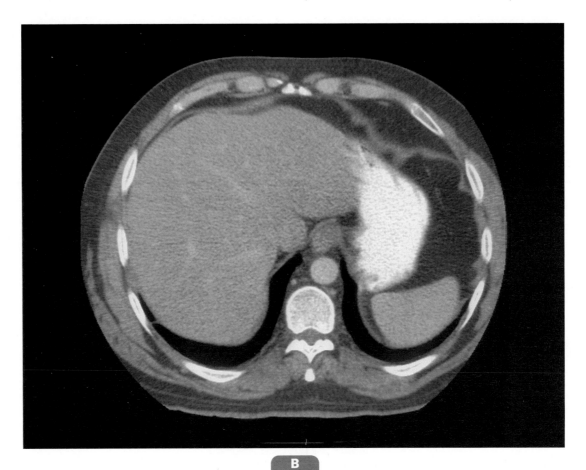

B

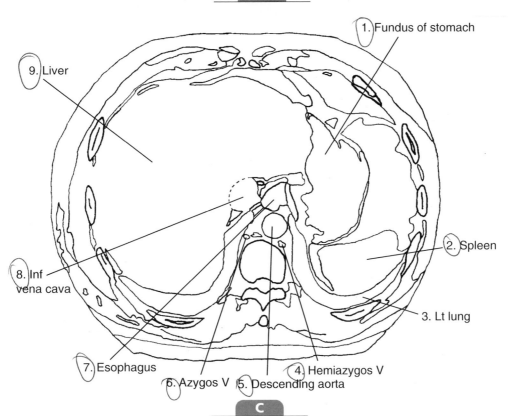

1. Fundus of stomach

9. Liver

8. Inf vena cava

2. Spleen

3. Lt lung

7. Esophagus

4. Hemiazygos V

6. Azygos V

5. Descending aorta

C

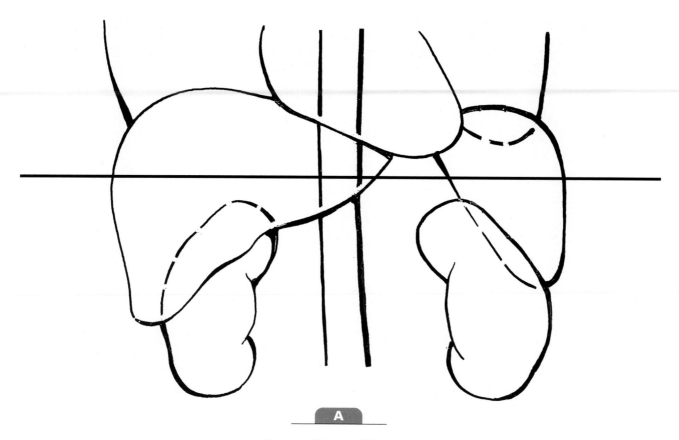

A

Figure 3-21 Axial CT image 4.

Figure 3-21 (A,B,C). Similar to the previous image, the liver is occupying the majority of the abdominal cavity. The right and left lobes of the liver can now be identified. In this section, the esophagus is joining the stomach, marking the middle portion of the stomach (the body). The inferior vena cava cannot be clearly distinguished from the liver and is separated from the descending aorta by the right crus of the diaphragm. On either side of the descending aorta, the hemiazygos and azygos veins are clearly seen anterior to the vertebral body. Along the posterior wall of the thoracic cage, the costodiaphragmatic recesses of the lungs form a narrow margin around the liver and spleen.

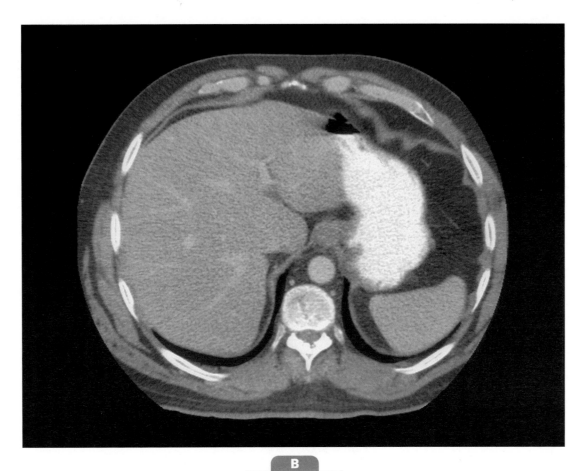

B

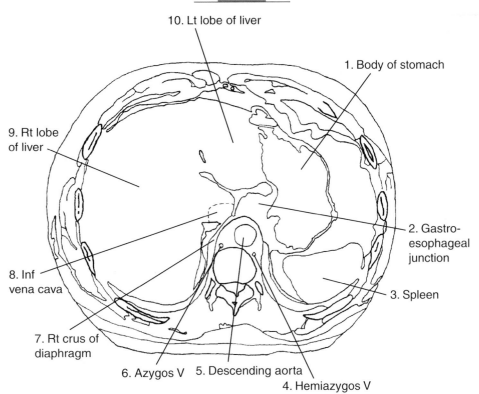

10. Lt lobe of liver

1. Body of stomach

9. Rt lobe
of liver

8. Inf
vena cava

2. Gastro-
esophageal
junction

3. Spleen

7. Rt crus of
diaphragm

6. Azygos V   5. Descending aorta

4. Hemiazygos V

C

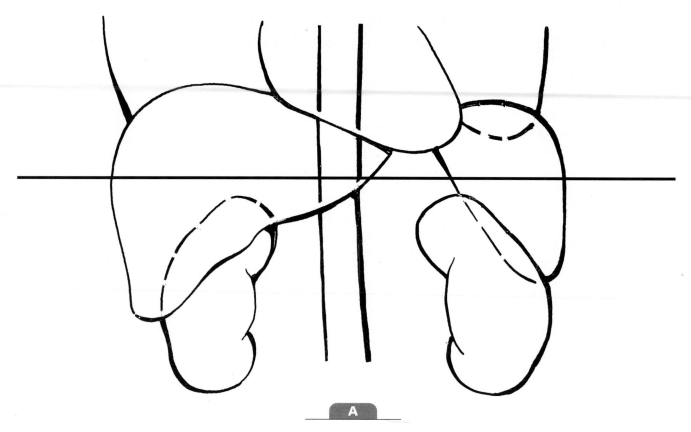

Figure 3-22 Axial CT image 5.

Figure 3-22 (A,B,C). The liver is limited to the right side of the abdomen and is divided into right and left lobes by the fossa for the ligamentum teres. The portal vein is within the porta hepatis, as described earlier, forming the transverse part of the H on the visceral surface of the liver. The caudate lobe of the liver is between the porta hepatis and the inferior vena cava. As in the previous image, the inferior vena cava is separated from the descending aorta by the right crus of the diaphragm. Behind the descending aorta, the azygos and hemiazygos veins are traversing through the diaphragm and are bordered by crural fibers. On the left side, an air–fluid level is shown in the contrast-filled stomach. Lateral to the stomach, the splenic flexure of the colon is now anterior to the spleen.

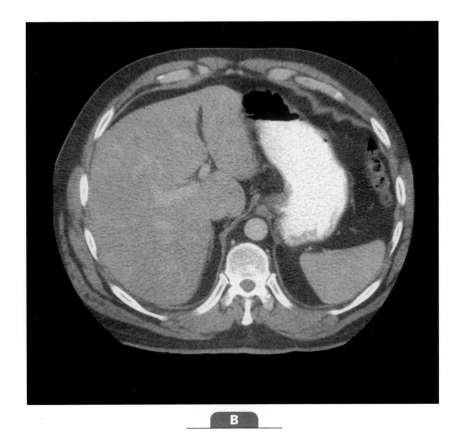

B

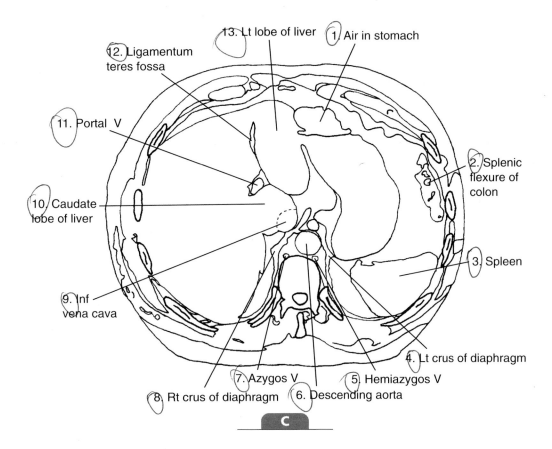

13. Lt lobe of liver

1. Air in stomach

12. Ligamentum teres fossa

11. Portal V

2. Splenic flexure of colon

10. Caudate lobe of liver

3. Spleen

9. Inf vena cava

4. Lt crus of diaphragm

7. Azygos V

5. Hemiazygos V

8. Rt crus of diaphragm

6. Descending aorta

C

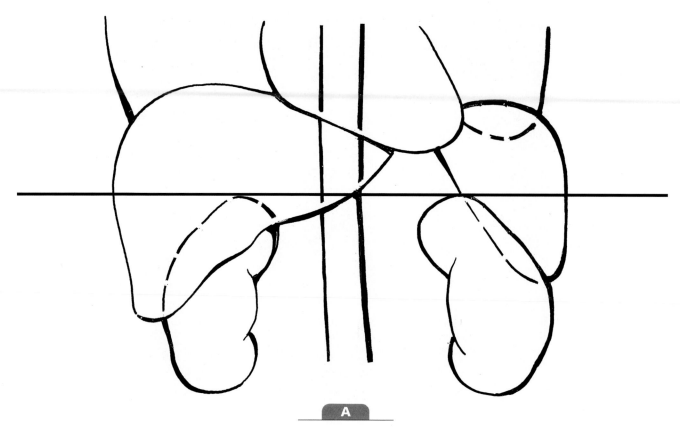

A

Figure 3-23 Axial CT image 6.

Figure 3-23 (A,B,C). Although the liver fills most of the right side of, it has decreased in size compared to the previous image, indicating the section is through the visceral surface. Within the liver, the gallbladder appears as a darkened area, with the tapered end pointing toward the porta hepatis, which contains the portal vein and the proper hepatic artery. On the visceral surface of the liver, the gallbladder marks the borders of the quadrate lobe. Posteriorly, the inferior vena cava marks the separation of the caudate lobe from the remaining right lobe of the liver. Just behind the inferior vena cava, the right adrenal gland is shown extending toward the upper pole of the right kidney and is surrounded by fat. On the left side, the stomach, splenic flexure of the colon, and the spleen appear much the same as described in the previous image.

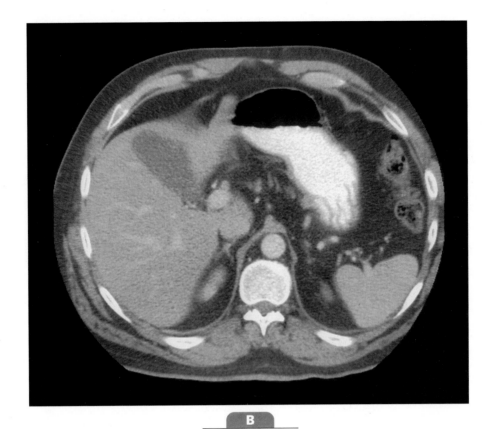

B

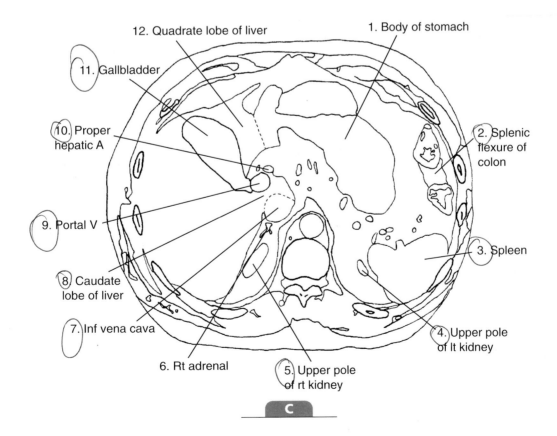

12. Quadrate lobe of liver

1. Body of stomach

11. Gallbladder

10. Proper hepatic A

2. Splenic flexure of colon

9. Portal V

3. Spleen

8. Caudate lobe of liver

7. Inf vena cava

4. Upper pole of lt kidney

6. Rt adrenal

5. Upper pole of rt kidney

C

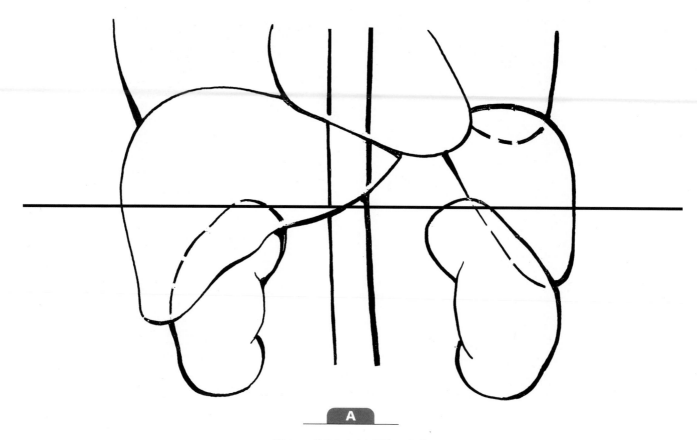

Figure 3-24 Axial CT image 7.

Figure 3-24 (A,B,C). Only the lower right lobe of the liver is shown, and the body of the stomach occupies a more central location. The gallbladder can clearly be discerned and appears as a darkened region within the liver, with the tapered end pointing posteriorly. At this lower level, the inferior vena cava and the portal vein are separated from the liver tissue, and the body of the pancreas is shown posterior to the stomach. To the left of the stomach, the splenic flexure of the colon has divided and given rise to the transverse colon and the descending colon. Adjacent to the posterior wall, the spleen is irregularly shaped, and the splenic vein is shown in longitudinal section as it extends toward the portal vein. On either side, the adrenal glands are found anterior to the upper poles of the kidneys.

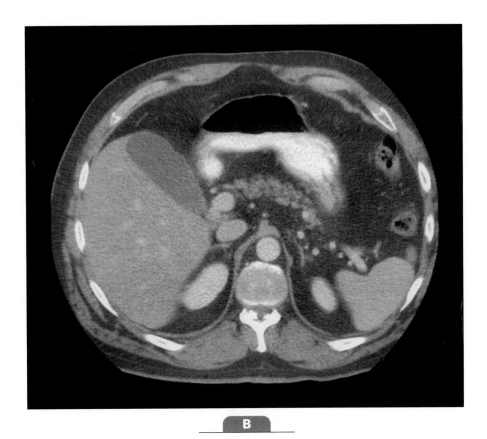

B

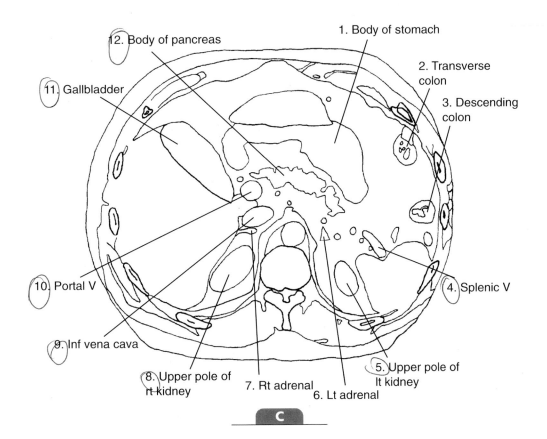

12. Body of pancreas

1. Body of stomach

2. Transverse colon

3. Descending colon

11. Gallbladder

10. Portal V

4. Splenic V

9. Inf vena cava

8. Upper pole of rt kidney

7. Rt adrenal

6. Lt adrenal

5. Upper pole of lt kidney

C

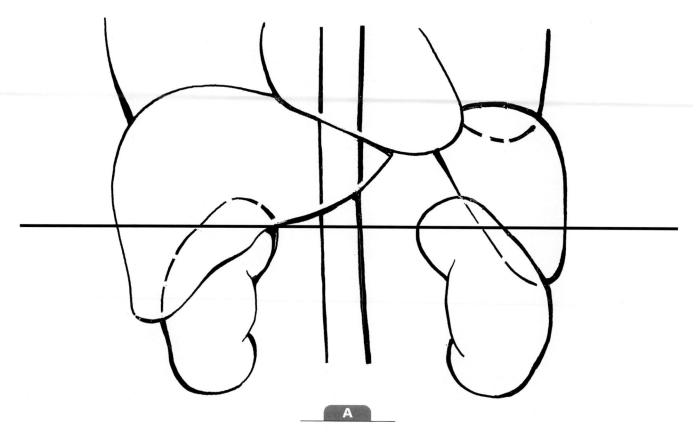

Figure 3-25 Axial CT image 8.

Figure 3-25 (A,B,C). The air–fluid level within the stomach is found centrally in front of the body of the pancreas in this figure. Within the glandular tissue of the body of the pancreas, the portal vein is next to the hepatic artery. Originating from the celiac trunk, both the hepatic artery and the splenic artery are shown within this section. Although the celiac trunk originates from the aorta, the arterial branches appear separated from the aorta by the crural ligaments of the diaphragm. The tail of the pancreas, extending in front of the left adrenal gland and kidney, points toward the spleen. This image clearly demonstrates the near linear course of the splenic vein beside the tortuous path of the splenic artery. Anterior to the spleen, the descending and transverse parts of the colon are labeled, because this section lies below the splenic flexure.

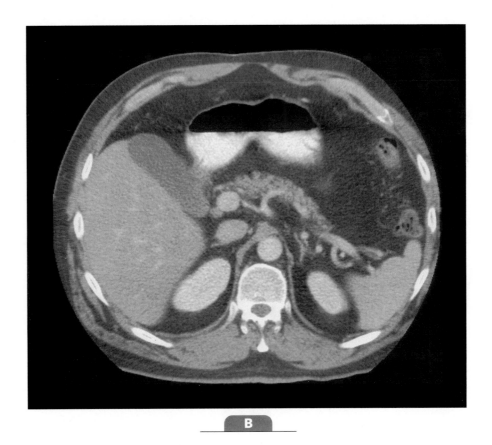

B

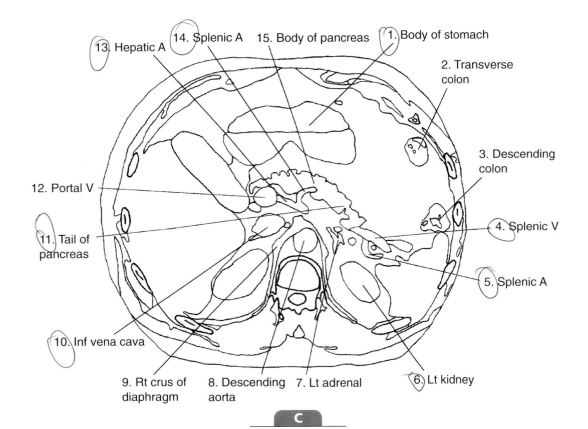

13. Hepatic A   14. Splenic A   15. Body of pancreas   1. Body of stomach

2. Transverse colon

3. Descending colon

12. Portal V

11. Tail of pancreas

4. Splenic V

5. Splenic A

10. Inf vena cava

9. Rt crus of diaphragm   8. Descending aorta   7. Lt adrenal   6. Lt kidney

C

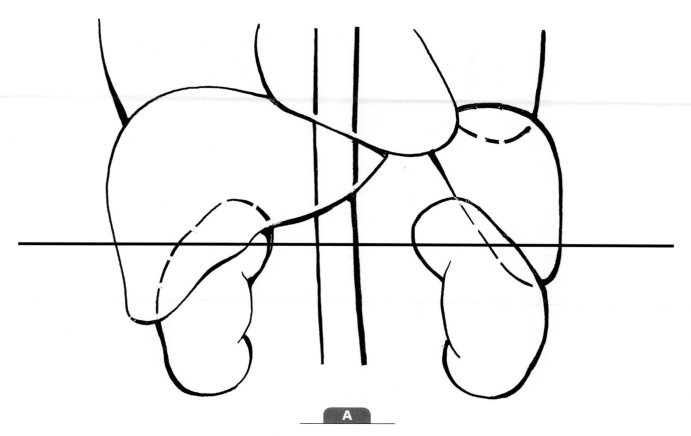

Figure 3-26 Axial CT image 9.

Figure 3-26 (A,B,C). The tapered end of the stomach, the pyloric antrum, is wrapping around the head of the pancreas that surrounds the common bile duct and the portal vein. Within the body of the pancreas, the near linear splenic vein is found in longitudinal section as it extends toward the portal vein. Posterior to the pancreas, the celiac trunk is shown originating from the abdominal aorta and extending through the crural ligaments. As described earlier, the celiac trunk usually gives rise to the splenic artery and the hepatic artery; however, 41% of individuals have aberrant hepatic arteries (commonly originate from the aorta or superior mesenteric artery). On the left side of the celiac trunk, the left adrenal gland is sectioned in front of the kidney. Much like the previous image, the transverse and descending parts of the colon are sectioned in front of the spleen.

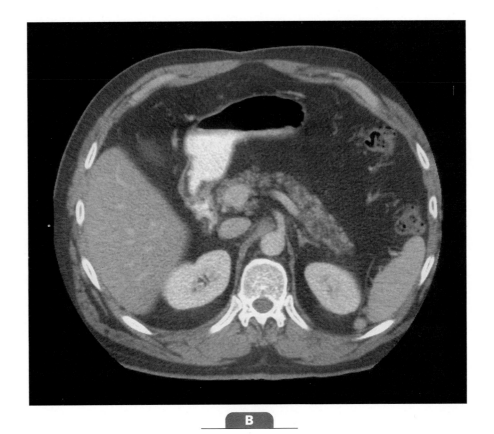

B

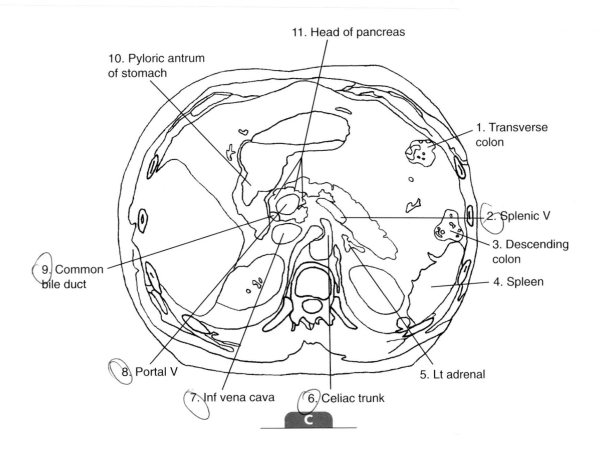

11. Head of pancreas

10. Pyloric antrum
of stomach

1. Transverse
colon

2. Splenic V

3. Descending
colon

9. Common
bile duct

4. Spleen

8. Portal V

5. Lt adrenal

7. Inf vena cava

6. Celiac trunk

C

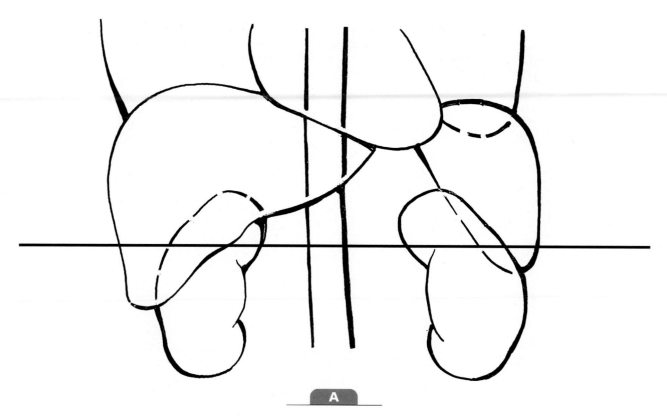

Figure 3-27 Axial CT image 10.

Figure 3-27 (A,B,C). The contrast within the pyloric antrum of the stomach is shown extending into the first part of the duodenum. Together, these structures wrap around the pancreas, which contains the portal and splenic veins. Posterior to the pancreas, the inferior vena cava is on the right side and the descending aorta is slightly to the left. Similar to the previous image, the transverse colon, descending colon, spleen, and liver are shown in the periphery of the abdominal cavity.

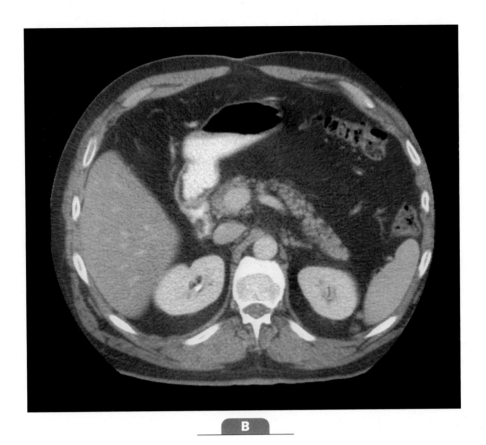

B

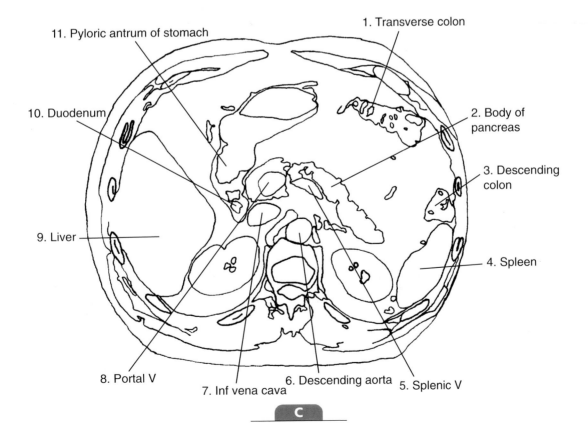

11. Pyloric antrum of stomach

1. Transverse colon

10. Duodenum

2. Body of pancreas

3. Descending colon

9. Liver

4. Spleen

8. Portal V

6. Descending aorta

5. Splenic V

7. Inf vena cava

C

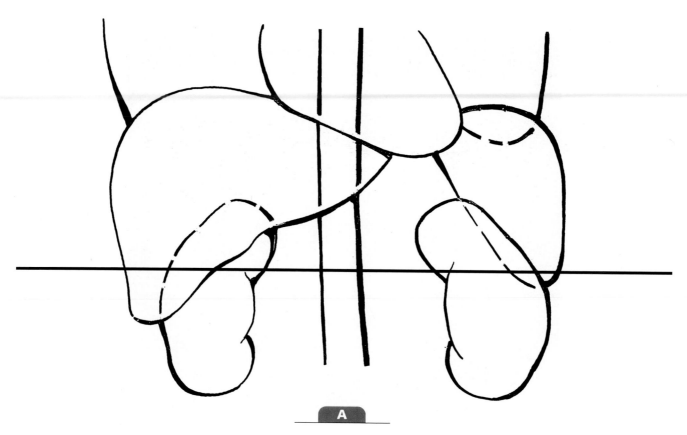

Figure 3-28 Axial CT image 11.

Figure 3-28 (A,B,C). At this level the lower stomach is seen as continuous with the duodenum and is found adjacent to the head of the pancreas. Although difficult to distinguish, the origin of the portal vein is included in this section. The portal vein originates from the joining of the superior mesenteric vein and the splenic vein. Behind the portal vein, an artery is shown arising from the abdominal aorta. The celiac trunk was described about 1 cm above, and the superior mesenteric artery is shown originating behind the head of the pancreas. The superior mesenteric artery will be shown in lower sections on the left side of the superior mesenteric vein. Like previous views, the descending and transverse parts of the colon are on the left side. At this level, the hepatic flexure of the colon is now found on the right side next to the visceral surface of the liver. Compared to the parts of the colon, the centrally located loops of small bowel are filled with contrast and are slightly smaller in diameter.

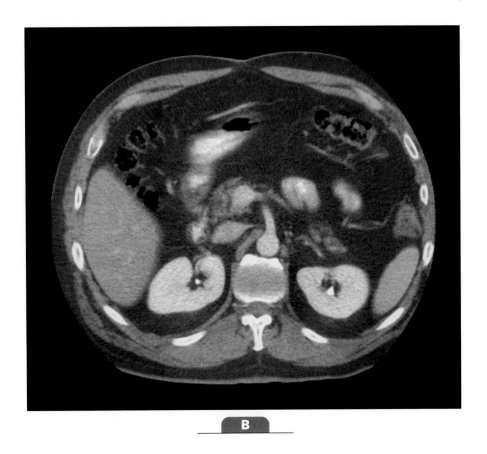

B

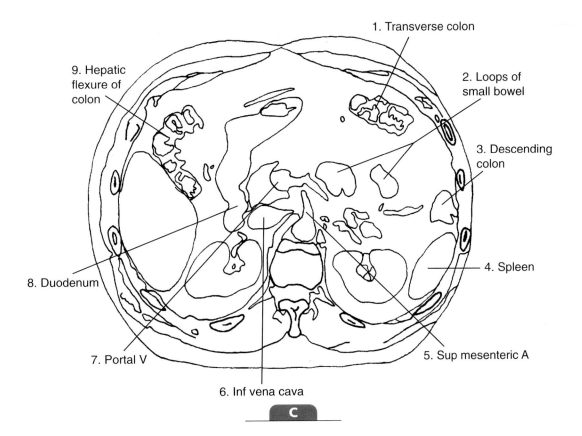

9. Hepatic
flexure of
colon

1. Transverse colon

2. Loops of
small bowel

3. Descending
colon

4. Spleen

8. Duodenum

7. Portal V

6. Inf vena cava

5. Sup mesenteric A

C

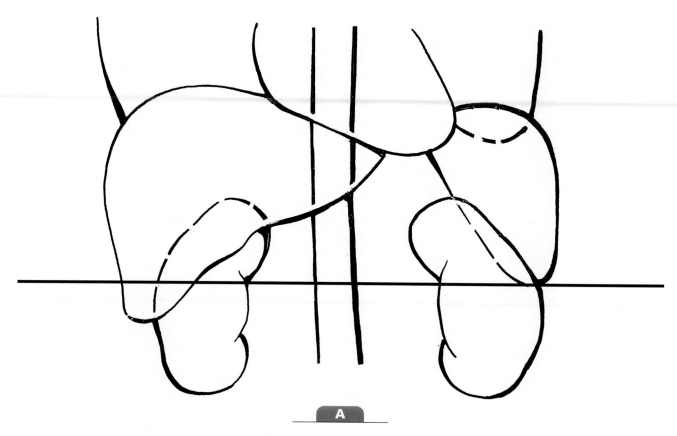

Figure 3-29 Axial CT image 12.

Figure 3-29 (A,B,C). Although the lower portions of the liver and spleen are shown, this section is below the level of the stomach. In the anterior abdominal cavity, the hepatic flexure is found in front of the liver and the descending colon is in front of the spleen. Extending between the two, the transverse colon is next to the anterior abdominal wall in front of the contrast-filled loops of small bowel. Centrally, the superior mesenteric artery and vein are traversing through the head of the pancreas. Posteriorly, the inferior vena cava is joining with the renal veins and the left renal vein is found passing in front of the descending aorta.

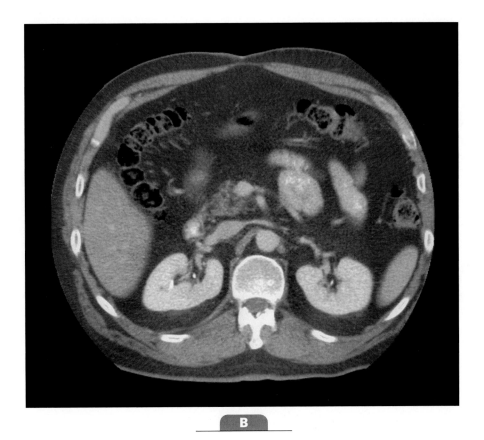

B

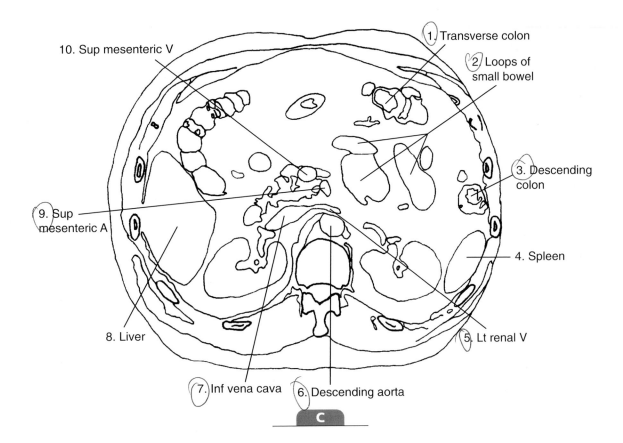

10. Sup mesenteric V

1. Transverse colon

2. Loops of small bowel

3. Descending colon

9. Sup mesenteric A

4. Spleen

8. Liver

5. Lt renal V

7. Inf vena cava

6. Descending aorta

C

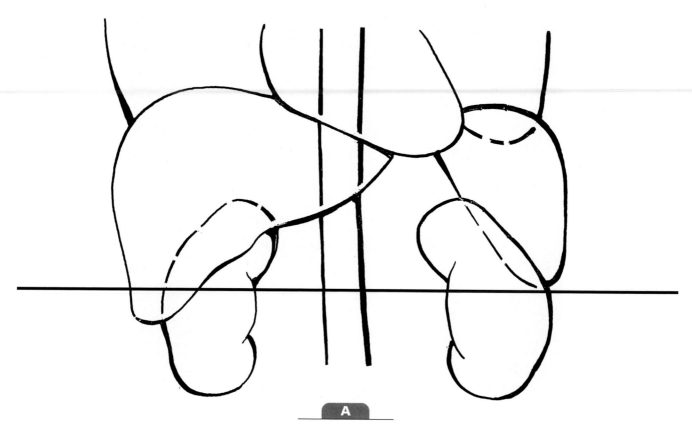

Figure 3-30 Axial CT image 13.

Figure 3-30 (A,B,C). This image clearly demonstrates the hepatic flexure of the colon near the liver, the transverse colon near the anterior abdominal wall, and the descending colon near the left abdominal wall. Between the parts of the colon, loops of contrast-filled small bowel are loosely organized on the left side of the abdomen. Given that the section is in the upper abdomen, the loops of small bowel are most likely the middle part of the small intestine (the jejunum). On the right side, vessels within the mesentery are seen along with the larger superior mesenteric artery and vein. Near the posterior wall, both kidneys are shown sectioned through the region of the hilum, demonstrating renal vessels. The left renal vein is again shown in front of the abdominal aorta, and the renal arteries are sectioned on either side behind the veins.

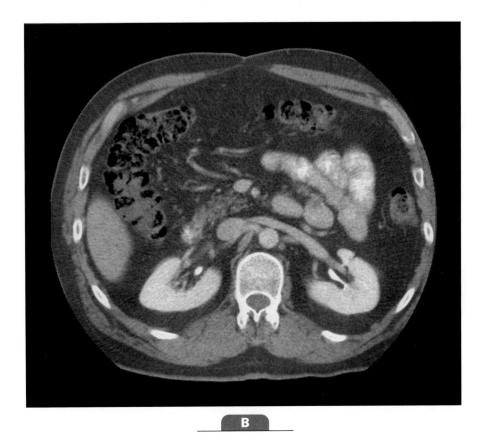

B

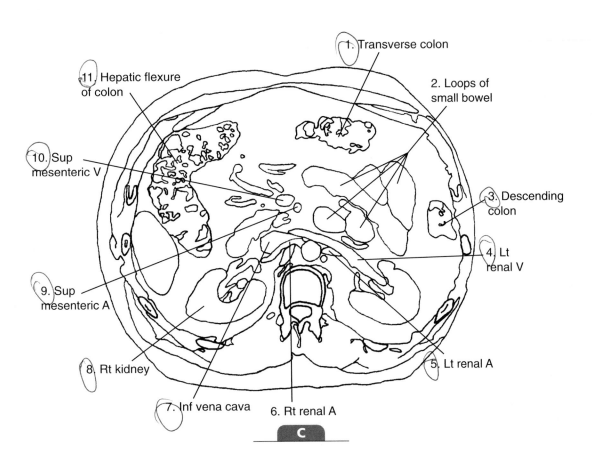

1. Transverse colon

11. Hepatic flexure of colon

2. Loops of small bowel

10. Sup mesenteric V

3. Descending colon

9. Sup mesenteric A

4. Lt renal V

8. Rt kidney

5. Lt renal A

7. Inf vena cava

6. Rt renal A

C

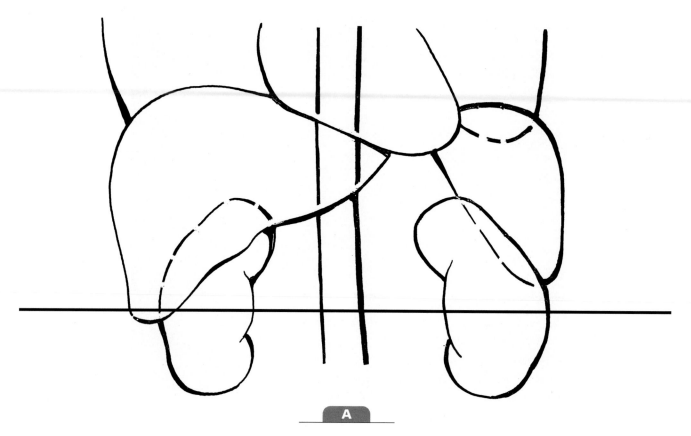

Figure 3-31 Axial CT image 14.

Figure 3-31 (A,B,C). Similar to the previous image, this image shows the hepatic flexure of the colon near the liver, the transverse colon near the anterior abdominal wall, and the descending colon near the left abdominal wall. Loops of small bowel are on the left side, and vessels within the mesentery are again shown on the right side. The kidneys, located behind the peritoneum on either side of the vertebral body, are sectioned through the lower hilar region, demonstrating the contrast-enhanced renal pelves. Between the kidneys, the descending aorta and inferior vena cava are cross-sectioned in front of the vertebral body. Behind the descending aorta, the hemiazygos vein is found on the left side, even though the azygos vein cannot be clearly delineated on the right.

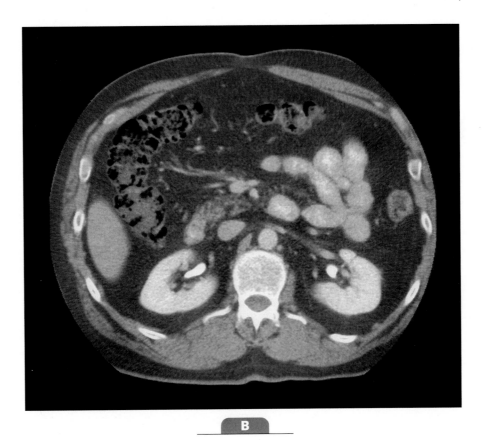

B

10. Mesenteric vessels

1. Transverse colon

9. Hepatic flexure of colon

2. Loops of small bowel

3. Descending colon

8. Liver

4. Hemiazygos V

7. Rt renal pelvis

6. Inf vena cava

5. Descending aorta

C

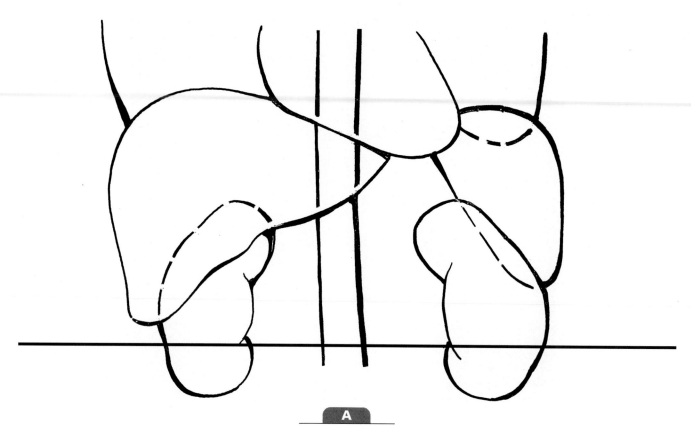

Figure 3-32 Axial CT image 15.

Figure 3-32 (A,B,C). This section, taken below the liver, includes the lower part of the transverse colon next to the anterior abdominal wall. On the right side, the ascending colon is separated from the kidney by the peritoneum and the fat pad surrounding and protecting the kidney. Within the fat, the contrast-enhanced ureter is medial to the kidney. Between the kidneys, the inferior vena cava and abdominal aorta are sectioned behind the loops of small bowel. The loops of small bowel, the jejunum, are wrapped with mesentery, containing branches of the superior mesenteric vessels. As in previous images, the descending colon is near the left abdominal wall.

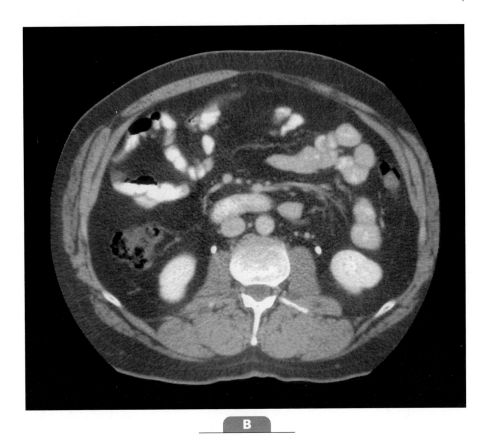

B

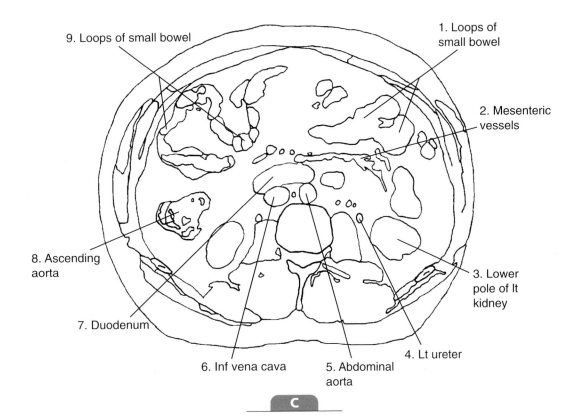

9. Loops of small bowel

1. Loops of small bowel

2. Mesenteric vessels

8. Ascending aorta

3. Lower pole of lt kidney

7. Duodenum

4. Lt ureter

6. Inf vena cava

5. Abdominal aorta

C

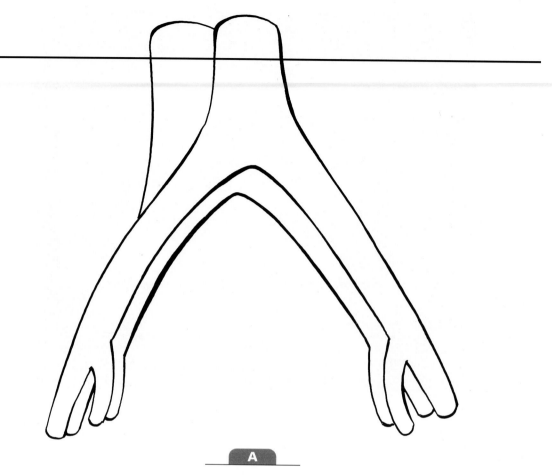

Figure 3-34 Axial CT image 17.

Figure 3-34 (A,B,C). Similar to the previous image, this image shows the contrast-enhanced loops of the small bowel are loosely organized in the anterior abdominal cavity. The location and size can be used to distinguish the segments of small bowel from those of the nearby colon. By comparison, the ascending and descending colon are larger in diameter and are adjacent to the abdominal wall, because both segments are retroperitoneal. In the posterior abdomen, the inferior vena cava, the abdominal aorta, and the ureters are also found retroperitoneal.

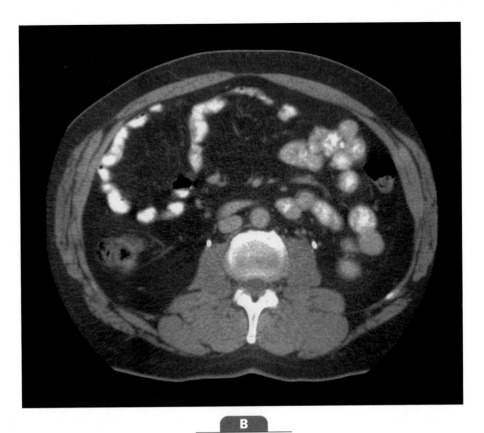

B

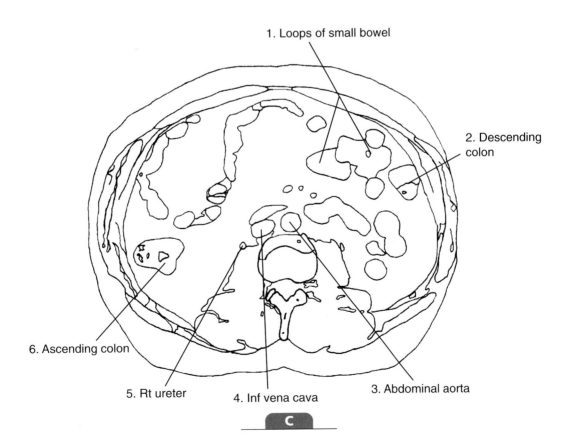

1. Loops of small bowel

2. Descending colon

6. Ascending colon

5. Rt ureter

4. Inf vena cava

3. Abdominal aorta

C

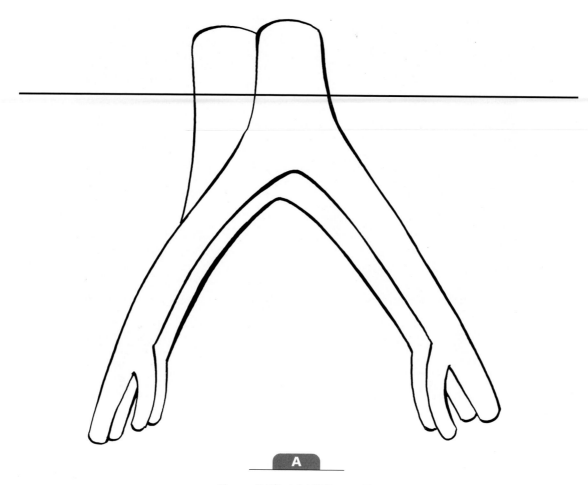

Figure 3-35 Axial CT image 18.

Figure 3-35 (A,B,C). This section, below the level of the ribs, was taken through the level of the third lumbar vertebra. Because lumbar vertebrae are responsible for supporting much of the individual's weight, their bodies are larger than those of other vertebrae. On either side of the vertebral body, the psoas muscles are shown originating from the transverse processes of the lumbar vertebrae. On the anterior surface of the psoas muscles, the ureters appear as "bright spots," owing to contrast enhancement. Between the ureters, the inferior vena cava and the abdominal aorta are next to the vertebral body. Originating on the anterior surface of the abdominal aorta, the inferior mesenteric artery is sectioned as it descends to supply blood to the last half of the large intestine. Similar to the images just described, the ascending and descending parts of the colon are shown behind the peritoneum and mesentery surrounding the loosely organized small bowel.

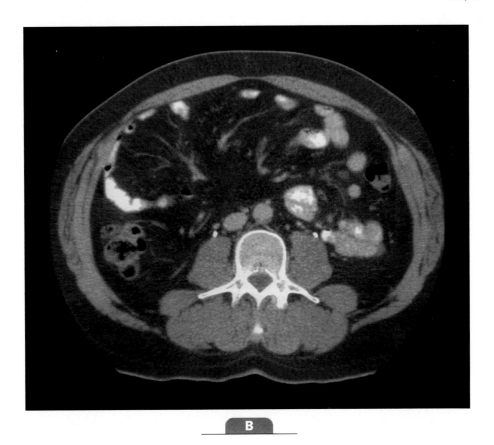

B

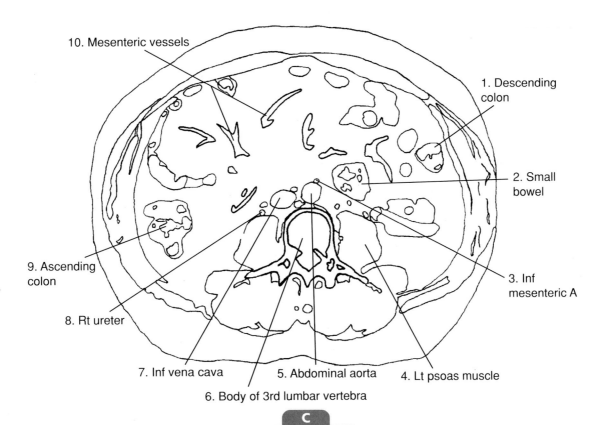

10. Mesenteric vessels

1. Descending colon

2. Small bowel

9. Ascending colon

3. Inf mesenteric A

8. Rt ureter

7. Inf vena cava

5. Abdominal aorta

4. Lt psoas muscle

6. Body of 3rd lumbar vertebra

C

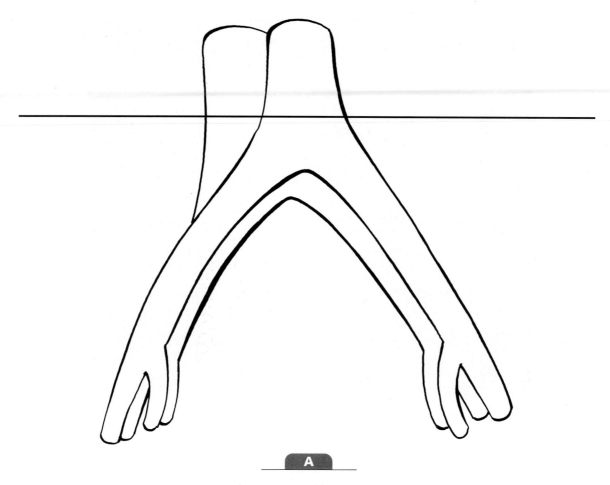

A

Figure 3-36 Axial CT image 19.

Figure 3-36 (A,B,C). The ascending and descending segments of the colon are on either side of the centrally situated loops of small bowel. Behind the small bowel, the inferior vena cava and the abdominal aorta are sectioned in front of the intervertebral disk between L3 and L4. Unlike the previous image, which showed the inferior mesenteric artery directly anterior to the abdominal aorta, the vessel is now shown on the left side of the aorta as it travels toward the left half of the large intestine.

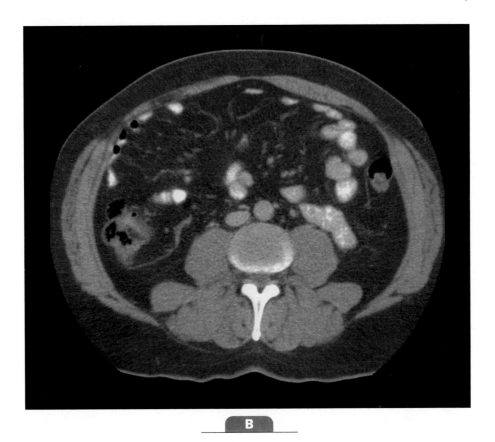

B

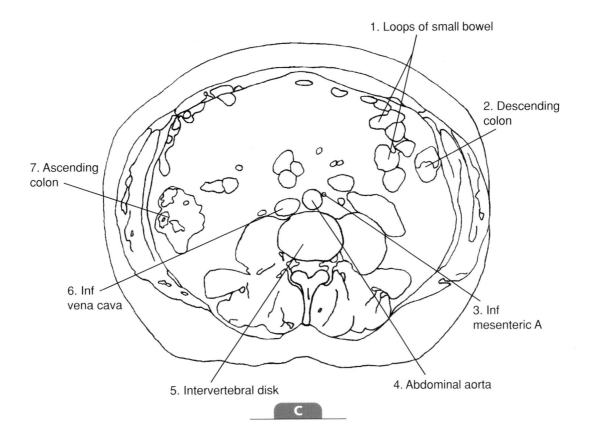

1. Loops of small bowel

2. Descending colon

7. Ascending colon

6. Inf vena cava

3. Inf mesenteric A

5. Intervertebral disk

4. Abdominal aorta

C

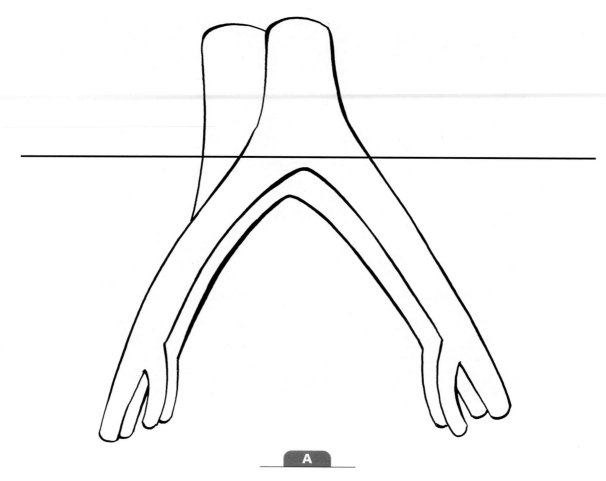

Figure 3-37 Axial CT image 20.

Figure 3-37 (A,B,C). This image shows the loops of small bowel as loosely organized in most of the anterior abdominal cavity. Even though the descending colon is still on the left side, the cecum is now found in the position previously occupied by the ascending colon. Beside the cecum, the ileum is sectioned near the terminal end of the small bowel. In the posterior abdomen, the inferior vena cava is still found on the right. The abdominal aorta, however, is splitting into two vessels, the right and left common iliac arteries. Lateral to the vessels, the contrast-filled ureters are lying on the anterior surfaces of the psoas muscles.

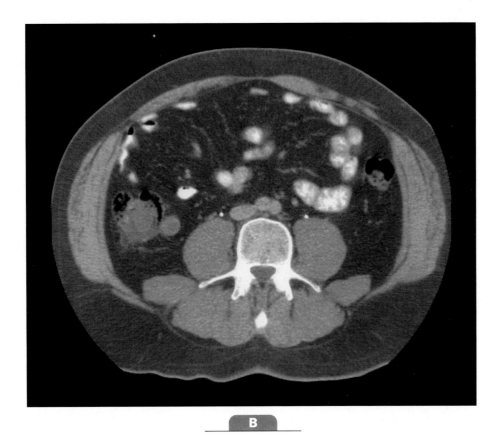

B

8. Ileum

1. Small bowel

2. Descending colon

7. Cecum

3. Lt psoas muscle

6. Inf vena cava   5. Bifurcation of common iliac A   4. Lt ureter

C

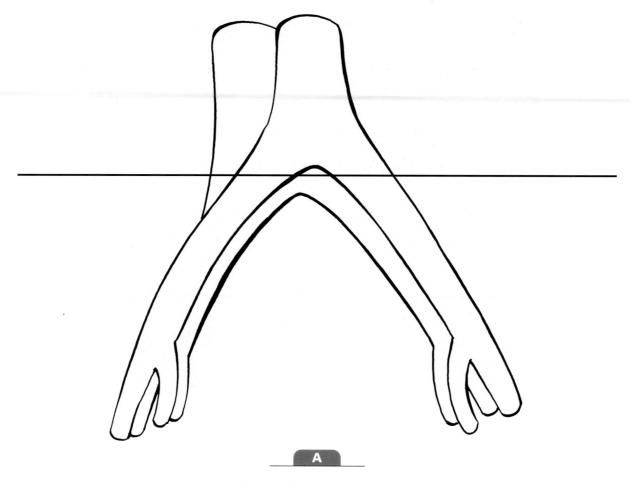

Figure 3-38 Axial CT image 21.

Figure 3-38 (A,B,C). The contrast-filled small bowel occupies most of the anterior abdomen, with large intestine on either side. By comparison, the large intestine can be distinguished from the small bowel by the larger diameter and location beside the abdominal wall. Although most of the small bowel is filled with contrast in this patient, the cross-section through the distal ileum shows it to be filled with fecal material and to be considerably smaller than the adjacent cecum. Behind the peritoneal cavity, three vessels are now distinguishable in front of the vertebral body. The inferior vena cava is on the right, and the right and left common iliac arteries are on the left, because they merge to form the origin of the abdominal aorta.

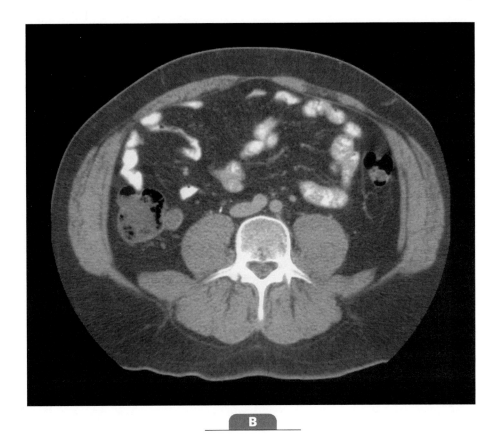

B

8. Ileum

1. Small bowel

2. Descending colon

7. Cecum

6. Rt ureter

5. Inf vena cava

4. Rt common iliac A

3. Lt common iliac A

C

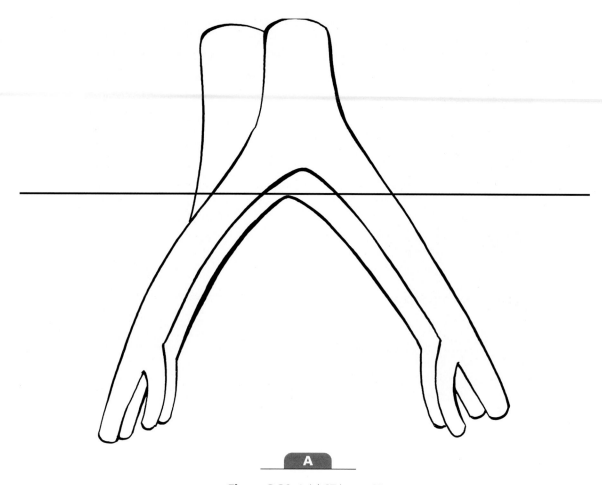

A

Figure 3-39 Axial CT image 22.

Figure 3-39 (A,B,C). The iliac crest is sectioned on either side of the vertebral column at the level of the intervertebral disk between L4 and L5. On both sides of the intervertebral disk, the large psoas muscles form much of the remaining posterior abdominal wall. Adjacent to the posterior wall, the inferior vena cava appears flattened and is shown bifurcating into the right and left common iliac veins. Compared to the previous image, the right and left common iliac arteries have diverged, and the right common iliac artery lies in front of the inferior vena cava. Similar to previous images, the large intestine is near the abdominal wall on either side of the small bowel, which occupies most of the peritoneal cavity.

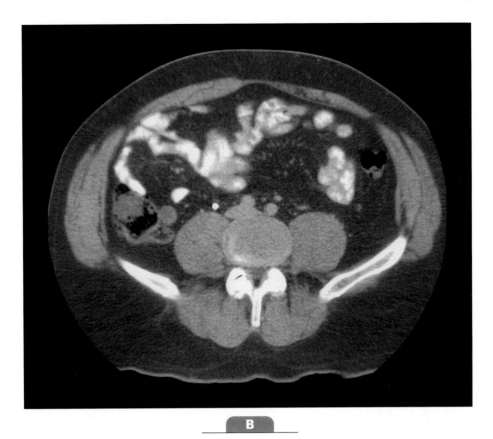

B

11. Rt common iliac A

1. Small bowel

10. Ileum

2. Descending colon

9. Cecum

3. Lt psoas muscle

8. Rt ureter

7. Iliac crest

4. Lt common iliac A

6. Bifurcation of inf vena cava

5. Intervertebral disk

C

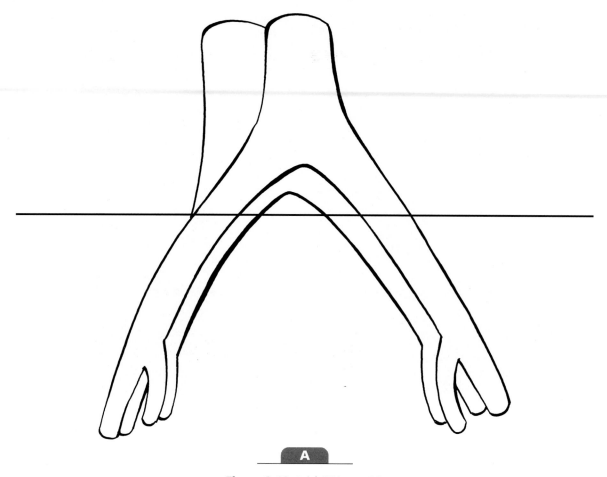

Figure 3-40 Axial CT image 23.

Figure 3-40 (A,B,C). Due to the proximity of the iliac crests to the vertebral body this section is through the lower abdomen at the level of the L5 vertebra. In this image, four vessels can be distinguished in front of the vertebral body and can be labeled as the right and left common iliac arteries and veins. In the last section, the right common iliac artery was in front of the inferior vena cava. Consequently, the right and left common iliac arteries are more anteriorly situated than the corresponding veins, which are adjacent to the vertebral body of L5. In the anterior abdominal cavity, loops of small bowel are found separating the descending colon and the cecum.

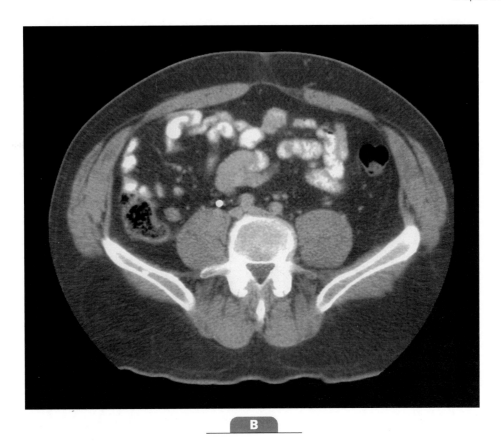

B

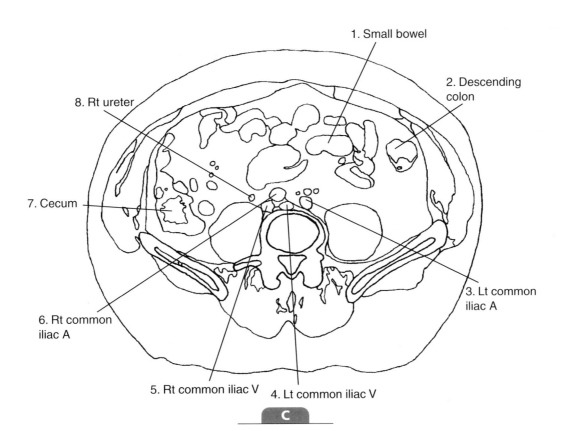

1. Small bowel

2. Descending colon

8. Rt ureter

7. Cecum

3. Lt common iliac A

6. Rt common iliac A

5. Rt common iliac V   4. Lt common iliac V

C

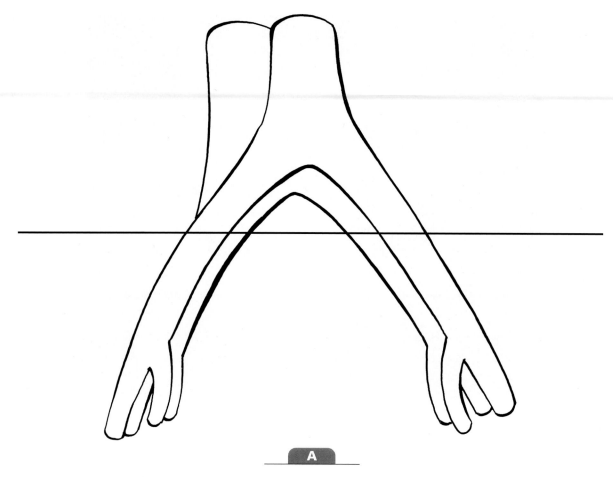

Figure 3-41 Axial CT image 24.

Figure 3-41 (A,B,C). The iliac bones are separate from the vertebral body, indicating the level of the section to be above the sacrum.
The round psoas muscles located on either side of the L5 vertebral
body are posterior to the contrast-enhanced ureters. Between the
ureters, the four vessels have diverged and paired on either side. As
seen above, the right and left common iliac arteries are in front of
the corresponding veins. Anteriorly, the small bowel fills most of the
central abdominal cavity. Because the section is within the greater
pelvis, this part of the small bowel would most likely be the ileum.
On either side of the small bowel, the retroperitoneal cecum and
descending colon are shown next to the abdominal wall.

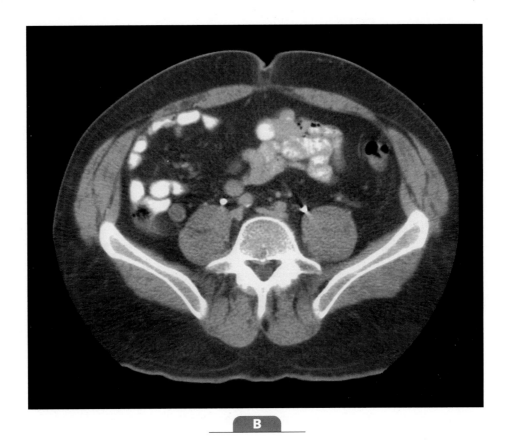

B

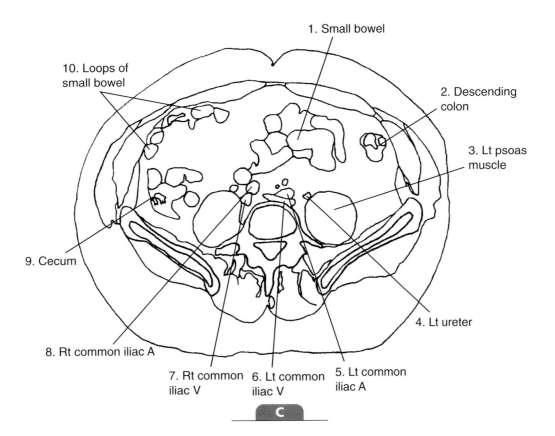

1. Small bowel

10. Loops of
small bowel

2. Descending
colon

3. Lt psoas
muscle

9. Cecum

4. Lt ureter

8. Rt common iliac A

7. Rt common
iliac V

6. Lt common
iliac V

5. Lt common
iliac A

C

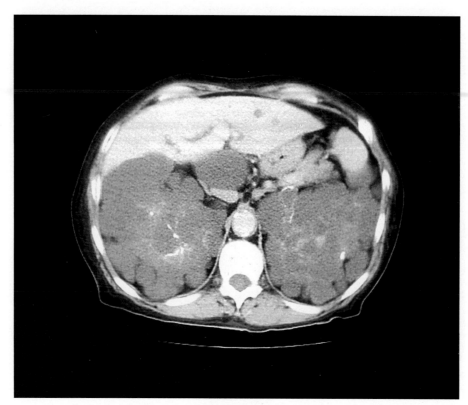

Figure 3-42

Supplement 3-1. *Figure 3-42 shows a CT scan of a 74-year-old woman with advanced polycystic kidney disease. Within the kidneys, the renal parenchyma has been replaced with numerous large cysts, and calcification is seen within some of the cysts. The enlarged kidneys compress the liver and spleen and displace both organs anteriorly. Despite the large size of the kidneys, the absence of normal renal parenchyma results in impaired renal function. The symptoms of autosomal dominant polycystic kidney disease usually don't appear before age 40 and advance slowly throughout life. Eventually, the disease will be fatal without renal dialysis or renal transplantation.*

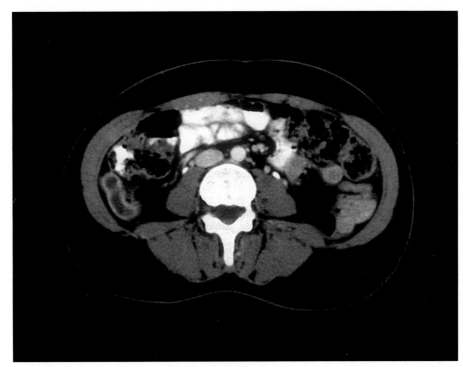

Figure 3-43

Supplement 3-2. *Figure 3-43 shows a 38-year-old woman who had acute abdominal pain in her lower right abdominal quadrant. Her physician ordered a CT examination of the abdomen, which demonstrates an obviously enlarged appendix. The appendix—a term commonly used to refer to the vermiform appendix, a worm-like appendage to the cecum that is usually 8 cm (3 inches) to 16 cm (6 inches) long and 1 cm (0.5 inch) in diameter—is attached to the posterior cecum. Directly behind the cecum, this appendix is approximately double its normal size. The appendix appears much like small bowel, except it is filled with a low-attenuation material that may be mucous. Much like the small bowel, the inflamed wall appears smooth and no rupture can be seen, although strands of inflammation are seen within the surrounding mesentery. Immediately after the CT scan, an appendectomy was performed, because it is safer to operate than to risk the possibility of rupture, resulting in peritonitis.*

REVIEW QUESTIONS

1. The boundary of the upper abdomen is formed by the_____, and the lower abdomen extends into the_____.

2. In an axial section through the hilum of the kidneys, which of the following would be most anterior? The right renal artery or the right renal vein.

3. Describe the location of the spleen and its relationship with adjacent structures.

4. Which of the following is located most superiorly?
   A. Transverse colon
   B. Hepatic flexure
   C. Splenic flexure
   D. Jejunum

5. List the three major structures found within the porta hepatis.

6. Which of the following is not supplied by the inferior mesenteric artery?
   A. Sigmoid colon
   B. Ascending colon
   C. Transverse colon
   D. Descending colon

7. On the visceral surface of the liver, which lobe is located most posteriorly? Caudate or Quadrate.

8. Describe where the portal vein lies in relationship to the stomach and pancreas.

9. List in order, from superior to inferior, the major branches of the abdominal aorta.

10. Which of the following structures is not considered retroperitoneal?
    A. Ileum
    B. Cecum
    C. Descending colon
    D. Kidneys

11. Which of the following structures is located most posteriorly as it passes through the diaphragm?
    A. Esophagus
    B. Inferior vena cava
    C. Celiac trunk
    D. Descending aorta

12. As the superior mesenteric vessels traverse through the head of the pancreas, is the artery or vein located farther to the right?

13. Describe function and structure of the small intestine.

14. The_____lies just below the anterior surface of the liver and the tapered end points toward the porta hepatis.

15. The stomach can be divided into three parts from superior to inferior:_____

16. The smooth connective tissue membrane covering the viscera within the abdomen is called the_____, and the_____is found lining the abdominal cavity.

17. Compared to the abdominal aorta, is the inferior vena cava on which side? Right or left?

18. The_____vein drains nutrient-rich blood from the rectum, sigmoid colon, and ascending colon to the_____vein.

19. Describe the structure and function of the mesentery.

20. Which of the following would be located most anteriorly?
    A. Jejunum
    B. Spleen
    C. Transverse colon
    D. Pancreas

Chapter 4

Male and Female Pelvis

OBJECTIVES

Upon completion of this chapter, the student should be able to:

1. Describe the boundaries of the greater and lesser parts of the pelvis.
2. Describe the three bones making up the pelvic girdle.
3. Identify the contents of the lower abdominal cavity found within the greater pelvic space.
4. Describe the pelvic peritoneum separating the contents of the abdominal cavity from the other structures within the greater pelvic cavity.
5. Correctly identify the major vessels on sectional images.
6. Identify and describe the alimentary structures within the pelvis.
7. Follow the course of urine as it passes through the pelvis.
8. Describe the major genitourinary structures in the male pelvis.
9. Describe the major genitourinary structures in the female pelvis.
10. Correctly identify anatomical structures on patient axial and coronal images of the pelvis.

ANATOMICAL OVERVIEW

The term *pelvis,* meaning "basin," describes the irregularly shaped opening created by the two hip bones: the sacrum, and the coccyx (Fig. 4-1 A,B). The pelvis is a skeletal feature that differs markedly between males and females; the male pelvis is typically narrower, and the female pelvis is wider and the alae or wings of the ilia are more open.

The opening within the pelvis is often separated into greater and lesser segments, sometimes called the false and true pelves, by an oblique plane at the pelvic inlet. The inlet is a flat plane extending from the sacral promontory to the superior border of the pubic symphysis and the middle of the pelvic brim. Above the pelvic inlet, the greater pelvic space or false pelvis is irregular in shape; and the boundaries are formed posteriorly by the lower lumbar vertebrae, laterally by the alae or wings of the ilia, and anteriorly by the anterior abdominal wall. Below the pelvic inlet, the lesser or true pelvis is the short, curved pelvic space located within the bony pelvis. The size and shape of this space are of great importance in birthing, because the newborn must pass through this space in vaginal deliveries. In general, the functions of the pelvis are to transmit the weight of the upper body to the lower limbs and to form the lower part of the abdominal cavity.

Skeletal

Pelvic girdle. Also called the innominate (*i-NOM-i-nāt*). A large, irregular shaped bone with a centrally located socket, the acetabulum (*as-ĕ-TAB-yū-lŭm*), for articulation with the head of the femur (Fig. 4-2). It is divided into three parts—ilium, pubis, and ischium—which are connected by cartilage in the young and fused in the adult.

Ilium (IL-ē-ŭm). Forms the upper part of the pelvic girdle. The most superior edge, the iliac crest, can easily be palpated along the lateral side. If the iliac crest is followed anteriorly, the termination (the anterior superior iliac spine) can also be felt on the anterior aspect of the hip. Below the superior spine, is a second, less prominent, spine (the anterior inferior iliac spine), which also extends from the anterior margin of the ilium. Similarly, on the posterior ilium, the iliac crest ends at the posterior superior iliac spine, and the posterior inferior iliac spine extends more inferiorly. Between the iliac spines, the central wing-shaped region of the ilium, the ala (*A-lă*), is located above the acetabulum.

Pubis (PŪ-bis). The lower anterior part of the pelvic girdle, which is divided into three parts: the body, the inferior ramus, and the superior ramus. The body is found most medially near the opposite pubis and forms the symphysis pubis joint. The inferior ramus is the projection of bone that

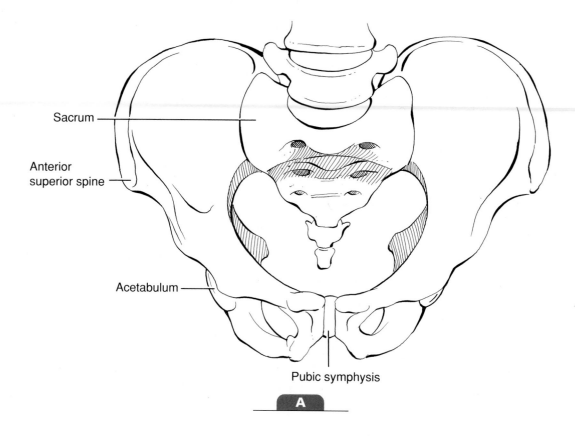

Sacrum

Anterior
superior spine

Acetabulum

Pubic symphysis

A

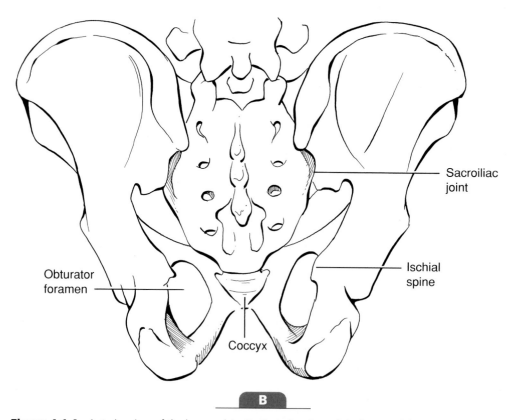

Sacroiliac
joint

Obturator
foramen

Ischial
spine

Coccyx

B

Figure 4-1 A. Anterior view of the bony pelvis. **B.** Posterior view of the bony pelvis.

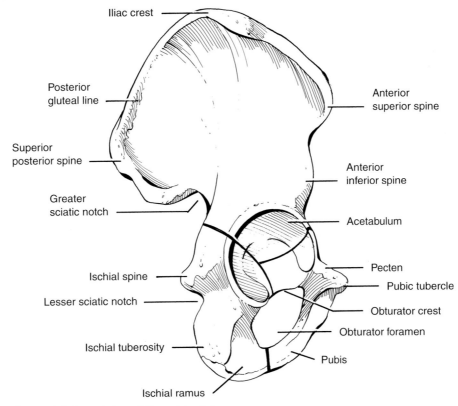

Figure 4-2 Lateral view of the pelvic girdle.

joins with the ischium and forms the lower boundary for the obturator foramen. The superior ramus projects upward to form the upper boundary of the obturator foramen and the anterior part of the acetabulum.

Symphysis (SIM-fi-sis) pubis. The amphiarthrodial joint where the pubic bones meet each other in the median plane. The thick articular cartilage between the pubic bones is held in place by surrounding ligaments and is generally larger in females than in males. Although this joint is usually capable of only slight movement, separation or rotation may occur during childbirth and pelvic trauma.

Ischium (IS-kē-ŭm). The lower, most inferior, posterior part of the pelvic girdle. It possesses an enlarged roughened area, the ischial tuberosity, which is the bony structure the body rests on in the seated position. Extending anteriorly from the tuberosity, the ischial rami joins the inferior pubic ramus, and together they form the lower boundary of the obturator foramen. Above the tuberosity, the ischial spine projects posteriorly forming the lower border of the greater sciatic notch.

Obturator foramen (OB-tū-rā-tŏr fō-RĀ-men). Within the lower aspect of the pelvic girdle, this opening is formed between the pubis and ischium.

Sacrum (SĀ-krŭm). Composed of five fused vertebral segments. This triangular bone forms the posterior portion of

the pelvis (Fig. 4-1). Because it articulates with the fused ilia on either side, the vertebral foramina for the sacral spinal nerves are on both its anterior and its posterior surfaces.

Sacroiliac joints (SĀ-krō-IL-ē-ak). Between the sacrum and the ilia, the slightly moveable joints (amphiarthrodial) found on either side of the sacrum.

Coccyx (KOK-siks). Formed by the fusion of three to five vertebral segments, this small, triangular bone is the most inferior portion of the vertebral column.

Femora (FEN-ŏ-rǎ). The longest, strongest, and heaviest bones in the body located within the thighs (Fig. 4-3 A,B) The femur (FĒ-mŭr) can be subdivided into three parts: proximal extremity, shaft, and distal extremity. The latter will be described in the region of the knee and is omitted from this chapter.

Proximal extremity. The greater trochanter (trō-KAN-ter) appears much like an extension of the shaft and is on the superior, lateral aspect. By comparison, the lesser trochanter is an expansion of bone more inferiorly located on the posterior, medial aspect. On the posterior view, the intertrochanteric crest is a ridge of bone between the greater and lesser trochanters. Next to the trochanters, the narrowed region of the neck extends toward the rounded head with the indention of the fovea capitis. The angle between the shaft

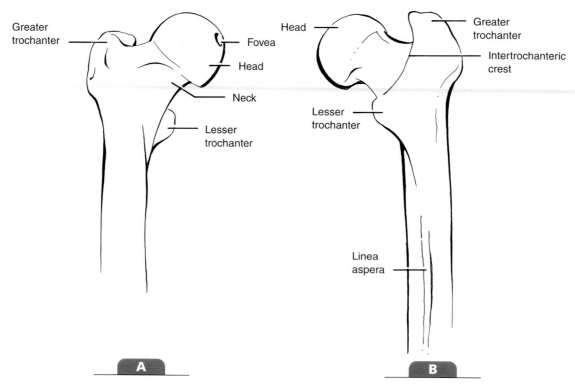

Figure 4-3 A. Anterior surface of the femur. **B.** Posterior surface of the femur.

and neck averages 120° to 125° but is larger in children and smaller in females.

Shaft. The long slender portion of the bone, or body, with the posteriorly situated roughened area, the linea aspera, delineated by medial and lateral lips.

Viscera (*VIS-er-ă*)

Sigmoid colon. S-shaped structure at the terminal end of the descending colon on the lower left side of the abdominal cavity; it begins at the pelvic brim (Fig. 4-4). Within the pelvis, this segment of the colon descends and curves toward the midline to cross the sacrum, where it turns downward to end in front of S3 at the rectum.

Rectum. Extending from the level of S3 through the lower opening of the pelvis, it lies just in front of the sacrum and coccyx and stops at the anal canal.

Ischiorectal fossae (*IS-kē-ō-REK-tăl FOS-ăē*). The wedge-shaped, fat-filled spaces containing rectal vessels and nerves on either side of the rectum between the ischium and the rectum.

Arteries

Internal iliac (*IL-ē-ak*) **arteries.** Originating in the greater pelvis, the internal branches of the common iliac arteries terminate as they travel through the posterior bony pelvis to give rise to the gluteal arteries in the region of the buttocks. Within the pelvis, the posteriorly situated arteries are the major blood supply for the pelvis.

Gluteal (*GLŪ-tē-ăl*) **arteries.** As branches of the internal iliac arteries, the superior and inferior gluteal arteries originate within the true pelvis. The arteries extend out of the posterior pelvis through the greater sciatic foramen to supply the gluteal muscles within the region of the buttocks.

External iliac arteries. Originating in the greater pelvis, the external branches of the common iliac arteries travel anteriorly to exit the pelvis above the pubic bones. Once the arteries have passed out of the pelvis, they continue as the femoral arteries and are the major source of blood supply for the legs.

Femoral (*FEM-ŏ-răl*) **arteries.** As continuations of the external iliac arteries, they originate as the vessels pass out of the pelvis to enter the region of the anterior thigh. Although the artery lies in close proximity to the femoral vein, the artery can be discerned in sectional images by its position lateral to the femoral vein.

Veins

Gluteal veins. Found by the corresponding arteries, these veins drain venous blood from the gluteal muscles. Originating within the buttocks, the veins extend through the greater sciatic notch to enter the bony pelvis and empty into the internal iliac veins.

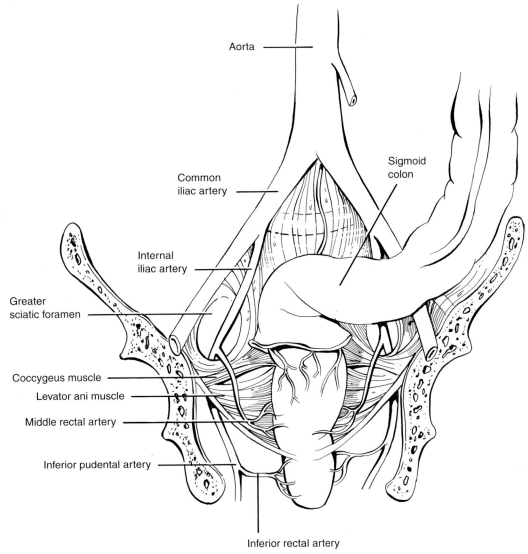

Figure 4-4 Sketch of the major arteries of the pelvis after removal of the anterior half of the pelvis.

Internal iliac veins. Originating from the gluteal veins in the region of the buttocks, the vessels travel through the posterior pelvis to drain into the common iliac veins (Fig. 4-5). During their course through the pelvis, the veins receive many branches draining venous blood from the pelvic viscera.

Femoral veins. Similar to the arteries, the veins are located in the anterior thighs. Originating from smaller vessels within the thigh, the femoral vein extends through the thigh to terminate in the external iliac vein as it passes over the pubic bone to enter the pelvis.

External iliac veins. Bilateral vessels formed at the termination of the femoral veins. The veins begin at the pubic bone and extend through the pelvis adjacent to the iliacus muscle to end at the common iliac veins.

Muscles

Iliacus (*il-i-ă-kŭs*). Originating from the inner iliac crest, they join with the psoas (*SŌ-as*) muscles and insert on the lesser trochanters of the femurs and act to flex the thighs (Fig. 4-6). In sectional images, the muscles are thin and flat on the inner surfaces of the iliac crests.

Pelvic diaphragm (*DĪ-ă-fram*). A group of muscles that form a sling across the pelvic cavity (Fig. 4-7). Similar to the diaphragm that forms the floor of the thoracic cavity, the pelvic diaphragm forms a floor that holds and supports the pelvic viscera (bladder, prostate, uterus, etc.)

Levator ani (*le-VĀ-ter Ā-ni*). Arising from the ischium, pubis, and coccyx, it attaches with its counterpart behind the rectum, forming a sling. This group of muscle fibers is

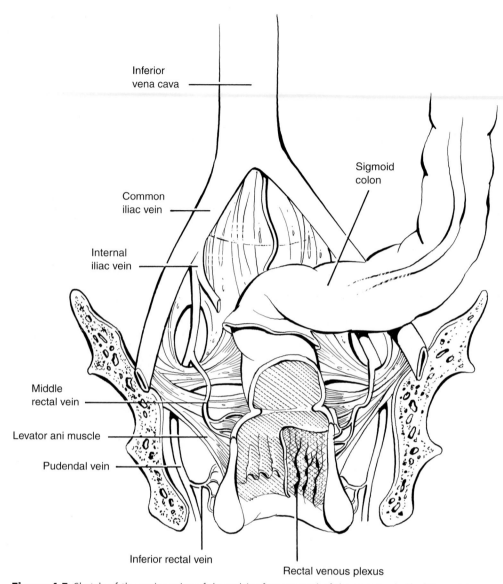

Figure 4-5 Sketch of the major veins of the pelvis after removal of the anterior half of the pelvis.

primarily responsible for controlling defecation. When they contract or shorten, they pull the rectum forward closing the alimentary opening.

Coccygeus (kok-si-JĒ-ŭs). Inserting on the sacrum and the coccyx, it arises from the ischial spine and forms the posterolateral portions of the pelvic diaphragm.

Male Urogenital System

Bladder. Roughly pyramidal in shape, its apex points downward between the pubis and the rectum (Fig. 4-8). Its upper surface normally appears flattened; but when the bladder becomes distended with urine, the upper surface becomes rounded and extends upward along the anterior abdominal wall. Located below the abdominal cavity, its upper surface

is draped with peritoneum; the bladder shifts in position as its volume changes.

Urethra *(yū-RĒ-thră).* Situated below the bladder, it extends for approximately 20 cm (8 in.) through the prostate, pelvic diaphragm, and penis. Besides draining urine from the bladder, it also transmits sperm to the exterior during ejaculation.

Prostate *(PROS-tāt).* A chestnut-size gland that surrounds the upper urethra that is between the bladder and the pelvic diaphragm. It is one of the most dense glands owing to the high concentrations of connective tissue and smooth muscle. During ejaculation, it secretes an alkaline fluid into the prostatic urethra that contributes to sperm motility.

Seminal vesicles *(SEM-i-năl VES-i-kls).* Glands located above the prostate and found between the bladder and the

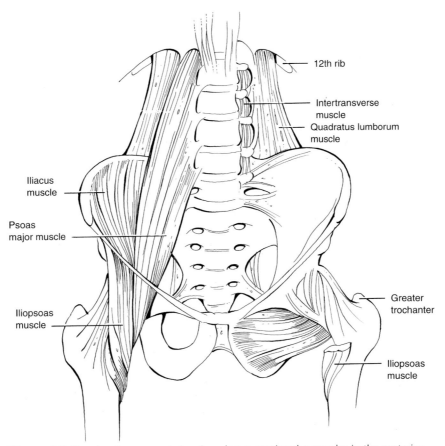

12th rib

Intertransverse muscle

Quadratus lumborum muscle

Iliacus muscle

Psoas major muscle

Iliopsoas muscle

Greater trochanter

Iliopsoas muscle

Figure 4-6 Drawing from an anterior view demonstrating the muscles in the posterior pelvis.

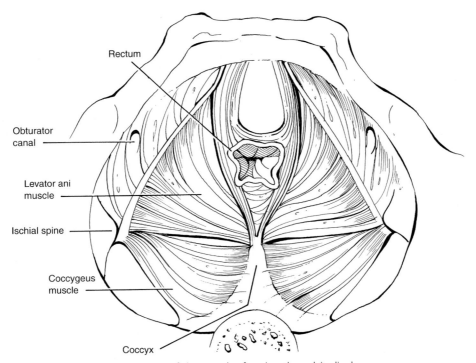

Rectum

Obturator canal

Levator ani muscle

Ischial spine

Coccygeus muscle

Coccyx

Figure 4-7 An inferior view of the muscles forming the pelvic diaphragm.

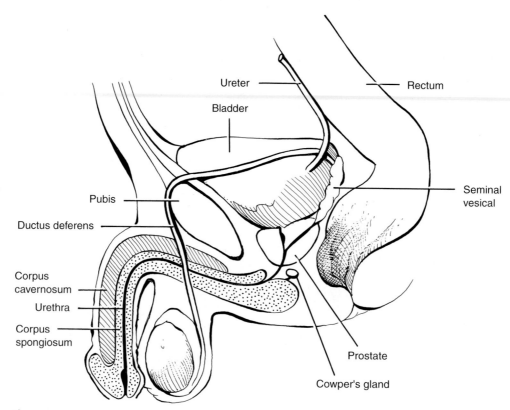

Figure 4-8 Median sagittal view of the male pelvis.

rectum on either side of the ductus (vas) deferens. Within the prostate, the seminal vesicle ducts join with the ductus (vas) deferens to join the prostatic urethra. During ejaculation, the seminal vesicles secrete an alkaline fluid rich in sugar that contributes to sperm viability.

Corpus cavernosum (*KOR-pûs kav-er-NO-sum*). Made up of erectile tissue surrounded by a strong fibrous capsule with tendon-like attachments to the ischiopubic rami. It forms the anterior three-quarters of the penis.

Corpus spongiosum (*spŭn-jē-O-sum*). An irregular-shaped bundle of erectile tissue that contains the penile urethra in the posterior part of the penis.

Spermatic cords. Bilateral structures consisting of the ductus (vas) deferens surrounded by thin layers of connective tissue and muscle that connect the testis with the anterior abdominal wall. During embryonic development, the testis, which are formed inside the abdominal cavity, are pulled through the anterior abdominal wall into the scrotum. As a result, the spermatic cords travel over the top of the pubic bones to enter the abdomen.

Female Urogenital System

Bladder. Roughly pyramidal in shape, with the apex pointing downward between the pubis and the vagina (Fig. 4-9). When nearly empty, it rests on the posterior surface of the pubis. Located below the abdominal cavity, the upper surface of the bladder and the uterus are draped with peritoneum.

Urethra. Situated below the bladder, it lies directly behind the symphysis pubis and is embedded in the anterior wall of the vagina. As it extends through the pelvic diaphragm, the adult urethra travels obliquely for roughly 4 cm (1.5 in.) to open exteriorly.

Uterus (*YU-ter-ŭs*). Located between the bladder and the rectum, it is shaped like an inverted pear and can be described in three parts: fundus, body, and cervix.

Fundus (*FŬN-dŭs*). The dome-shaped roof of the uterus found above the uterine tubes.

Body. The largest part of the uterus, it is centrally located and is tapered in shape.

Cervix (*SER-viks*). The most inferior constricted region of the uterus that opens into the vagina.

Rectouterine (*rek-tō-YU-ter-in*) **pouch.** Also referred to as the pouch of Douglas or the posterior cul-de-sac. Found within the peritoneum lining the abdominal cavity on the upper surface of the uterus and the rectum. The depressed area between the uterus and the rectum forms the lowest part of the abdominal cavity in the upright and supine positions. As such, the opening is closely evaluated to

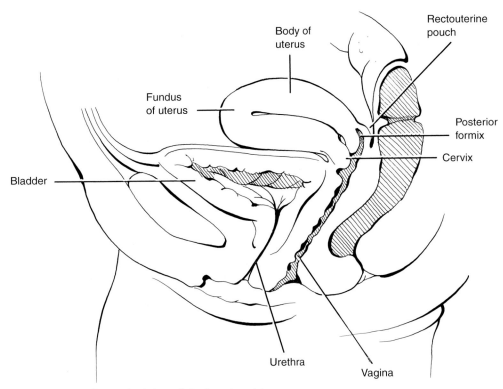

Figure 4-9 Median sagittal view of the female pelvis.

determine if excessive fluid is present within the peritoneal cavity.

Vagina (*vă-JĪ-nă*). Situated below the uterus, this organ can be generally described as a muscular tube, lined with a mucous membrane, that connects the uterine cavity with the exterior. Extending approximately 10 cm (4 in.) in length, it is situated between the bladder and the rectum. Although the vagina is described as a hollow organ, a tampon is necessary to clearly delineate the vaginal margin in sectional images.

Fornix (*FOR-niks*). At the juncture of the vagina with the cervix, a recess is formed around the portion of the cervix extending into the vagina. Although the recess is on all sides, the posterior fornix is usually deeper than the other sides.

Labia majora (*LĀ-bē-ă mă-JOR-ă*). Folds of pigmented skin containing pubic hair and covering layers of loose connective tissue and fat found on either side of the labia minora (small, longitudinal folds of skin around the vestibule).

Vestibule (*VES-ti-būl*). Located between the labia minora, this area has the openings of both the vagina and urethra.

Broad ligaments. As the peritoneum extends across the upper surface of the pelvis containing the uterus, oviducts, ligaments, etc., the folds of connective tissue form mesometrium, or the broad ligaments (Fig. 4-10 A,B). Lateral to the uterus, the peritoneum drapes over smaller structures, forming the anterior and posterior layers that attach and support the pelvic organs.

Adnexal (*ad-NEK-săl*) **areas.** The uterine appendages including the ovaries, oviducts, ligaments, etc., found within the broad ligaments on either side of the uterus.

Ovaries (*Ō-vă-rēz*). The two almond-shaped glands located in the upper pelvis on either side of the uterus within the adnexal areas. They are on the posterior side of the broad ligament and produce ova as well as hormones partially responsible for regulating the female reproductive cycle.

Oviducts (*Ō-vi-dŭkts*). Also called uterine tubes. Found in the free or upper margin of the broad ligament, extending from the ovaries to the uterus. They transport the ova produced by the ovaries to the uterus.

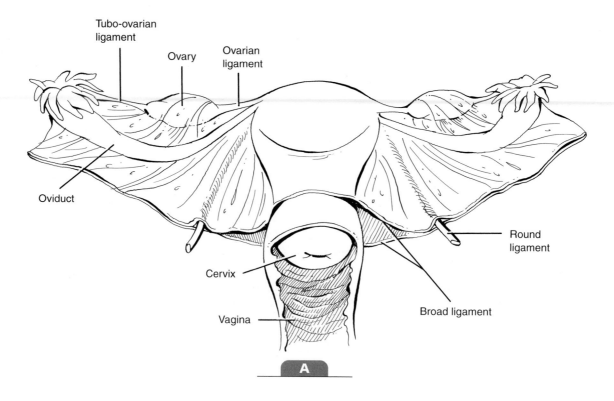

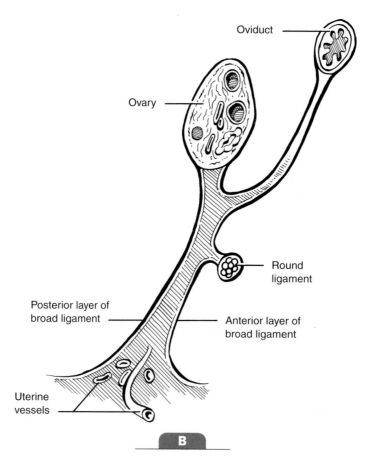

Figure 4-10 A. Anterior view of the broad ligament. **B.** Sagittal section through the broad ligament at the level of the ovary.

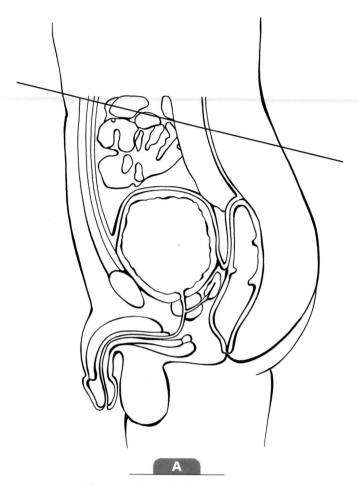

Figure 4-11 Axial CT image 1—male.

AXIAL CT IMAGES: MALE

The following 21 axial CT images of the male pelvis are described at 8.0 mm intervals from superior to inferior. The images were generated immediately after the administration of 100 mL venous contrast at the following technical factors: 120 kVp and 150 mA-s. Abbreviations: kVp = kilovolt peak, mA-s = milliampere-second.

Figure 4-11 (A,B,C). In the first image, the intervertebral disk occupies a central location in front of the vertebral foramen. At this level, the iliac crests are not yet seen, indicating the section is slightly above the pelvis and representing the appropriate location for the first image in an examination of the pelvis. On either side of the intervertebral disk, the psoas muscles appear as large round areas with a density similar to that of the intervertebral disk. Along the anteromedial surface of the psoas muscles, the ureters can be seen because of the contrast enhancement. Medial to the ureters, three major vessels can be discerned within the pelvis. The largest vessel on the right side, the inferior vena cava, has yet to bifurcate; and the two vessels on the left side, the right and left common iliac arteries, have originated from the bifurcation of the abdominal aorta. In the abdominal cavity, the most notable structure is the enlarged area of the intestine on the far right side. Given the large size of this part of the intestine, especially compared to the loops of the small bowel, it can be identified as the cecum.

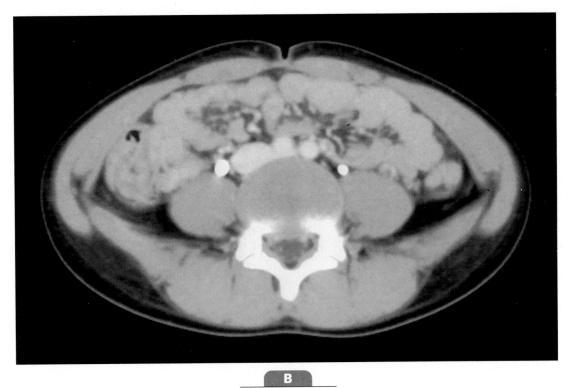

B

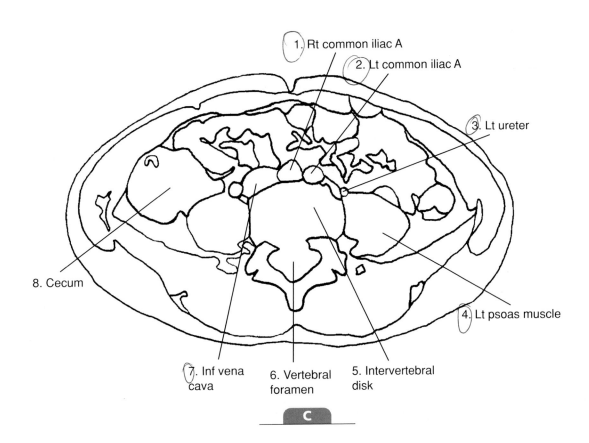

1. Rt common iliac A

2. Lt common iliac A

3. Lt ureter

8. Cecum

4. Lt psoas muscle

7. Inf vena cava

6. Vertebral foramen

5. Intervertebral disk

C

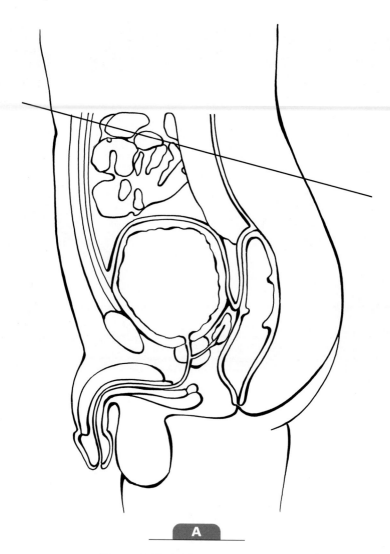

Figure 4-12 Axial CT image 2—male.

Figure 4-12 (A,B,C). The largest vertebra of the body, L5, is shown in this image between the upper iliac crests. Because the iliac crest is now visible, this section would be the first image showing pelvic structures. Similar to the previous image, the major vessels of the pelvis are shown sectioned just anterior to the body of L5. The three distinct major vessels seen in the previous image have changed at this level; it is now difficult to tell if there are three or four vessels. Because the common iliac arteries were identified on the previous section, they are also present at this level; and the inferior vena cava is shown bifurcating into the right and left common iliac veins. Lateral to the major vessels, the ureters can be seen as bright vessels anteromedially located next to the psoas muscles. Although most intestinal structures are located within the peritoneum, the cecum, identified on the right side, and the descending colon, found on the left side, are retroperitoneal in location.

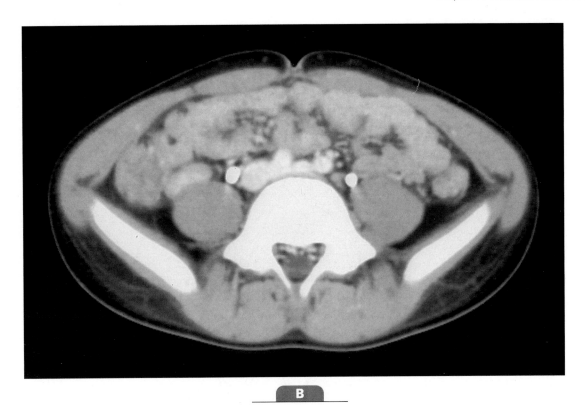

B

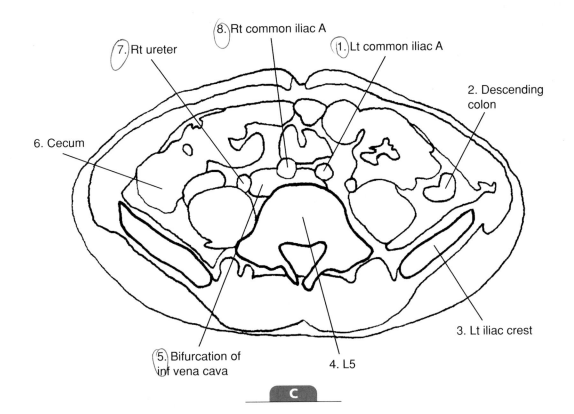

8. Rt common iliac A

7. Rt ureter

1. Lt common iliac A

2. Descending colon

6. Cecum

3. Lt iliac crest

5. Bifurcation of inf vena cava

4. L5

C

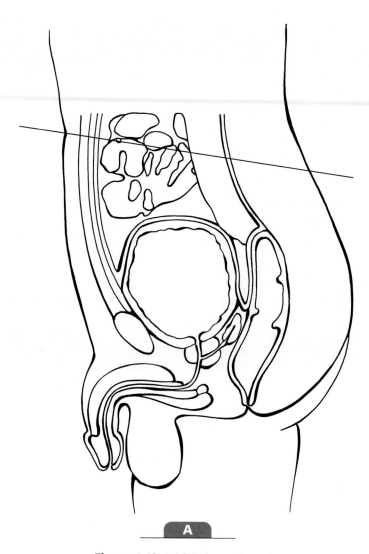

Figure 4-13 Axial CT image 3—male.

Figure 4-13 (A,B,C). Sectioned through the lower end of the vertebral body of L5, this image demonstrates the inferior vertebral notches between the vertebral body and the lamina. The vertebral notches are the location of the spinal nerves exiting between L5 and S1. Anterior to the vertebra, the major vessels of the abdomen now appear as four distinct vessels. On the right side, the right common iliac artery occupies a more anterior location than the right common iliac vein, which is slightly larger. On the left side, the left common iliac artery is more anterior than the left common iliac vein, which is longitudinally sectioned near the bifurcation of the inferior vena cava. Lateral to the major vessels, the right and left ureters are demonstrated and are clearly visualized owing to their bright contrast enhancement.

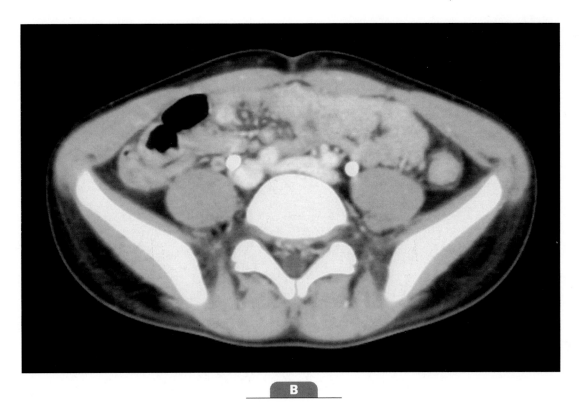

B

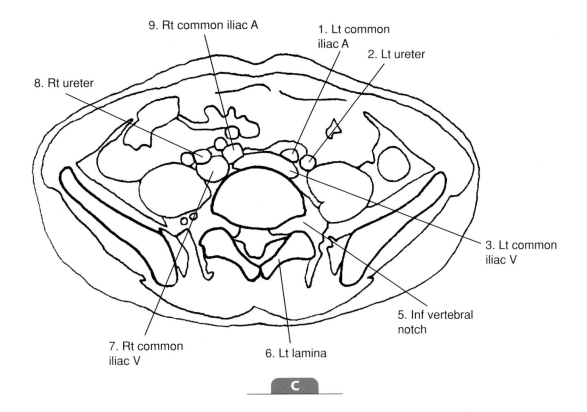

9. Rt common iliac A

1. Lt common iliac A

2. Lt ureter

8. Rt ureter

3. Lt common iliac V

5. Inf vertebral notch

7. Rt common iliac V

6. Lt lamina

C

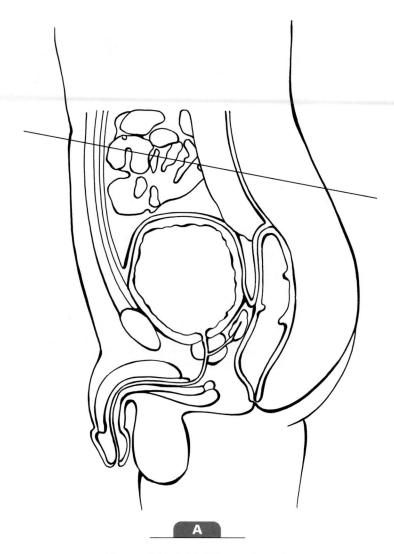

Figure 4-14 Axial CT image 4—male.

Figure 4-14 (A,B,C). The unique shape of the vertebra indicates that this image is at the level of the sacrum. Compared to previous vertebral bodies, the sacral vertebrae have a distinct "bat" shape, because the transverse processes are fused to form lateral parts that articulate with the iliac bones. In this section, the intervertebral disk can be seen separating the vertebral bodies of L5 and S1. Anterior to the vertebral column, four major vessels are demonstrated in the pelvis. On the right side, the right common iliac artery lies adjacent to the right common iliac vein; and on the left side, the left common iliac artery and vein are seen together. As demonstrated previously, the arteries are somewhat smaller than the veins and occupy a more anterior position. On either side of the vertebrae, the psoas muscles are shown in cross-section and serve as landmarks for other structures in the area. Lateral to the psoas muscles, the descending colon and cecum are demonstrated fixed to the posterior abdominal wall.

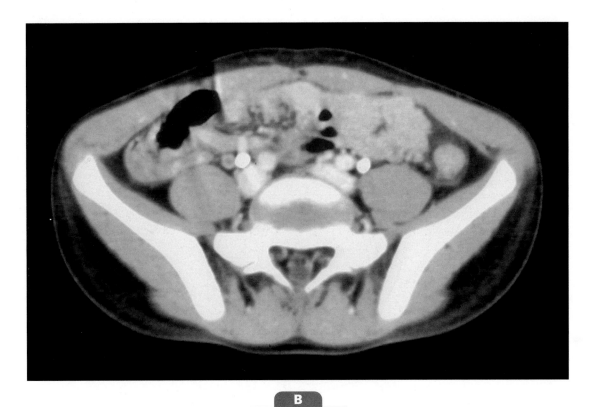

B

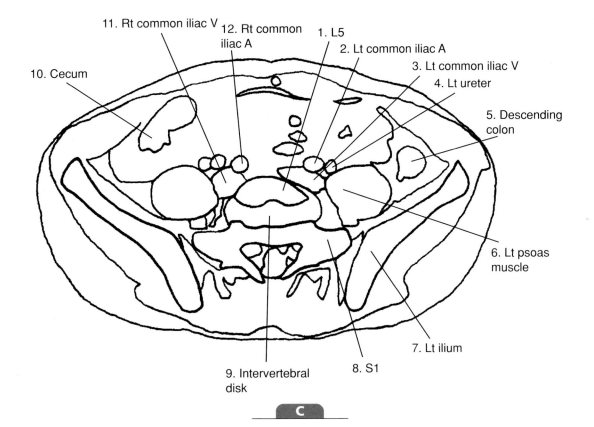

11. Rt common iliac V   12. Rt common   1. L5
                        iliac A   2. Lt common iliac A

10. Cecum   3. Lt common iliac V
                                          4. Lt ureter

                                          5. Descending
                                          colon

                                          6. Lt psoas
                                          muscle

                                          7. Lt ilium

9. Intervertebral   8. S1
disk

C

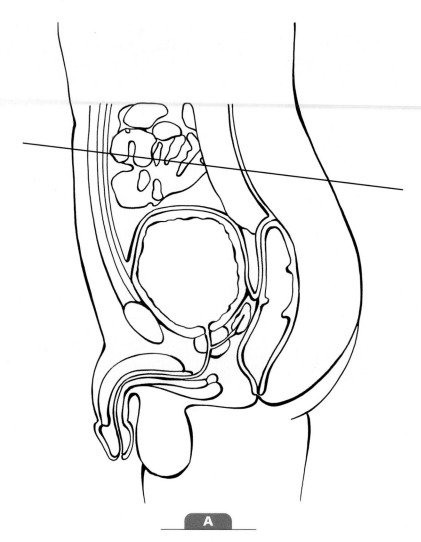

Figure 4-15 Axial CT image 5—male.

Figure 4-15 (A,B,C). The characteristic appearance of the sacral vertebra is more evident in this section through the body of S1. The lateral parts of S1 are shown articulating with the iliac bones on either side. On the anterior part of S1, a small part of the intervertebral disk can still be seen. On the back side of S1, the first pair of vertebral foramina are emerging from the sacral canal. Within the greater pelvis, the iliacus and psoas muscles are shown lining the posterior wall of the pelvic cavity. Similar to previous images, the ureters appear as bright, contrast-enhanced vessels near the psoas muscles and are in close proximity to the major vessels of the pelvis. As in the previous image, the common iliac veins are continuing in a posterior location adjacent to the vertebral body; however, the common iliac arteries have bifurcated and given rise to the internal and external iliac arteries. In the anterior pelvic cavity, numerous loops of small bowel are loosely organized centrally, and the descending colon is seen on the left side occupying a position near the iliacus muscle.

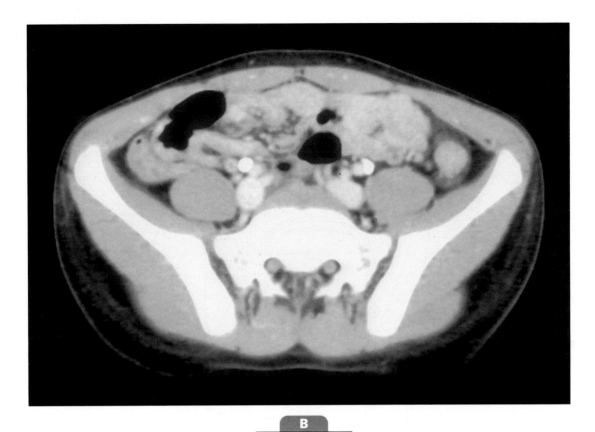

B

1. Loops of small bowel

2. Descending colon

10. Rt iliacus muscle

3. Lt ureter

9. Rt psoas muscle

4. Lt common iliac V

8. S1

7. Int & ext iliac A

6. Sacral canal

5. Lt vertebral foramen

C

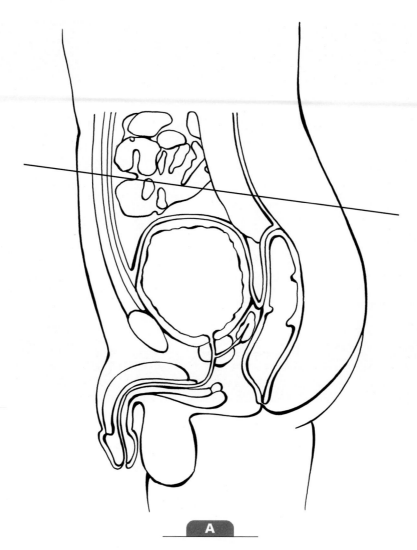

Figure 4-16 Axial CT image 6—male.

Figure 4-16 (A,B,C). The sacral foramina are separated by bone from the sacral canal at this level. Lining the posterior pelvic wall, the iliacus and psoas muscles are shown in cross-section adjacent to the iliac bones. In this image, the external and internal iliac arteries are shown on either side of the left ureter and in front of the larger common iliac vein. Like previous images, the descending colon and the cecum are on opposite sides of the randomly organized loops of small bowel distributed within the peritoneal cavity.

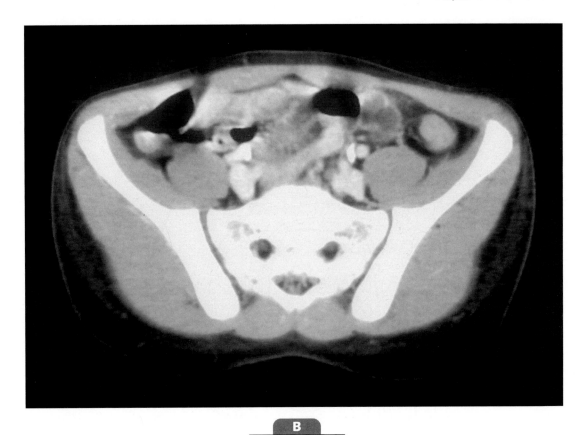

B

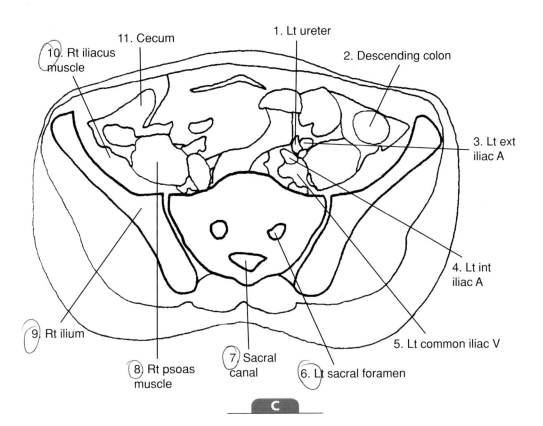

10. Rt iliacus
muscle

11. Cecum

1. Lt ureter

2. Descending colon

3. Lt ext
iliac A

4. Lt int
iliac A

5. Lt common iliac V

6. Lt sacral foramen

7. Sacral
canal

8. Rt psoas
muscle

9. Rt ilium

C

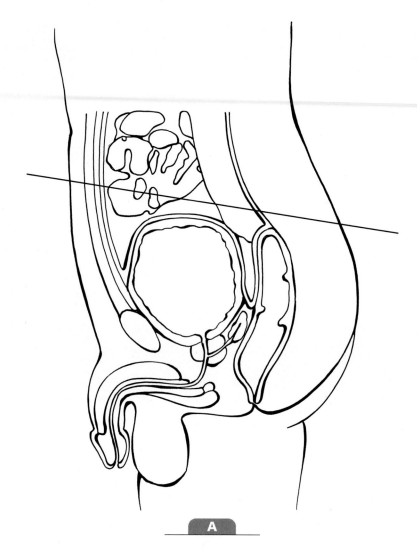

A

Figure 4-17 Axial CT image 7—male.

Figure 4-17 (A,B,C). This oblique section through the sacrum shows two pairs of sacral foramina, the first and second. Although the first pair of sacral foramina are near the point of exit from the sacrum, the second pair are just emerging from the sacral canal. On either side of the sacrum, the iliac bones form the sacral iliac joints where they articulate with the lateral parts of the sacrum. Within the greater pelvis, the left ureter is enhanced and lies near the medial border of the psoas muscle. Beside the ureter, the external and internal iliac arteries are diverging; the external iliac artery is moving to a more anterior position, and the internal iliac artery is occupying a more posterior position. Seen between the iliac arteries, the common iliac vein is still larger. Within the peritoneal cavity, the loops of small bowel occupy most of the anterior pelvis. Because this part of the small bowel is within the pelvis, the ileum is probably the part of the small bowel shown.

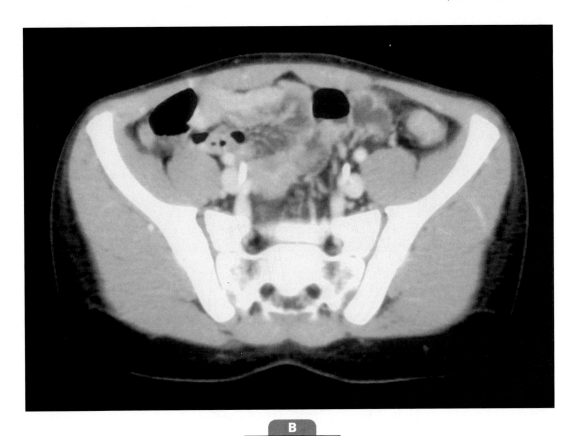

B

1. Loops of small bowel

2. Lt ext iliac A

3. Lt ureter

4. Lt common iliac V

5. Lt int iliac A

6. Lt sacral foramina

7. Sacral canal

8. Rt sacroiliac jt

C

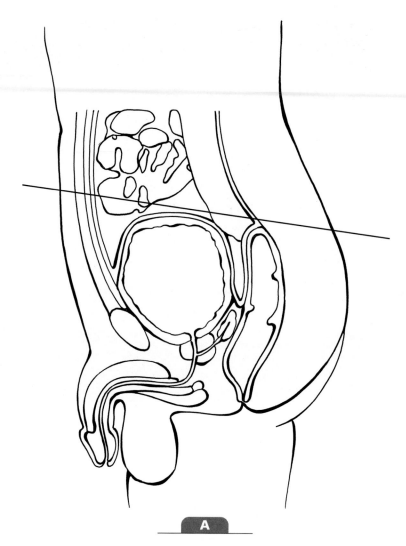

Figure 4-18 Axial CT image 8—male.

Figure 4-18 (A,B,C). The sacrum, iliac bones, iliacus muscles, and psoas muscles are shown in cross-section forming the posterior wall of the pelvic cavity. Compared to previous images, the psoas and iliacus muscles are not as clearly separable as they join to form the iliopsoas muscles in the lower pelvis. Near the psoas muscles, the ureters are readily visible as contrast-enhanced structures between the external and internal iliac vessels. The intestinal structures are similar to previous views, with the small bowel occupying most of the peritoneal cavity. Posterior to the peritoneum, the lower edge of the cecum is shown on the right and the descending colon is demonstrated on the left. Although the descending colon ends in the sigmoid colon, the irregular shape of the sigmoid colon moves upward so that it is also included within this section.

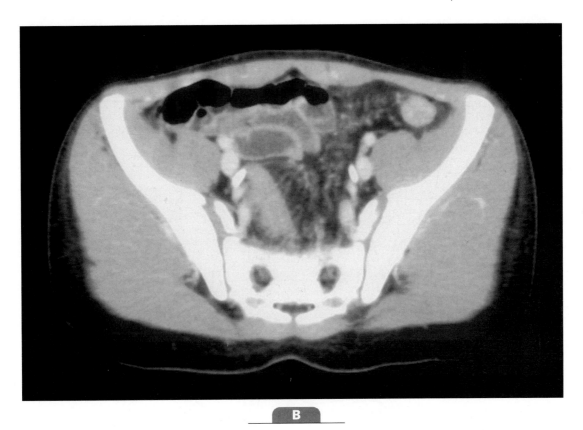

B

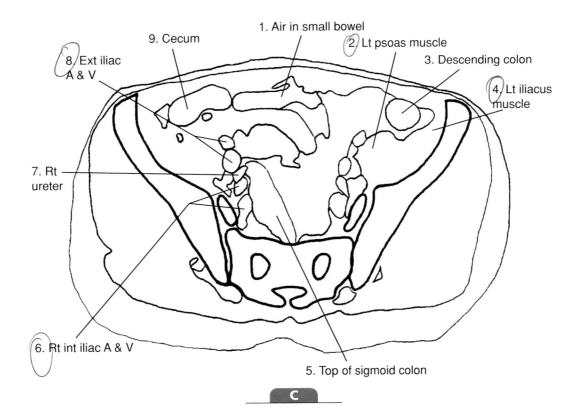

1. Air in small bowel
9. Cecum
2. Lt psoas muscle
8. Ext iliac A & V
3. Descending colon
4. Lt iliacus muscle
7. Rt ureter
6. Rt int iliac A & V
5. Top of sigmoid colon

C

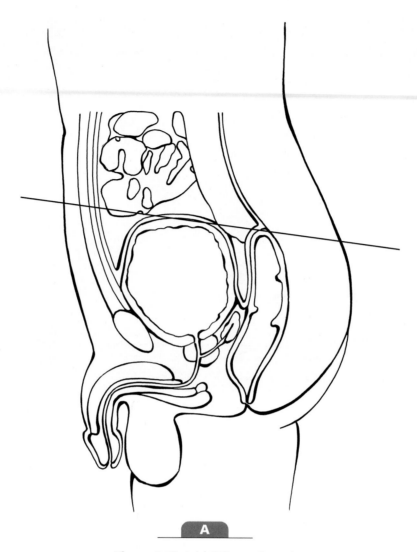

Figure 4-19 Axial CT image 9—male.

Figure 4-19 (A,B,C). The sacrum is smaller than in the previous images. This image includes the bottom of the sacroiliac joint. Although the ilium is shown in cross-section similar to previous views, the central portion of the ilium is beginning to expand, indicating the section is nearing the acetabulum. Within the pelvic cavity, the sigmoid colon is more clearly seen in its characteristic S-shape as it extends toward the descending colon on the left side. Owing to contrast enhancement, the ureters are easily identified between the iliac vessels. Anterior to the ureter, the external iliac vessels are medial to the psoas muscle, and the artery is more anterior and slightly smaller than the corresponding vein. Posterior to the left ureter, the left internal iliac vessels are between the sigmoid colon and the left ilium. Although some small bowel can be seen in this section, much of the anterior pelvic cavity is occupied by the top of the bladder, which appears as a dense structure between loops of small bowel.

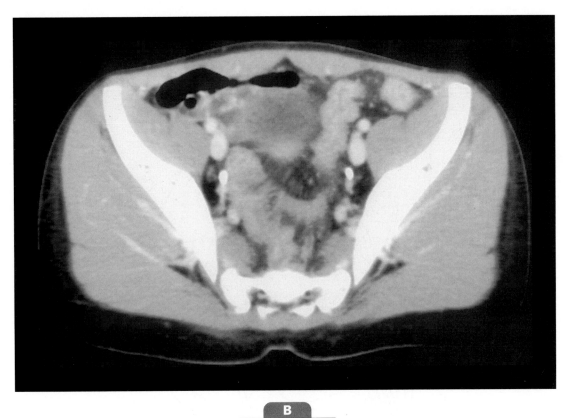

B

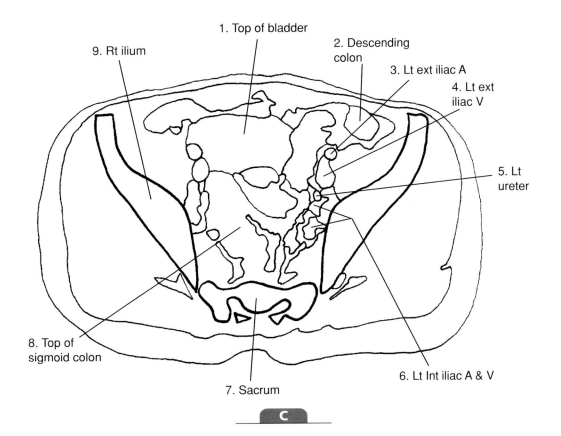

9. Rt ilium

1. Top of bladder

2. Descending colon

3. Lt ext iliac A

4. Lt ext iliac V

5. Lt ureter

8. Top of sigmoid colon

6. Lt Int iliac A & V

7. Sacrum

C

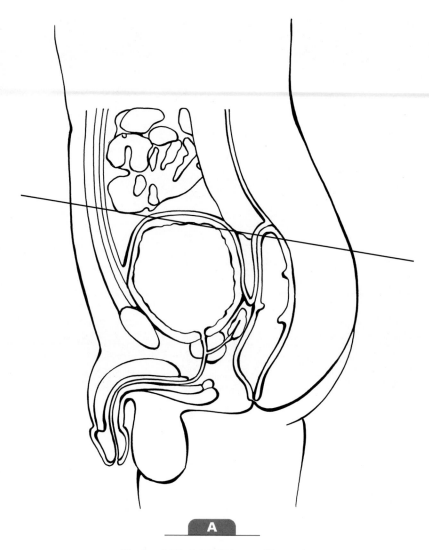

Figure 4-20 Axial CT image 10—male.

Figure 4-20 (A,B,C). At this level, the sacrum and iliac bones are separated and the bladder is easily recognized occupying most of the anterior pelvic cavity. Within the bladder, a contrast-fluid level is demonstrated, because part of the fluid within the bladder is contrast enhanced. Around the bladder, small bowel can be seen anteriorly, and the characteristic S-shape of the sigmoid colon is between the bladder and the sacrum. On either side of these visceral structures, the ureters are seen along with the external and internal iliac vessels.

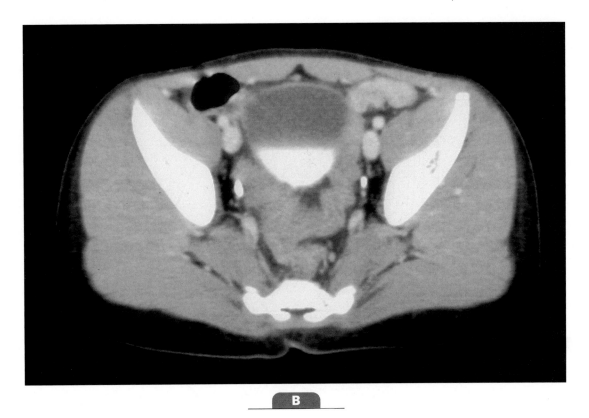

B

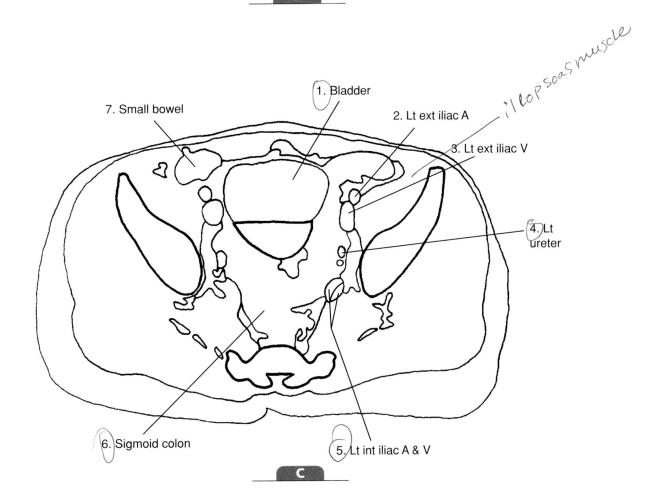

7. Small bowel

1. Bladder

2. Lt ext iliac A

3. Lt ext iliac V

iliopsoas muscle

4. Lt ureter

6. Sigmoid colon

5. Lt int iliac A & V

C

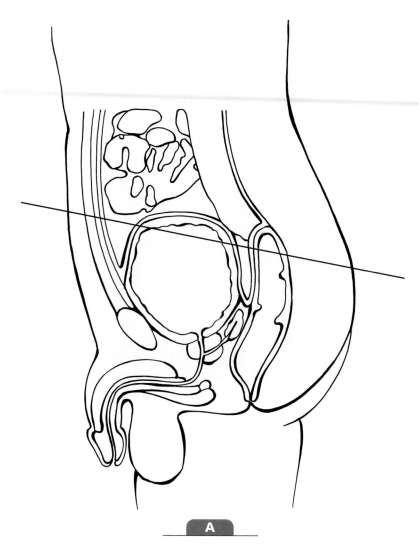

Figure 4-21 Axial CT image 11—male.

Figure 4-21 (A,B,C). The iliac bones appear shortened and thicker because they are near the level of the acetabula. Although the bladder occupies most of the pelvic cavity, the ureters are demonstrated in cross-section between the iliac bones as they extend toward the lower bladder. On either side of the bladder, the external iliac artery and vein are seen, and the artery is more anterior and slightly smaller in size. Posterior to the bladder, the S-shaped sigmoid colon has been replaced by the top of the rectum, found just in front of the lower sacrum. At this point, the internal iliac vessels have branched and are difficult to discern other than as a group of contrast-enhanced vessels.

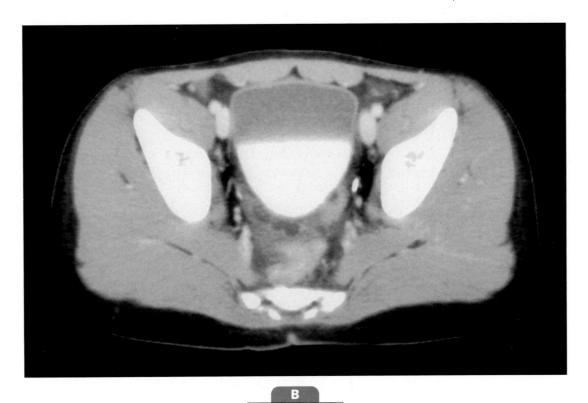

B

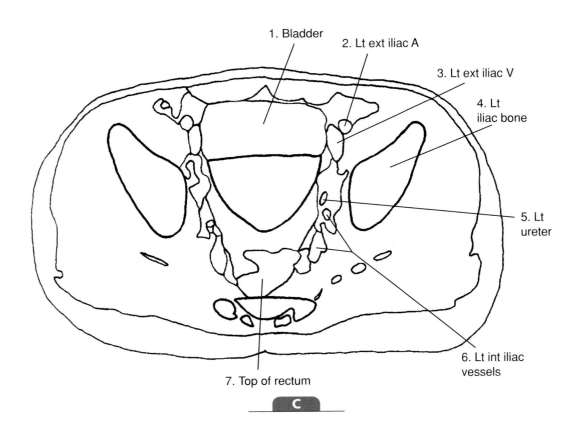

1. Bladder
2. Lt ext iliac A
3. Lt ext iliac V
4. Lt iliac bone
5. Lt ureter
6. Lt int iliac vessels
7. Top of rectum

C

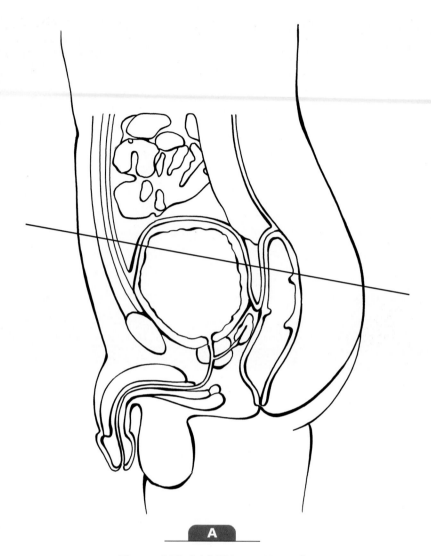

Figure 4-22 Axial CT image 12—male.

Figure 4-22 (A,B,C). The iliac bones are shortened and thicker, because they are forming the roof of the acetabula. Between the iliac bones, the contrast- and urine-filled bladder occupies most of the pelvic cavity. On either side of the bladder, the external iliac vessels are found; the arteries are more anterior and smaller in size. Between the bladder and the sacrum, the rectum is shown in cross-section along with the internal iliac vessels, which are difficult to distinguish at this low level.

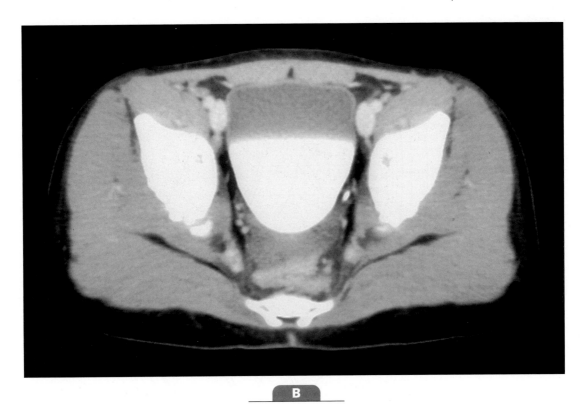

B

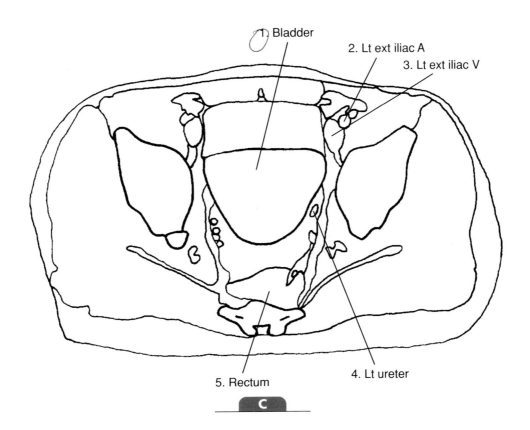

1. Bladder
2. Lt ext iliac A
3. Lt ext iliac V
4. Lt ureter
5. Rectum

C

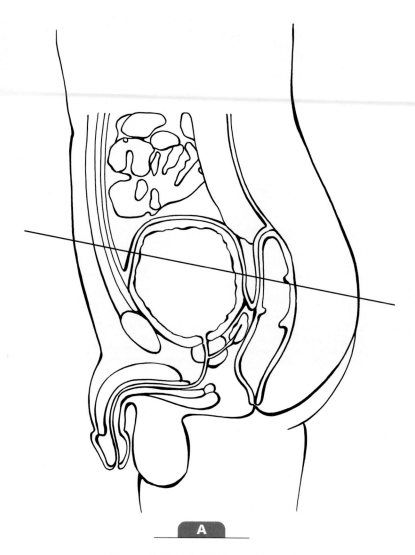

A

Figure 4-23 Axial CT image 13—male.

Figure 4-23 (A,B,C). The upper part of the femoral heads are articulating with the iliac part of the acetabula. Similar to previous images, the bladder occupies most of the pelvic cavity and clearly shows a contrast–fluid level. In the anterior pelvic cavity, the left external iliac artery and vein are shown in cross-section lateral to the bladder. Posterior to the bladder, the rectum is found just anterior to the tip of the sacrum.

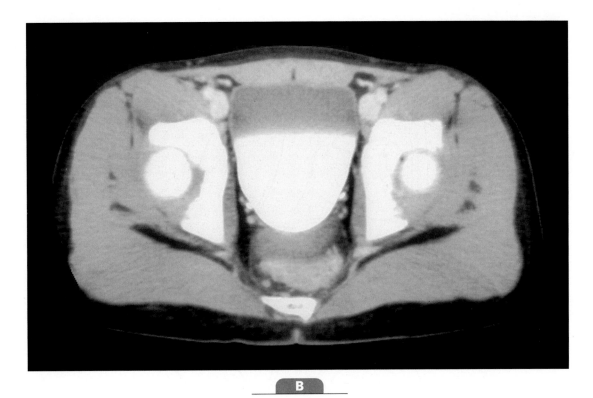

B

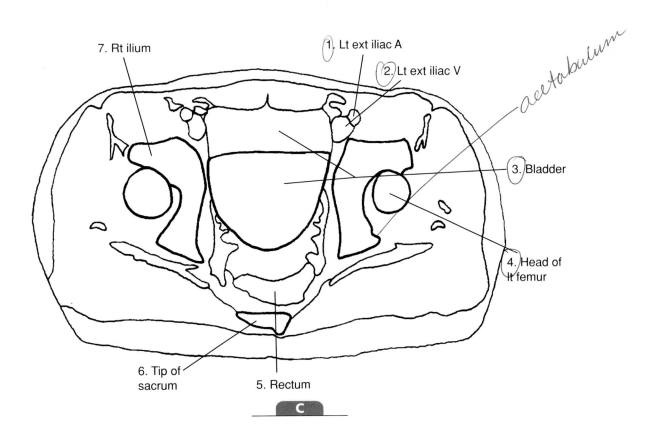

7. Rt ilium

1. Lt ext iliac A

2. Lt ext iliac V

acetabulum

3. Bladder

4. Head of lt femur

6. Tip of sacrum

5. Rectum

C

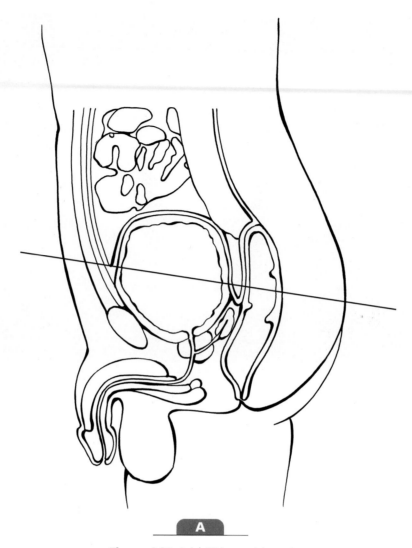

A

Figure 4-24 Axial CT image 14—male.

Figure 4-24 (A,B,C). The heads of the femurs are easily identified on either side articulating with the acetabula. Although previous images labeled the bone forming the upper acetabulum as the ilium, the lower half of the acetabulum is formed by the ischial and pubic bones. Similar to previous images, the bladder occupies most of the pelvic cavity, and the rectum is located more posteriorly. In contrast to previous images, the external iliac vessels on either side of the anterior bladder are now labeled as the femoral artery and veins, because they are outside of the bony pelvic cavity.

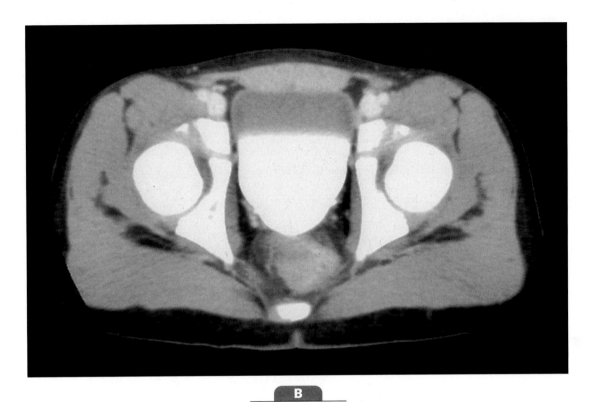

B

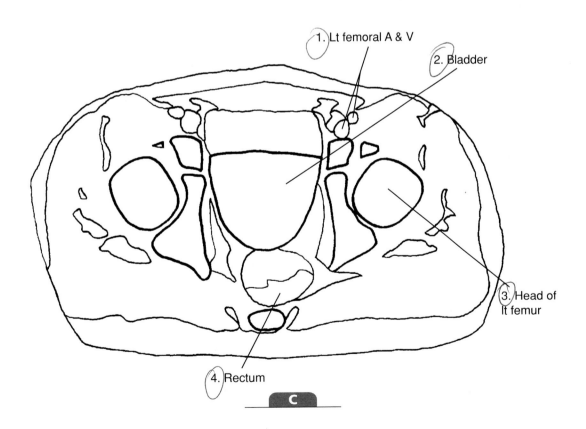

1. Lt femoral A & V

2. Bladder

3. Head of lt femur

4. Rectum

C

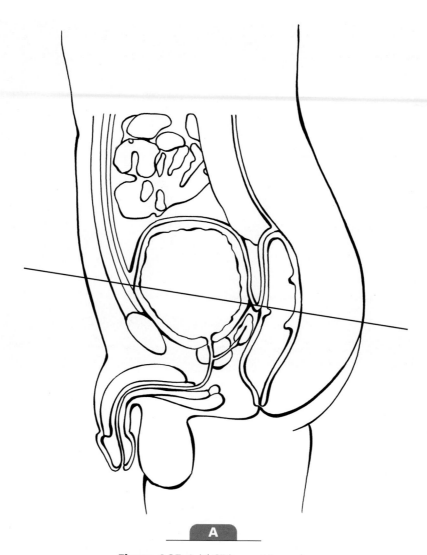

Figure 4-25 Axial CT image 15—male.

Figure 4-25 (A,B,C). The heads of the femurs are within the acetabula on either side of the lower bony pelvis. Anterior to the pelvic cavity, the femoral arteries and veins are clearly demonstrated outside of the bony pelvis. Within the pelvis, the bladder occupies most of the anterior cavity, and the rectum is the major structure in the posterior pelvic cavity. Lateral to the rectum, the pelvic diaphragm is shown sectioned as it forms a sling across the pelvic cavity. Posterior to the rectum, the sacrum has been replaced by the coccyx, which marks the posterior border of the bony pelvis.

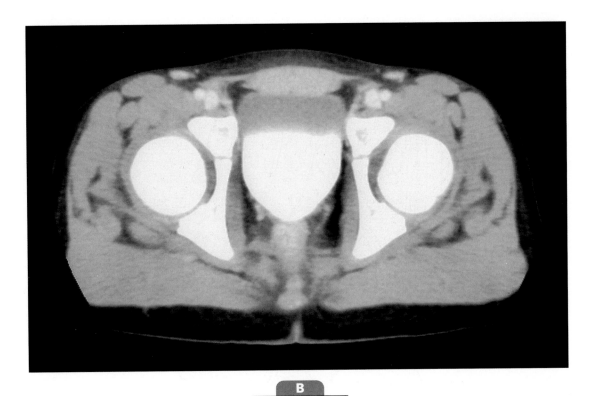

B

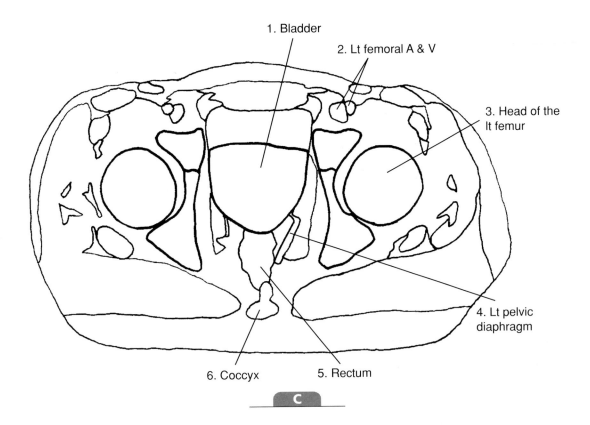

1. Bladder

2. Lt femoral A & V

3. Head of the
lt femur

4. Lt pelvic
diaphragm

6. Coccyx   5. Rectum

C

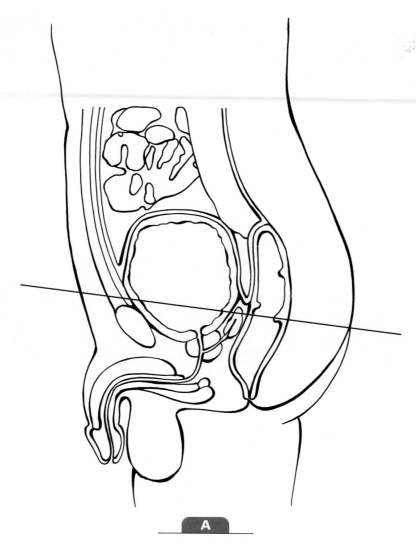

Figure 4-26 Axial CT image 16—male.

Figure 4-26 (A,B,C). The heads of the femurs can be readily identified as round bony structures on either side of the lower bony pelvis resting in the acetabula. Because this section is through the lower half of the acetabulum, the pubis forms the anterior part and the ischium forms the posterior part. Inside the bony pelvis, the bladder and the rectum are the major structures seen, as in the previous images. Unlike previous images, glandular structures, the seminal vesicles, are now apparent next to the posterior wall of the bladder. As described earlier, the seminal vesicles are located above the prostate gland and are posterior to the bladder. On either side of the rectum, the pelvic diaphragm is shown in cross-section as a thin muscular sheet attached to the bony pelvis forming a sling for the contents of the pelvic cavity. Lateral to the pelvic diaphragm, radiolucent areas representing fat within the ischiorectal fossae are demonstrated on either side. Outside the pelvis, the contrast-enhanced femoral artery and vein can be seen in the anterior thigh. As described earlier, the femoral artery is usually smaller and more laterally situated than the femoral vein.

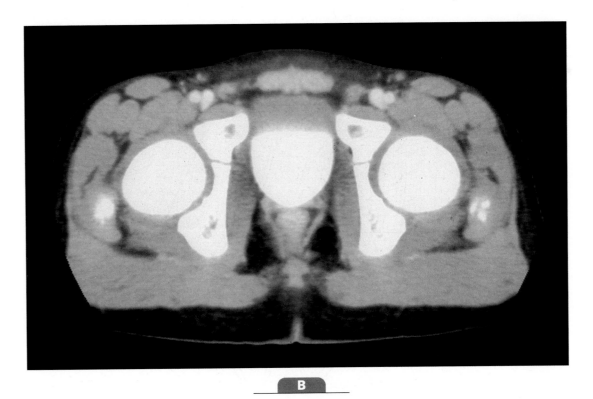

B

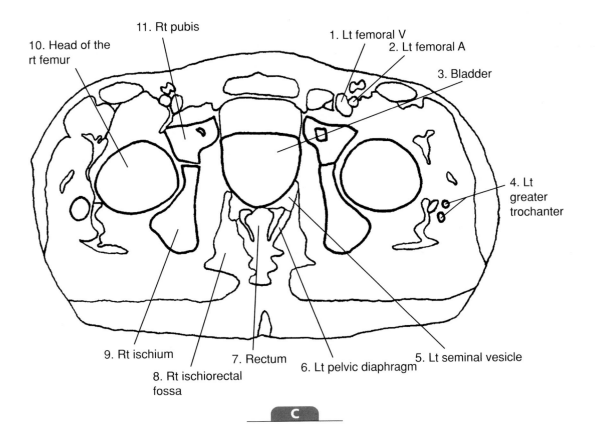

10. Head of the rt femur

11. Rt pubis

1. Lt femoral V

2. Lt femoral A

3. Bladder

4. Lt greater trochanter

5. Lt seminal vesicle

6. Lt pelvic diaphragm

7. Rectum

8. Rt ischiorectal fossa

9. Rt ischium

C

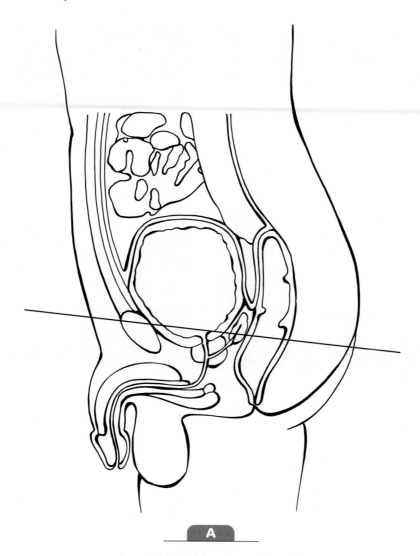

Figure 4-27 Axial CT image 17—male.

Figure 4-27 (A,B,C). Along with the lower part of the femoral heads, the greater trochanters now appear as large hook-like projections on the posterior femur. The heads of the femurs rest within the lower acetabula formed by the pubic and ischial bones. At this low level, the bladder is much smaller and appears behind the pubic bones. Posterior to the bladder, the seminal vesicles appear larger and are situated between the bladder and the rectum. Similar to the previous image, the pelvic diaphragm is shown in cross-section as a thin sheet of muscle projecting downward, separating the rectum from the fat-filled ischiorectal fossae. Much like previous views, the femoral artery and vein are clearly seen anterior to the pubic bones.

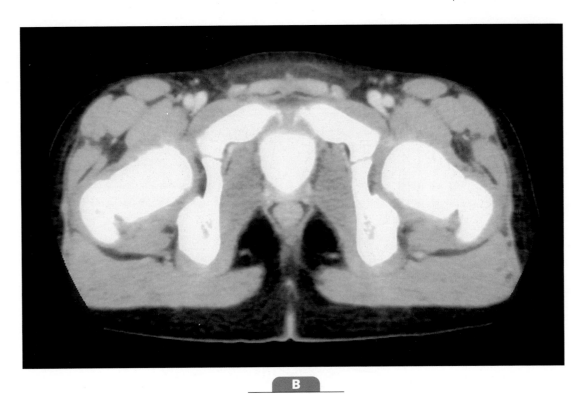

B

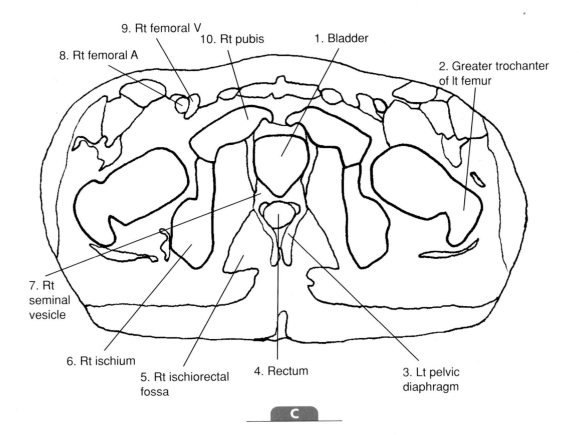

9. Rt femoral V

8. Rt femoral A

10. Rt pubis

1. Bladder

2. Greater trochanter of lt femur

7. Rt seminal vesicle

6. Rt ischium

5. Rt ischiorectal fossa

4. Rectum

3. Lt pelvic diaphragm

C

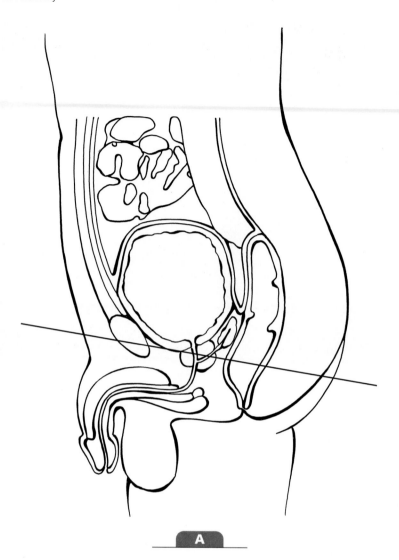

Figure 4-28 Axial CT image 18—male.

Figure 4-28 (A,B,C). The bony anatomy at the low level through the pelvis has a unique appearance, because none of the bones seems to be attached. The femoral head is no longer present and the neck is shown obliquely sectioned. In place of the acetabula, the obturator foramina are demonstrated between the pubic and ischial bones. Also, the right and left pubic bones are separated by thick articular cartilage forming the symphysis pubis. Posteriorly, the ischial bones appear expanded compared to previous images, indicating that the level is through the ischial tuberosities. Within the bony pelvis, the bladder is no longer seen and has been replaced by a dense gland, the prostate, which is nearly inseparable from the rectum. Outlining both of these structures, the pelvic diaphragm is shown in cross-section attaching to the pubic bones. Outside of the bony pelvis, the femoral artery and vein are again seen near the anterior surface. Medial to the femoral vessels, the spermatic cords are shown in cross-section as they extend up from the testes to travel over the pubic bones to enter the anterior abdominal wall.

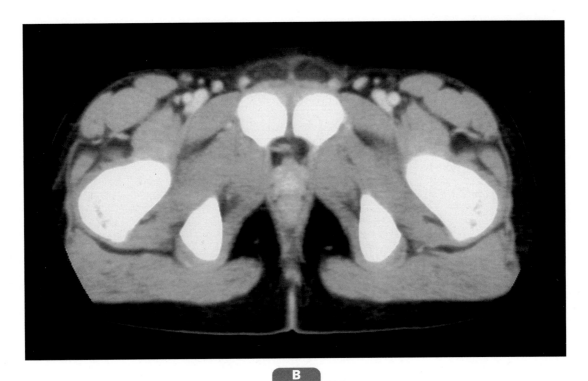

B

11. Symphysis
pubis

2. Lt femoral V

10. Rt spermatic cord

1. Lt pubis

3. Lt femoral A

4. Lt obturator
foramen

5. Neck of
the lt femur

9. Prostate

8. Rectum

7. Lt pelvic
diaphragm

6. Lt ischial
tuberosity

C

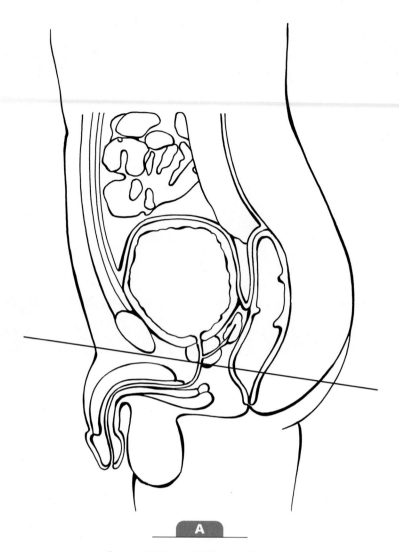

Figure 4-29 Axial CT image 19—male.

Figure 4-29 (A,B,C). The femurs on either side of the image appear oval shaped because the section is through the neck. Between the femurs, the enlarged part of the ischial bones, the ischial tuberosities, are separated from the slender inferior pubic rami by the obturator foramina. Within the bony pelvis, the prostate and rectum are surrounded by the pelvic diaphragm. Between the pelvic diaphragm and the ischial tuberosities, the fat-filled areas of the ischiorectal fossae are shown on either side and are continuous with the fat in the region of the buttocks. On the anterior aspect of the image, the spermatic cords appear near the surface, whereas the femoral arteries and veins have moved deeper into the musculature of the anterior thighs.

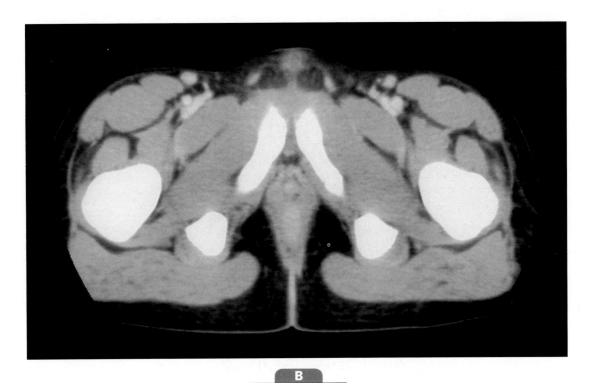

B

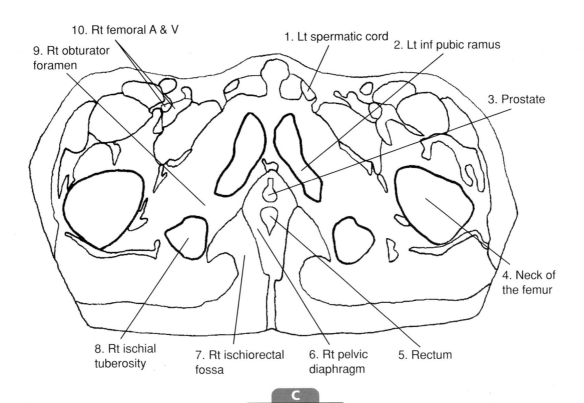

10. Rt femoral A & V

9. Rt obturator foramen

1. Lt spermatic cord

2. Lt inf pubic ramus

3. Prostate

4. Neck of the femur

8. Rt ischial tuberosity

7. Rt ischiorectal fossa

6. Rt pelvic diaphragm

5. Rectum

C

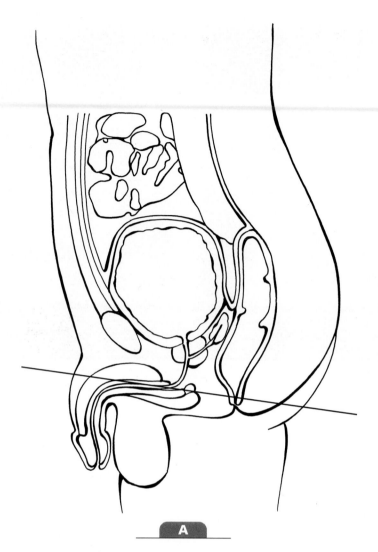

Figure 4-30 Axial CT image 20—male.

Figure 4-30 (A,B,C). The irregularly shaped femoral bones are shown in cross-section on either side of the image, and the ischial rami appear as long slender bones more centrally located. Between the ischial bones, the prostate and rectum are no longer seen and have been replaced by the corpus spongiosum surrounding the urethra. An erectile tissue of the posterior penis, the corpus spongiosum lies below the pelvic diaphragm and extends out into the penis. By comparison, the corpus cavernosum, forming the anterior erectile tissue of the penis, is sectioned anterior to the bony pelvis. On either side of the corpus cavernosum, the spermatic cords are shown in cross-section as they travel to the testes. The femoral arteries and veins, which previously occupied a superficial position, are found within the musculature of the thighs.

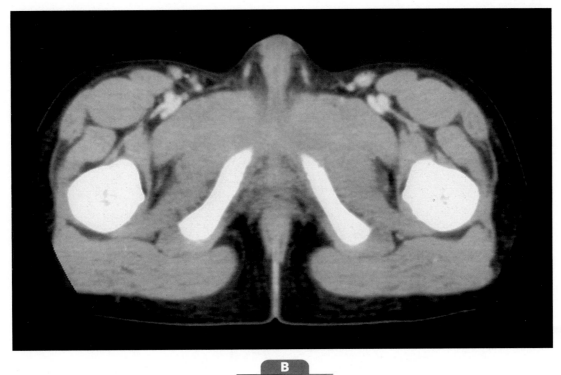

B

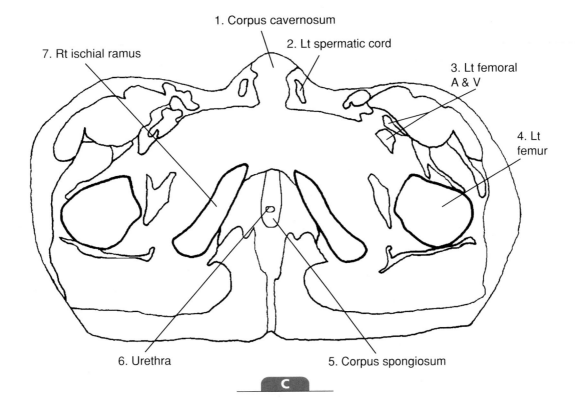

1. Corpus cavernosum

2. Lt spermatic cord

7. Rt ischial ramus

3. Lt femoral
A & V

4. Lt
femur

6. Urethra

5. Corpus spongiosum

C

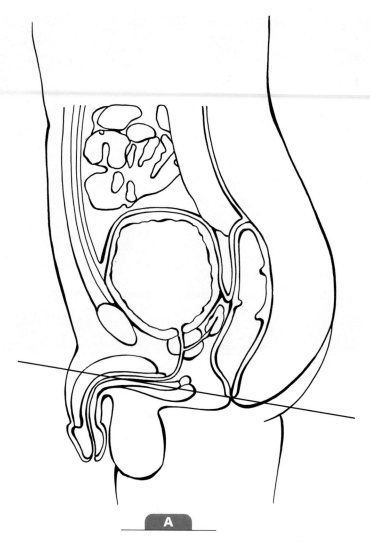

A

Figure 4-31 Axial CT image 21—male.

Figure 4-31 (A,B,C). The shafts of the femurs, readily identified on either side, and the absence of pelvic bones indicates that this image is below the level of the pelvis. Typically, this image would indicate the conclusion of an examination of the pelvis. The majority of the structures visualized are muscles in the thighs; however, the corpus spongiosum is demonstrated in longitudinal section extending toward the corpus cavernosum. Together, these two groups of erectile tissue form the penis. On either side, the spermatic cords can be seen superficially, and the femoral vessels are found embedded within the musculature of the anterior thighs.

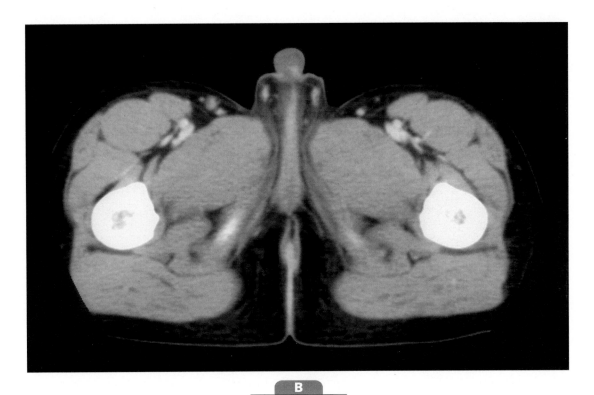

B

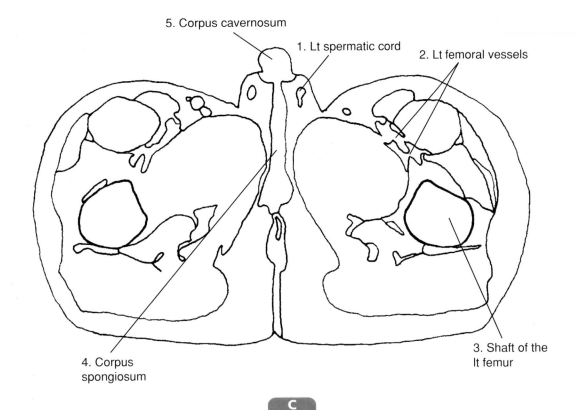

5. Corpus cavernosum

1. Lt spermatic cord

2. Lt femoral vessels

4. Corpus
spongiosum

3. Shaft of the
lt femur

C

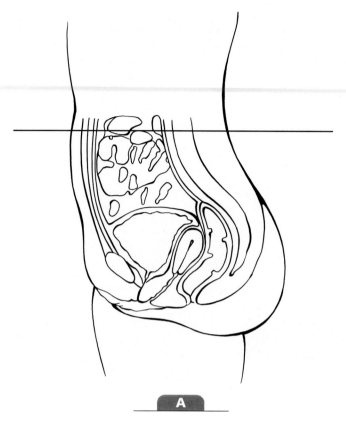

Figure 4-32 Axial CT image 1—female.

AXIAL CT IMAGES: FEMALE

The following 26 axial CT images of the female pelvis will be described at 8.0 mm intervals from superior to inferior. The patient was administered 1000 mL oral contrast over a 12 hour period; the images were generated immediately after the administration of 100 mL venous contrast at the following technical factors: 120 kVp and 150 mA-s. Abbreviations: kVp = kilovolt peak, mA-s = milliampere-second.

Figure 4-32 (A,B,C). The left iliac crest appears as a thin slice of bone and the right iliac crest is not yet seen, indicating this section is located at the upper border of the bony pelvis. Between the iliac crests, the vertebra would be the last of the lumbar, L5. In this image, all of the parts making up the border of the vertebral foramen can be identified, including the pedicles, the laminae, and spinous process. Anterior to L5, four major vessels are within the upper pelvis. On the right side, the right common iliac vein is slightly larger and more posteriorly situated than the right common iliac artery. On the left side, one round vessel can be distinguished, and the other appears to be in a longitudinal or oblique section. Based on the location, the round vessel can be identified as the left common iliac artery, and the longitudinally sectioned vessel originating from the inferior vena cava can be labeled the left common iliac vein. Lateral to the major vessels, the ureters are demonstrated in cross-section as well as parts of the large intestine. On the far left side, this part of the intestine can be identified as the descending colon by the retroperitoneal location and large size compared to the nearby small bowel. On the right side, the large intestine appears larger than the descending colon and represents the cecum.

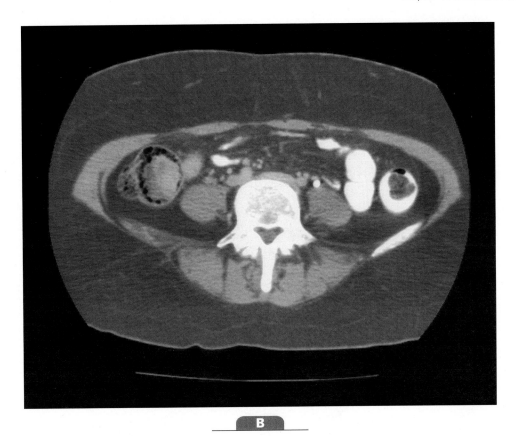

B

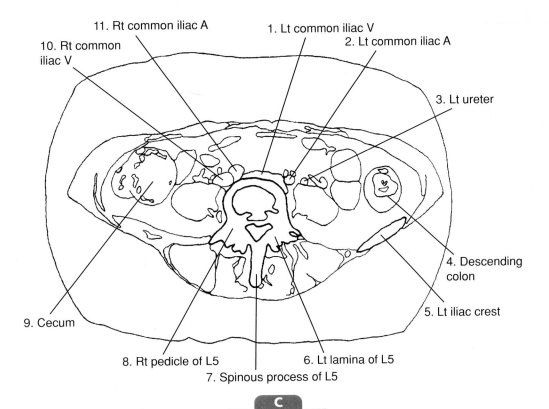

11. Rt common iliac A

10. Rt common
iliac V

1. Lt common iliac V

2. Lt common iliac A

3. Lt ureter

4. Descending
colon

5. Lt iliac crest

9. Cecum

8. Rt pedicle of L5

7. Spinous process of L5

6. Lt lamina of L5

C

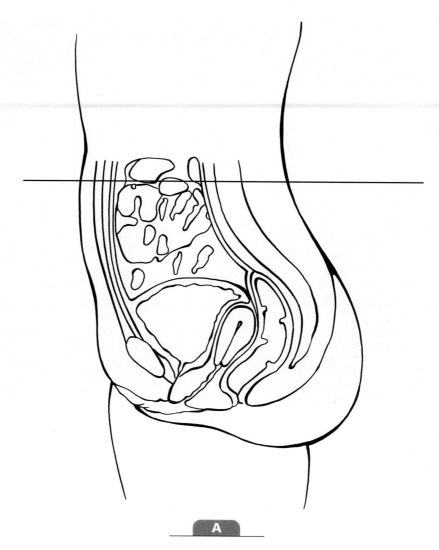

Figure 4-33 Axial CT image 2—female.

Figure 4-33 (A,B,C). The flat bones sectioned on either side of this image can be readily identified as the iliac crests. Similar to the previous image, the lower part of L5 is demonstrated centrally. Adjacent to the body of L5, four vessels can be distinguished at this level. On the right side, the two rounded vessels represent the right common iliac artery and vein. By comparison, the vein is more posteriorly situated and slightly larger in size. On the left side, the vein is obliquely sectioned as it extends across the vertebral body to the left side to lie adjacent to the common iliac artery. Near the vessels, the ureters can be distinguished owing to contrast enhancement from the other small vessels in the area. In regard to alimentary structures, the descending colon is again shown in a retroperitoneal location on the left side. In this section, the descending colon appears filled with contrast and fecal material. Occupying a similar position on the right side, the cecum appears as an enlarged part of the large intestine containing fecal material and air. Adjoining the cecum, the terminal part of the small bowel, the ileum, is shown in the anterior abdominal cavity.

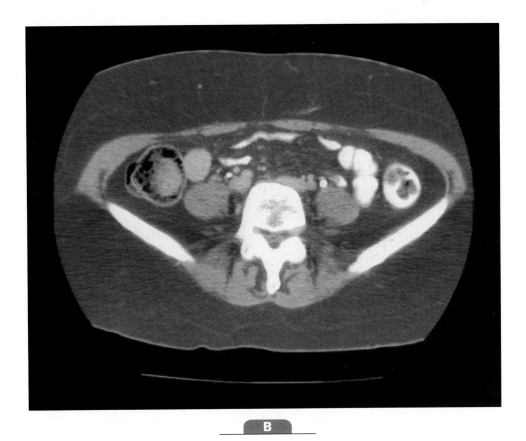

B

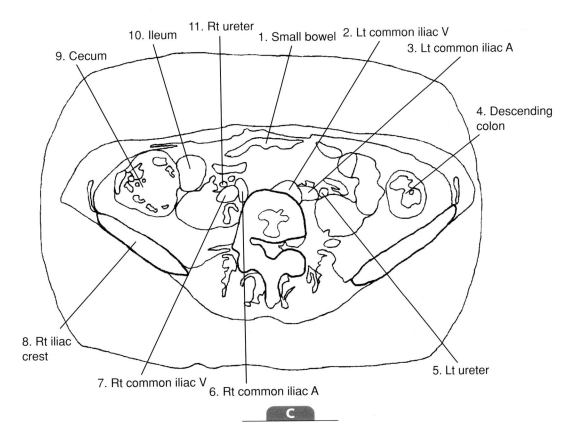

9. Cecum

10. Ileum

11. Rt ureter

1. Small bowel

2. Lt common iliac V

3. Lt common iliac A

4. Descending colon

5. Lt ureter

6. Rt common iliac A

7. Rt common iliac V

8. Rt iliac crest

C

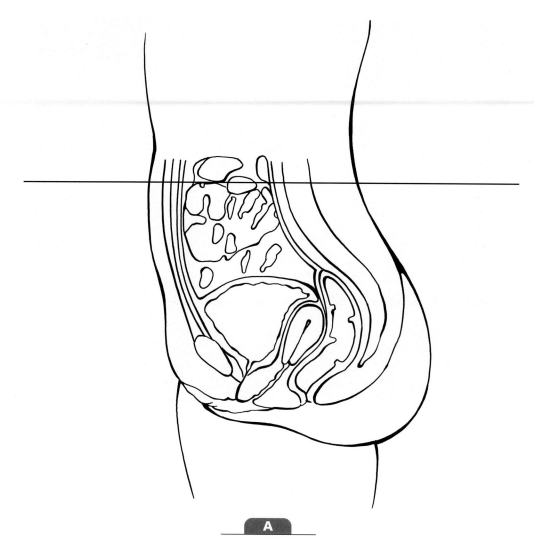

Figure 4-34 Axial CT image 3—female.

Figure 4-34 (A,B,C). This section demonstrates the right and left alae (wings) of the ilia on either side of upper parts of the sacrum. The sacrum can be distinguished from L5 by the larger size and the lateral parts formed by the fusion of the transverse processes. As described in previous images, the four major vessels can be identified near the body of S1. On the right side, the common iliac artery and vein can again be identified; the vein is more posterior and slightly larger in size. On the left, the vessels are more difficult to distinguish. However, with the aid of adjacent images, the left common iliac artery can be distinguished next to the ureter and the left common iliac vein is obliquely sectioned next to the vertebral body. On either side of the vertebral body, the psoas muscles are shown in cross-section as round muscles that are nearly the same size as the vertebral body. The alimentary structures are much the same as described in the previous section; the enlarged part of the large intestine, the cecum, is shown on the right side, and the contrast-filled small bowel is sectioned in a variety of planes.

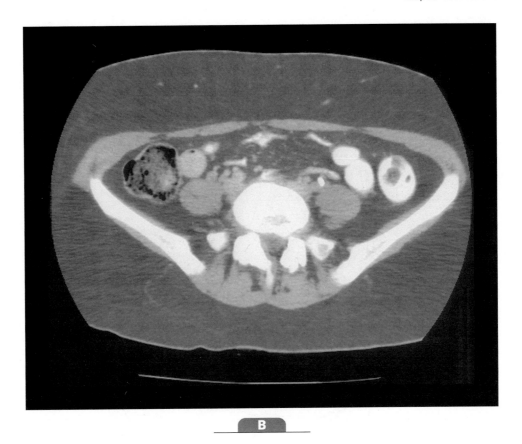

B

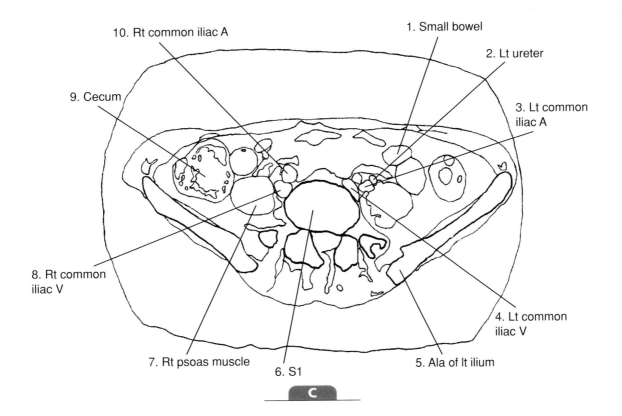

10. Rt common iliac A

1. Small bowel

2. Lt ureter

9. Cecum

3. Lt common iliac A

8. Rt common iliac V

4. Lt common iliac V

7. Rt psoas muscle

5. Ala of lt ilium

6. S1

C

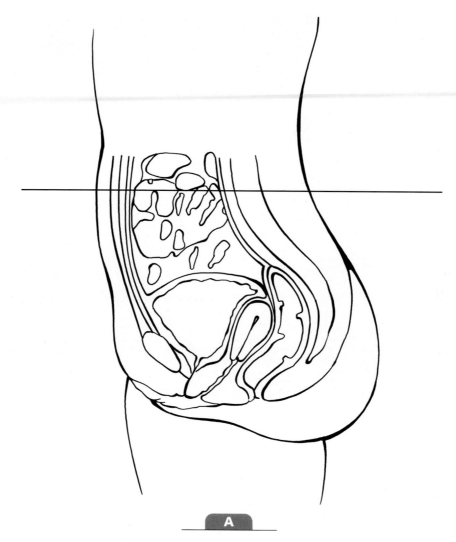

Figure 4-35 Axial CT image 4—female.

Figure 4-35 (A,B,C). The characteristic "bat" shape of the first sacral vertebra is shown in this image. Adjacent to the alae, the ilia- cus muscles are shown in cross-section as sheets of muscle covering the anterior surface of the iliac bones. More anteriorly, the psoas muscles are cross-sectioned and nearly equal in size to the vertebral body. Between the psoas muscles, the ureters and major vessels of the pelvis are found adjacent to the vertebral body. Although it is dif- ficult to distinguish the two vessels on the right side previously described, the left common iliac artery and vein are better distin- guished at this lower level. The contrast-enhanced ureter lies just anterior to the left common iliac artery and vein. As described pre- viously on the right side, the right common iliac artery is slightly smaller and more anteriorly situated than the common iliac vein. In the anterior pelvis, the descending colon can be labeled on the left side behind the peritoneal cavity owing to its large size and lateral location. The other part of the large intestine shown, the cecum, is seen on the far right side, with the adjoining terminal part of the ileum and various loops of small bowel occupying the anterior pelvis.

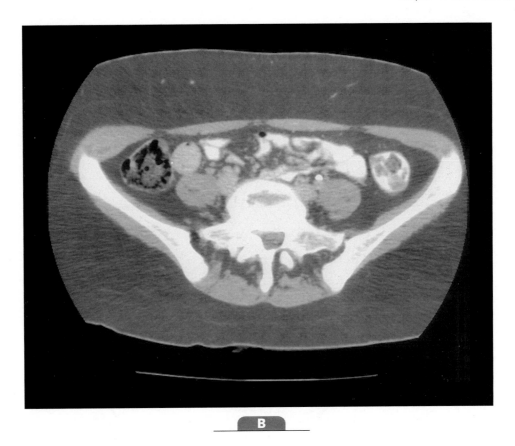

B

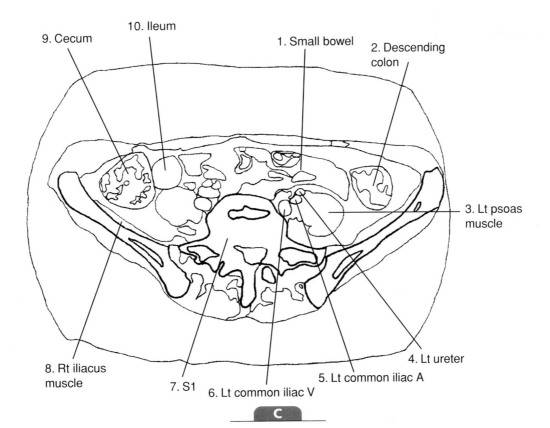

9. Cecum

10. Ileum

1. Small bowel

2. Descending colon

3. Lt psoas muscle

4. Lt ureter

5. Lt common iliac A

6. Lt common iliac V

7. S1

8. Rt iliacus muscle

C

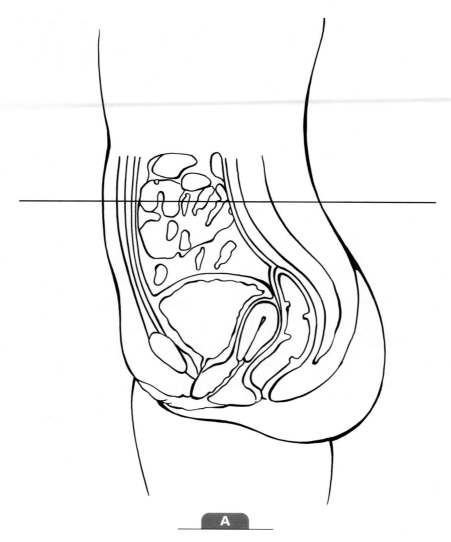

Figure 4-36 Axial CT image 5—female.

Figure 4-36 (A,B,C). This section passes through more of the sacrum and better demonstrates its unique appearance. Extending from either side of the vertebra, the lateral parts (fused transverse processes) extend to articulate with the iliac bones on either side forming the sacroiliac joints. Between the lateral parts of the sacrum, the sacral canal gives rise to the vertebral foramina that extend through both the anterior and posterior sacrum. Within the bony pelvis, the major vessels are again found adjacent to the vertebral body. However, at this level, four vessels can be identified on the right side. As demonstrated in the previous section, the common iliac artery lies anterior to the common iliac vein. Therefore, the two anterior vessels are labeled the external and internal iliac arteries and the two more posterior vessels are the right external and internal iliac veins. On the left side, two major vessels can be distinguished, the left common iliac artery and the left common iliac vein. Near the vessels, the left ureter can be distinguished because of the contrast enhancement. On the right side, the ureter is not enhanced with contrast in this image and is difficult to distinguish from the other small vessels in the area. Similar to previous images, the anterior part of the pelvis contains the cecum, the descending colon, and loosely organized loops of small bowel.

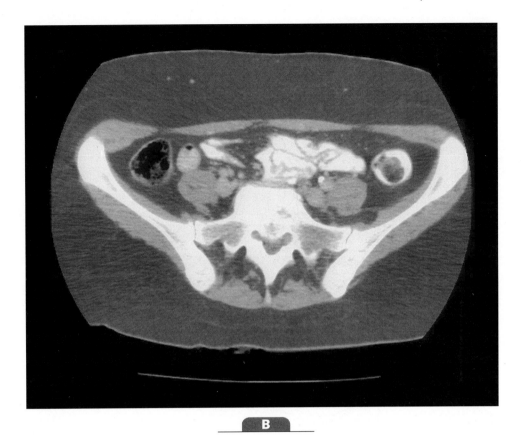

B

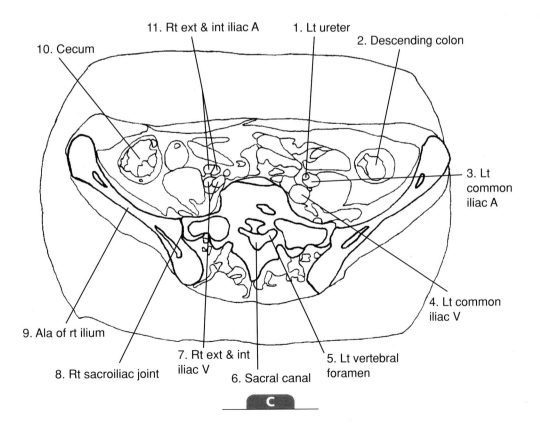

10. Cecum

11. Rt ext & int iliac A

1. Lt ureter

2. Descending colon

3. Lt common iliac A

4. Lt common iliac V

5. Lt vertebral foramen

6. Sacral canal

7. Rt ext & int iliac V

8. Rt sacroiliac joint

9. Ala of rt ilium

C

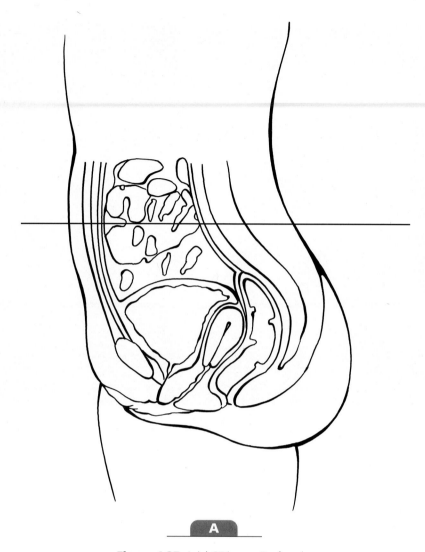

Figure 4-37 Axial CT image 6—female.

Figure 4-37 (A,B,C). The upper part of the sacrum is articulating with the iliac bones on either side to form the bony wall of the pelvic cavity. Within the pelvis, a large number of vessels are sectioned on either side of the vertebral body. On the right side, the four vessels previously described have altered in position, and the iliac arteries are now lying near the corresponding veins. Of the four vessels, the external iliac artery is the most anterior and the adjacent vessel represents the external iliac vein. More posteriorly, the internal iliac artery is found directly behind the right ureter, and the adjacent vessel is the right internal iliac vein. On the left side, three vessels can be distinguished; the most posterior vessel is considerably larger than the other two. Based on the previous image, the most posterior vessel would be the left common iliac vein and the other two vessels are the left external iliac artery and the left internal iliac artery. Because the arteries in the pelvis are generally located anterior to the corresponding veins, the iliac vessels on the right side are labeled accordingly. On either side, the contrast-enhanced ureters are adjacent to the iliac vessels. Although the descending colon and the cecum are seen in the upper pelvis, the small bowel previously seen between these structures has been replaced by the sigmoid colon, which is filled with contrast and air.

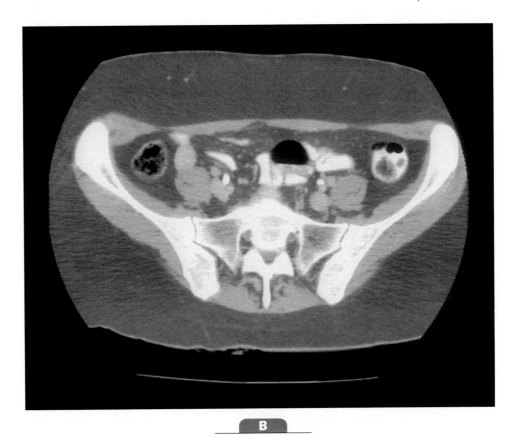

B

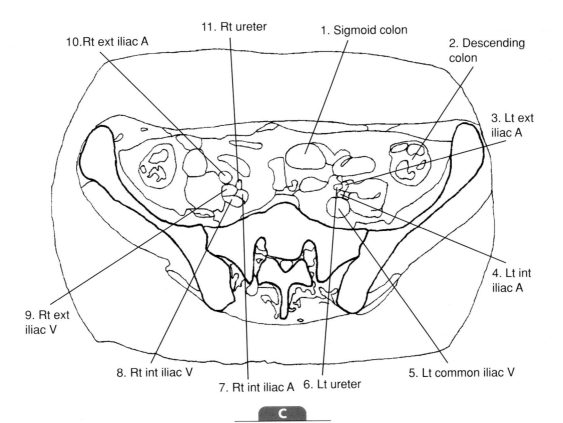

11. Rt ureter

1. Sigmoid colon

10.Rt ext iliac A

2. Descending colon

3. Lt ext iliac A

4. Lt int iliac A

9. Rt ext iliac V

8. Rt int iliac V

7. Rt int iliac A   6. Lt ureter

5. Lt common iliac V

C

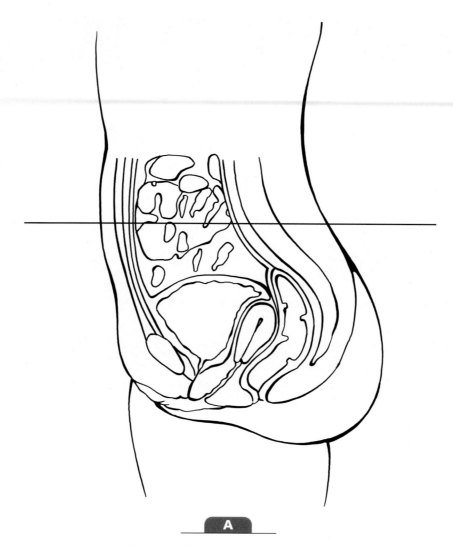

Figure 4-38 Axial CT image 7—female.

Figure 4-38 (A,B,C). This section is a good example of the bat-like appearance of the sacrum; the vertebral body resembles the head of the bat, the spinous process resembles the feet, and the lateral parts extending on either side resemble the wings. Between the lateral parts and the vertebral body, the anterior sacral foramina can be seen, which originate from the sacral canal. The lateral parts of the sacrum articulate with the iliac bones, and together they form the posterior bony wall of the pelvis. Within the pelvis, four major vessels can be distinguished on the right side. Because of the location of the vessels, from anterior to posterior, the vessels can be labeled as the right external iliac artery, right external iliac vein, right internal iliac artery, and right internal iliac vein. On the left side, only three major vessels can be identified: the left external iliac artery, the left internal iliac artery, and the left common iliac vein. In this section, the left common iliac vein has not yet divided into the internal and external iliac veins. Between the major vessels of the pelvis, the sigmoid colon is sectioned, demonstrating the contents to be air and contrast.

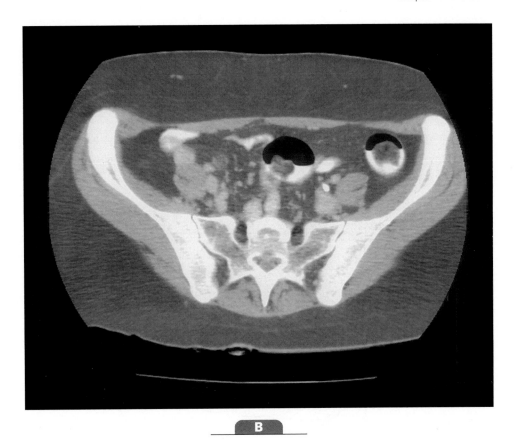

B

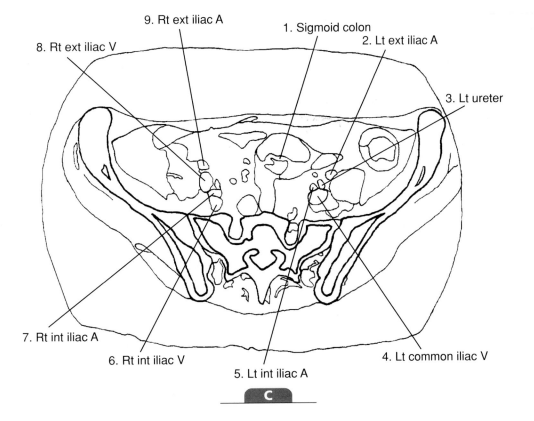

9. Rt ext iliac A

8. Rt ext iliac V

1. Sigmoid colon

2. Lt ext iliac A

3. Lt ureter

7. Rt int iliac A

6. Rt int iliac V

5. Lt int iliac A

4. Lt common iliac V

C

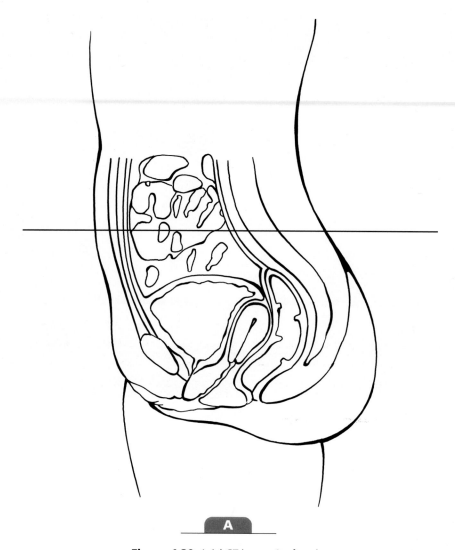

Figure 4-39 Axial CT image 8—female.

Figure 4-39 (A,B,C). As in the previous image the sacrum is articulating with the iliac bones on either side, which appear as irregularly shaped flat bones in axial section. Lining the anterior surface of the iliac bones, the iliacus muscles are on either side adjacent to the psoas muscles, originating from the transverse processes of the lumbar vertebrae. Together, the iliopsoas muscles travel downward through the pelvis to insert on the lesser trochanters of the femurs and act to flex the thighs. Medial to the psoas muscles, the major vessels of the pelvis can be seen in cross-section. Although there are four vessels that can be identified on the right side as the external and internal iliac arteries and veins, there are still only three vessels distinguishable on the left side. Based on location, the three vessels can be identified; the most anterior is the left external iliac artery, the most posterior is the left internal iliac artery, and the other is the larger left common iliac vein. Also within the pelvic cavity, the sigmoid colon is shown centrally and is a continuation of the descending colon sectioned on the left side of this image.

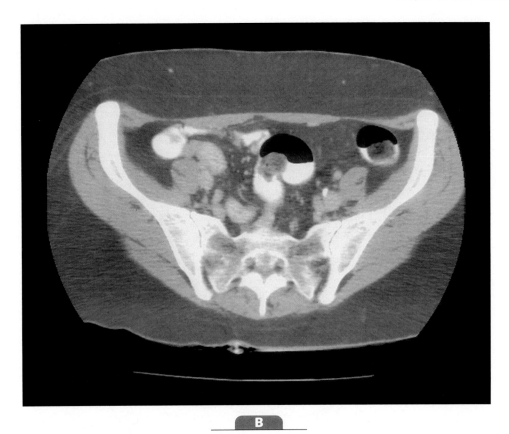

B

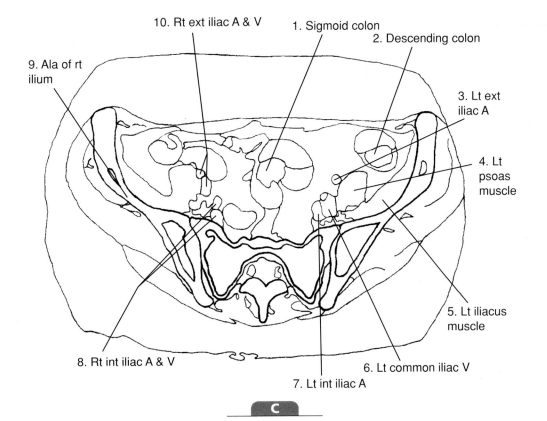

9. Ala of rt ilium

10. Rt ext iliac A & V

1. Sigmoid colon

2. Descending colon

3. Lt ext iliac A

4. Lt psoas muscle

5. Lt iliacus muscle

6. Lt common iliac V

7. Lt int iliac A

8. Rt int iliac A & V

C

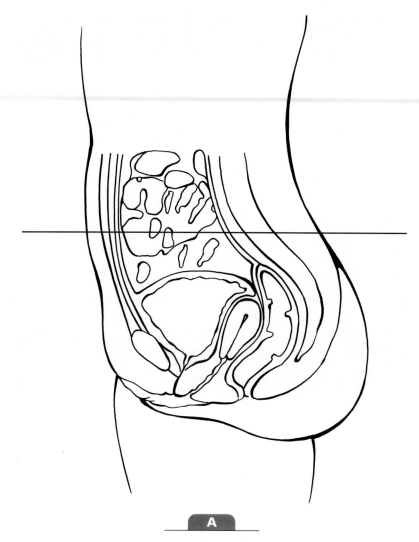

Figure 4-40 Axial CT image 9—female.

Figure 4-40 (A,B,C). The sacrum is adjoining the iliac bones on either side, forming the right and left sacroiliac joints. Within the sacrum, several foramina can be identified. The largest and centrally located foramen represents the sacral canal containing the cauda equina. The cauda equina is a collection of spinal roots that descend from the lower part of the spinal cord. On either side of the sacral canal, sacral foramina extend to both the anterior and posterior surfaces of the sacrum and transmit the sacral spinal nerves. Within the bony pelvis, the sigmoid colon occupies a central location. The sigmoid colon can be identified by its large diameter, characteristic S-shape, and location near the descending colon. Although the right ureter does not appear contrast enhanced in this section, the contrast-enhanced left ureter is easily identified between the left external and internal iliac arteries. Adjacent to the left ureter, the large vessel represents the point of bifurcation of the left common iliac vein into the internal and external iliac veins.

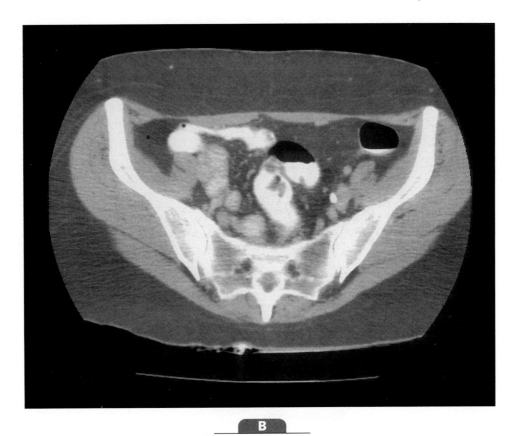

B

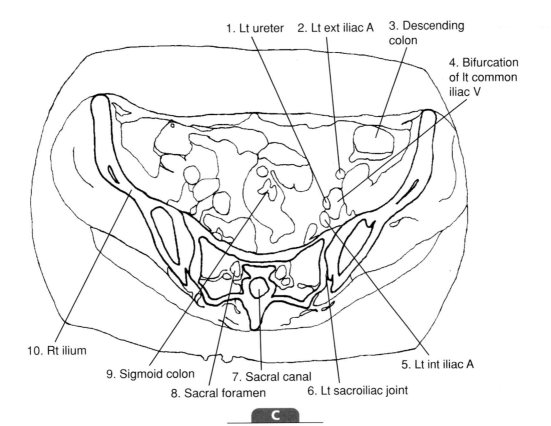

1. Lt ureter   2. Lt ext iliac A   3. Descending colon

4. Bifurcation of lt common iliac V

10. Rt ilium

9. Sigmoid colon   7. Sacral canal   5. Lt int iliac A

8. Sacral foramen   6. Lt sacroiliac joint

C

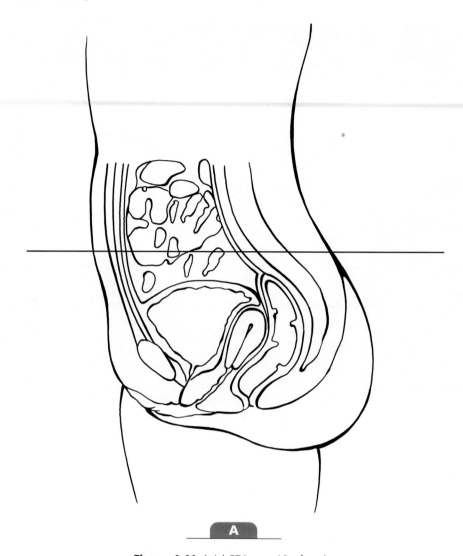

Figure 4-41 Axial CT image 10—female.

Figure 4-41 (A,B,C). The sacrum demonstrates its characteristic bat-like appearance. On either side of the sacrum, the sacroiliac joints are found between the sacrum with the long, flat iliac bones. Adjacent to the lateral part of the iliac bones, the iliacus and psoas muscles are shown in cross-section. At this level, both the iliacus and psoas muscles appear somewhat smaller than in previous views higher in the pelvis and occupy a more lateral location. Near the center of the pelvis, the contrast-filled sigmoid colon is shown originating from the terminal part of the descending colon. Based on previous images, four major vessels of the pelvis can be identified on the left side. From anterior to posterior the vessels are the left external iliac artery, left external iliac vein, left internal iliac vein, and left internal iliac artery. Unlike other parts of the body, like the neck or chest, the arteries in the pelvis tend to occupy a more anterior location than the corresponding veins.

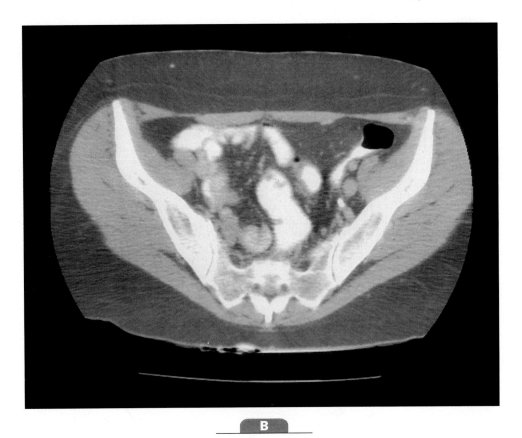

B

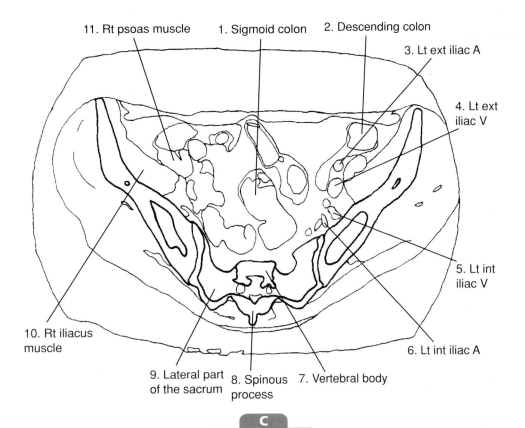

11. Rt psoas muscle   1. Sigmoid colon   2. Descending colon

3. Lt ext iliac A

4. Lt ext iliac V

5. Lt int iliac V

6. Lt int iliac A

10. Rt iliacus muscle

9. Lateral part of the sacrum   8. Spinous process   7. Vertebral body

C

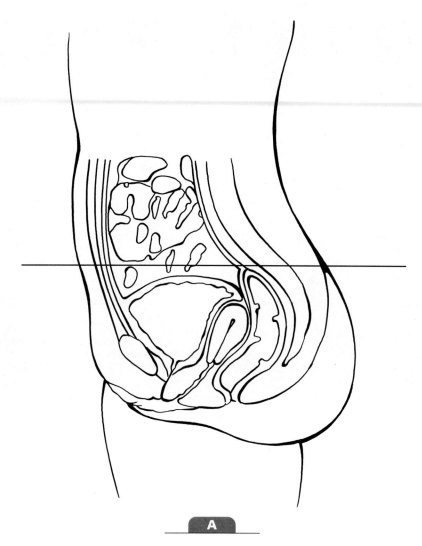

Figure 4-42 Axial CT image 11—female.

Figure 4-42 (A,B,C). Compared to previous images, the iliac bones appear to be shortened and thicker, and the sacrum is smaller in size. Although the lower sacroiliac joint is shown on the left side, the section lies below the level of the right sacroiliac joint. Within the pelvis, the centrally located sigmoid colon is demonstrated in two parts owing to its irregular S-shape. Aside from the sigmoid colon, the rectum is also shown filled with contrast in a more posterior location. Within the right anterior pelvic cavity, loops of small bowel are filled with contrast and air. Because they are within the lower right abdominal cavity, this part of the small bowel can be described as the ileum. (To spell the word ileum correctly, remember the e-shape of this part of the small bowel.) The vessels are labeled on the left side along with the contrast-enhanced left ureter. Between the first part of the sigmoid colon and the left psoas muscle, the external iliac vessels can be distinguished; the artery is slightly smaller and more anteriorly situated than the vein. Posterior to the ureter, lying adjacent to the left ileum, the internal iliac vessels can be distinguished; the artery is slightly smaller and more posterior.

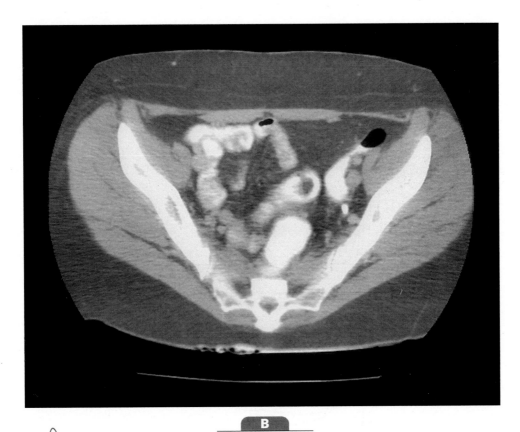

B

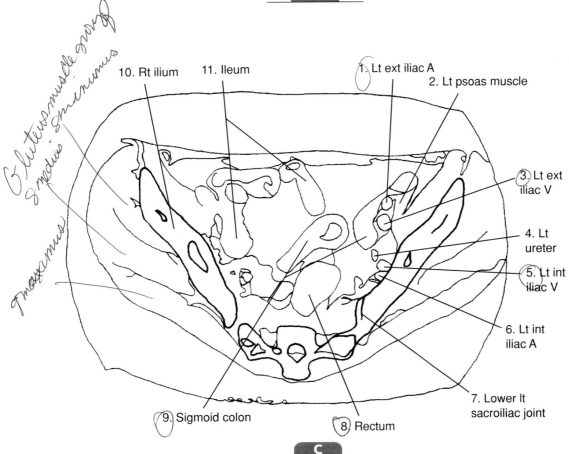

10. Rt ilium

11. Ileum

1. Lt ext iliac A

2. Lt psoas muscle

3. Lt ext iliac V

4. Lt ureter

5. Lt int iliac V

6. Lt int iliac A

7. Lower lt sacroiliac joint

9. Sigmoid colon

8. Rectum

*Gluteus muscle group
S. medius · S. minimus
g. maximus*

C

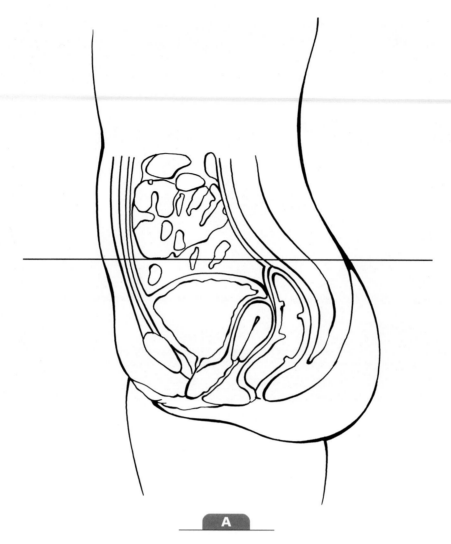

Figure 4-43 Axial CT image 12—female.

Figure 4-43 (A,B,C). This section is through the region of the lower pelvic girdle, because the iliac bones are shortened and thicker and are separate from the sacrum. Within the lower pelvis, the rectum is demonstrated as a large contrast-enhanced structure lying in front of the sacrum. Anterior to the rectum, the S-shaped sigmoid colon is sectioned in two parts and is filled with contrast and fecal material. A concentration of contrast-enhanced small bowel can be seen in the right anterior part of the pelvis. Based on location, this part of the small bowel can be labeled as the ileum. In later images, this concentration of small bowel will be found resting on the roof of the full bladder. Because this section is through the lower pelvis, the previously described psoas and iliacus muscles have now merged to form the right and left iliopsoas muscles. Medial to the left iliopsoas muscle, the external iliac vessels are shown in cross-section in the anterior pelvis, and the internal iliac artery and vein are shown nearing their point of exit through the posterior pelvis. Between the iliac vessels, the left ureter again appears contrast enhanced, although the right ureter is difficult to distinguish in this image.

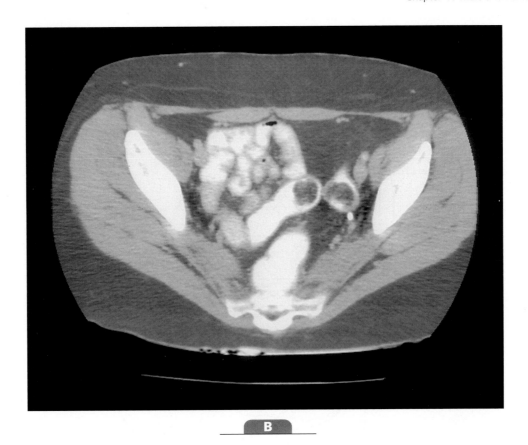

B

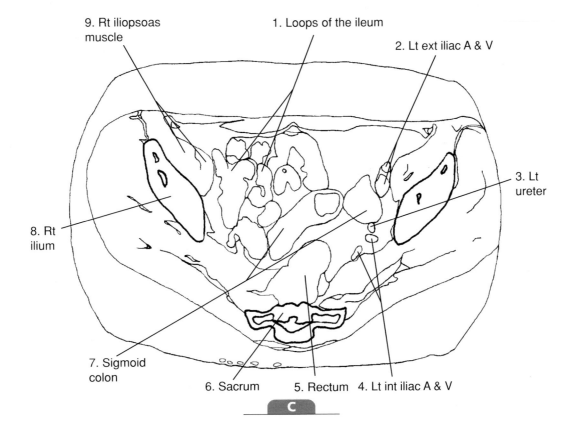

9. Rt iliopsoas muscle

1. Loops of the ileum

2. Lt ext iliac A & V

3. Lt ureter

8. Rt ilium

7. Sigmoid colon

6. Sacrum

5. Rectum

4. Lt int iliac A & V

C

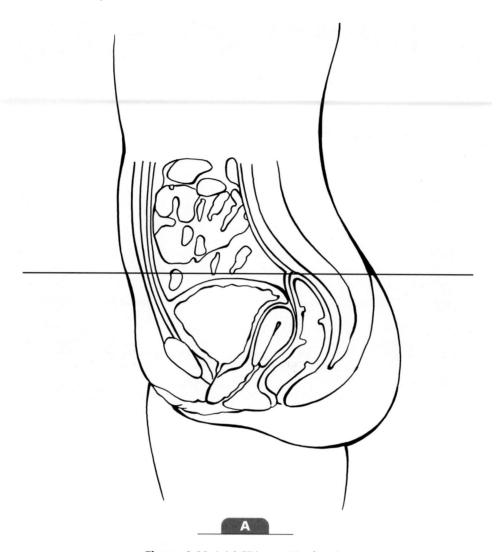

Figure 4-44 Axial CT image 13—female.

Figure 4-44 (A,B,C). The placement of this section would be slightly above the acetabula, because the iliac bones appear shortened and irregularly shaped. Also, the sacrum is smaller than in previous images. Within the pelvis, the contrast-enhanced rectum is between the sacrum and the sigmoid colon. In the anterior pelvis, numerous loops of the ileum are found on the right side and will be seen in the next image as resting on top of the bladder. In regard to the major vessels, the external iliac artery and vein are in the anterior pelvic cavity nearing the anterior thigh. More posteriorly, the internal iliac artery and vein are beside the posterior pelvic wall and will later be shown to be continuous with the gluteal vessels in the region of the buttocks.

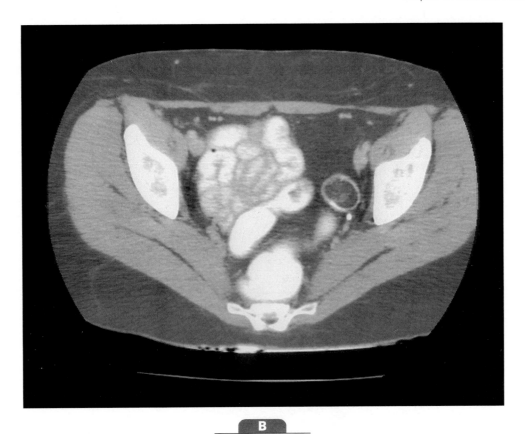

B

1. Loops of the ileum   2. Lt ext iliac A & V

3. Lt ureter

7. Rt ilium

6. Sigmoid colon

5. Rectum

4. Lt int iliac A & V

C

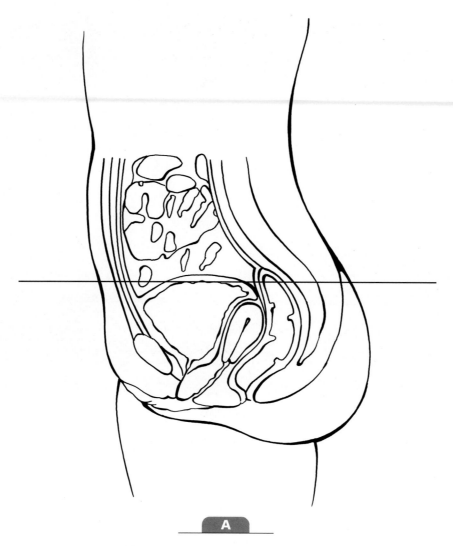

Figure 4-45 Axial CT image 14—female.

Figure 4-45 (A,B,C). The bony anatomy includes both the right and left iliac bones and the fifth segment of the sacrum. Owing to the short, irregular shape of the iliac bones, this section is located just above the acetabula. Although the sacrum was previously described as bat shaped, the terminal part of the sacrum, lower part of S5, has a unique appearance, because the sacral canal terminates at this level owing to the absence of a posterior border. The most notable feature of this image is the large contrast-enhanced structure occupying most of the pelvis formed by the top of the bladder. Typically, a contrast–fluid level can be distinguished within the bladder. However, in this patient, the bladder is completely filled with contrast-enhanced urine. Behind the bladder, the irregularly shaped sigmoid colon extends from the left anterior part of the pelvis to continue as the rectum. Although the right ureter is not enhanced with contrast in this image, it lies behind the bladder similar to the left ureter. Posterior to the ureters, the internal iliac vessels are found along the posterior wall of the pelvis. Anterior to the ureters, the external iliac vessels are found closer to the anterior abdominal wall than in previous images.

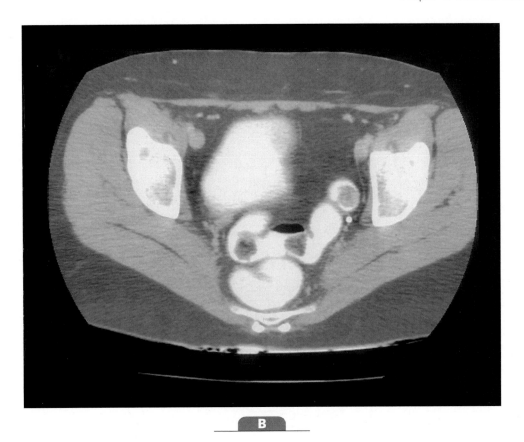

B

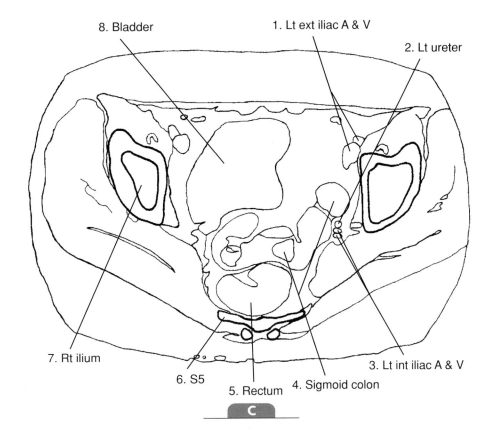

8. Bladder

1. Lt ext iliac A & V

2. Lt ureter

7. Rt ilium

3. Lt int iliac A & V

6. S5

5. Rectum

4. Sigmoid colon

C

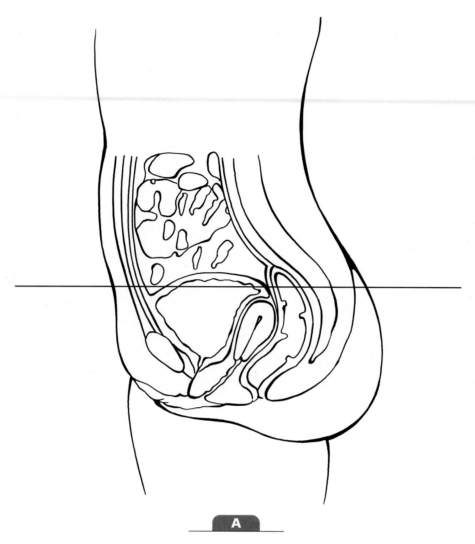

Figure 4-46 Axial CT image 15—female.

Figure 4-46 (A,B,C). Following the structures described in the previous image, the lower part of S5 and the right and left iliac bones make up the bony anatomy within this image. The most remarkable structure, the bladder, occupies most of the pelvic cavity. Posterior to the bladder, the sigmoid colon is longitudinally sectioned as it extends from the right anterior pelvis to a central location where it joins the rectum. In this patient, the central part of the sigmoid colon ascends to the level described in Figure 4-37. Anterior to approximately S3, the sigmoid colon continues as the rectum, which descends through the lower pelvis. Similar to previous images, the left ureter is enhanced with contrast and the right ureter is difficult to distinguish from other soft tissue vessels behind the right side of the bladder. At this level, it is difficult to distinguish the internal iliac vessels, because they are continuing as the gluteal vessels, which exit the pelvis to enter the region of the buttocks. However, the external iliac vessels can be discerned as they near the anterior abdominal wall and will be shown in lower sections to exit the pelvis to enter the anterior thigh.

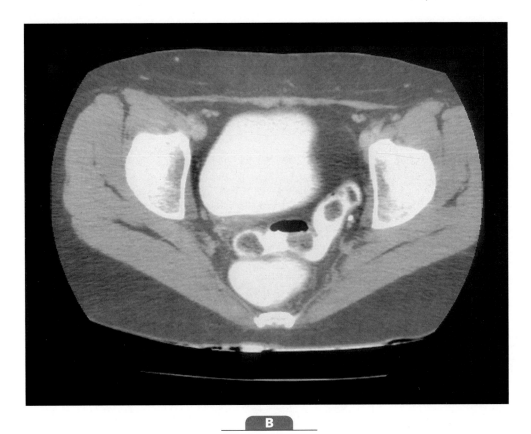

B

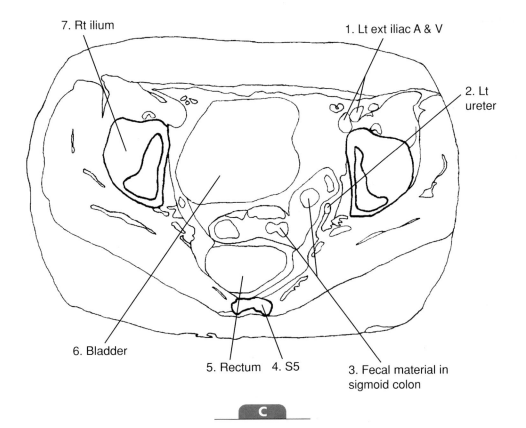

7. Rt ilium

1. Lt ext iliac A & V

2. Lt ureter

6. Bladder

5. Rectum   4. S5

3. Fecal material in sigmoid colon

C

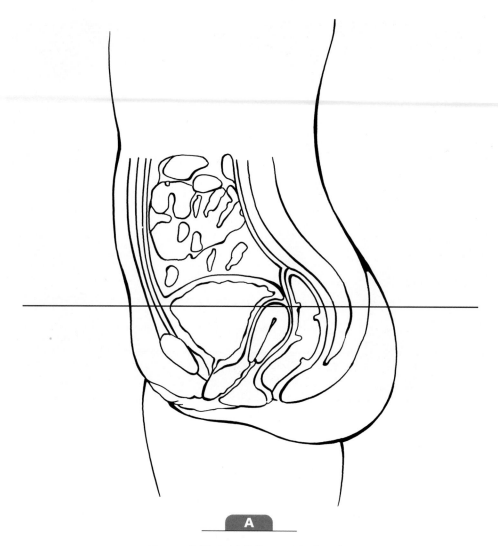

A

Figure 4-47 Axial CT image 16—female.

Figure 4-47 (A,B,C). The coccyx is shown at this level because the sacral foramen can no longer be seen. On either side, the heads of the femurs can be seen within the upper part of the acetabula, which are formed by the iliac bones. Within the pelvis, the full bladder occupies most of the anterior cavity and the contrast-enhanced rectum occupies much of the posterior cavity. Between these two structures in what was previously the location of the sigmoid colon, a soft tissue structure is shown, representing the fundus of the uterus. If the bladder were not full, the fundus would be more anteriorly situated within the pelvis.

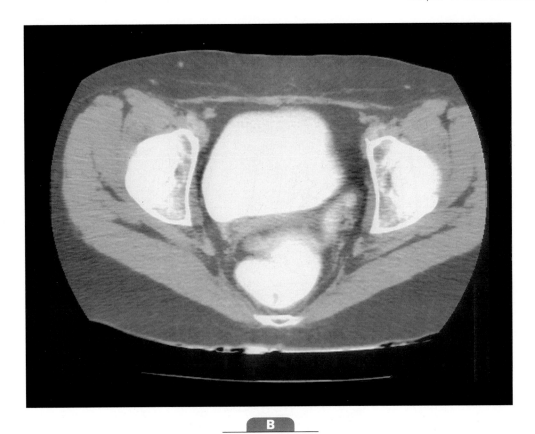

B

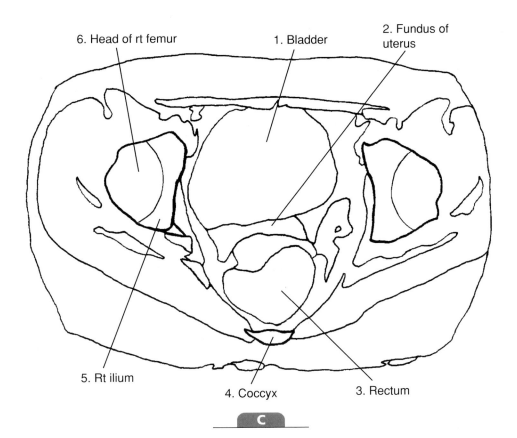

6. Head of rt femur   1. Bladder   2. Fundus of uterus

5. Rt ilium   4. Coccyx   3. Rectum

C

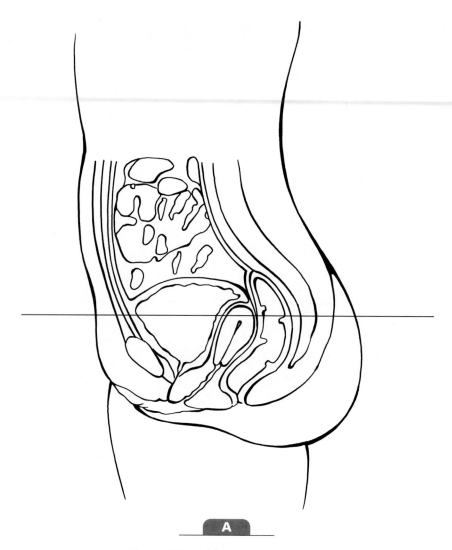

Figure 4-48 Axial CT image 17—female.

Figure 4-48 (A,B,C). Owing to the absence of the sacral foramen, the coccyx forms the posterior border of the bony pelvis. On either side, the heads of the femurs can be seen within the middle region of the acetabula where the three bones forming the pelvic girdle join (ilium, pubis, and ischium). Within the pelvis, the full bladder and contrast-enhanced rectum occupy most of the pelvic cavity. Between the bladder and the rectum, the body of the uterus is sectioned along with appendages extending to either side to form the right and left adnexal areas. As described earlier, the adnexal area is formed by uterine appendages, including the ovaries, oviducts, and other elements of the broad ligament. Because of contrast enhancement, the left ureter is shown obliquely sectioned near its point of entry into the bladder. The major vessels demonstrated in this cross-section are now outside of the bony pelvis, thus they are labeled as the femoral arteries and veins, which are continuations of the external iliac vessels.

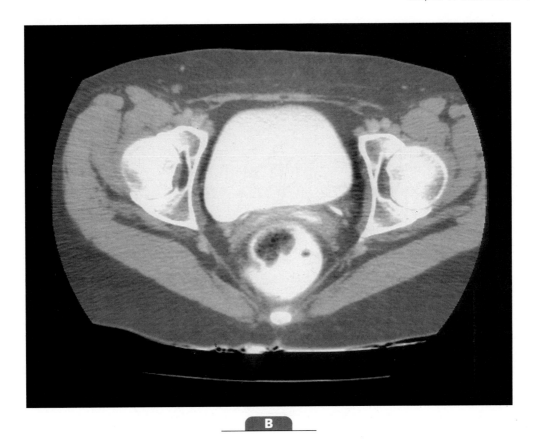

B

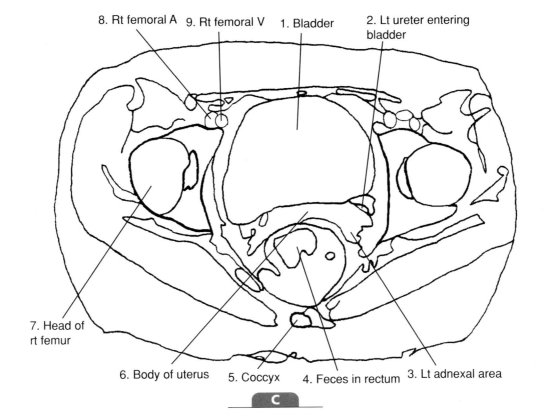

8. Rt femoral A   9. Rt femoral V   1. Bladder   2. Lt ureter entering bladder

7. Head of rt femur

6. Body of uterus   5. Coccyx   4. Feces in rectum   3. Lt adnexal area

C

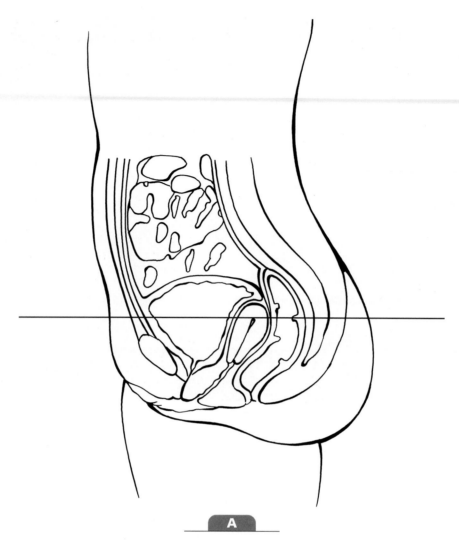

Figure 4-49 Axial CT image 18—female.

Figure 4-49 (A,B,C). Although very small, the tip of the coccyx is found posterior to the contrast- and fecal-filled rectum. On either side, the heads of the femurs are within the midregion of the acetabula. In the anterior pelvis, the urine-filled bladder occupies most of the pelvic cavity and appears to be extending out the anterior pelvic wall above the symphysis pubis. Posterior to the bladder, the body of the uterus is again demonstrated in cross-section, with its appendages, the left and right adnexal areas, on either side. Owing to the filled state of both the bladder and the rectum, the uterus is compressed in this image and appears to wrap around the anterior surface of the rectum. Extending from the pelvic girdle on either side to the coccyx, a thin muscular sheet, the pelvic diaphragm, is demonstrated in cross-section and appears to loop around the posterior rectum. Outside of the pelvic cavity, two vessels are sectioned on either side and can be labeled as the femoral arteries and veins. Because the femoral artery is found in a more lateral location and is slightly smaller than the femoral vein, the four vessels can be individually identified.

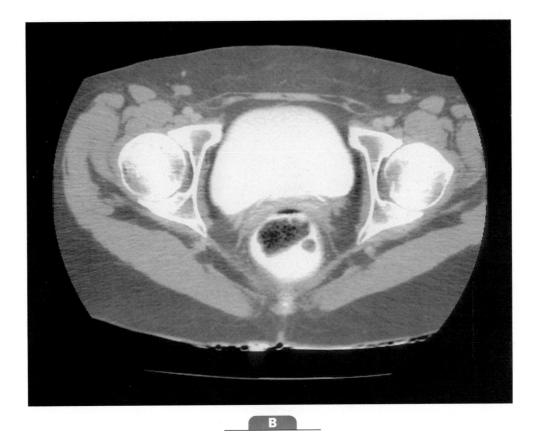

B

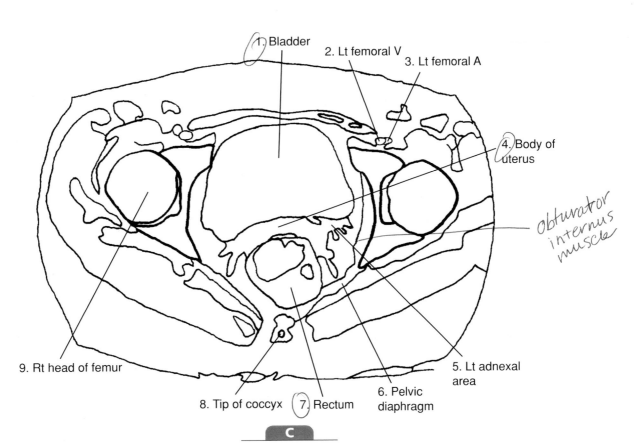

1. Bladder
2. Lt femoral V
3. Lt femoral A
4. Body of uterus
5. Lt adnexal area
6. Pelvic diaphragm
7. Rectum
8. Tip of coccyx
9. Rt head of femur

obturator internus muscle

C

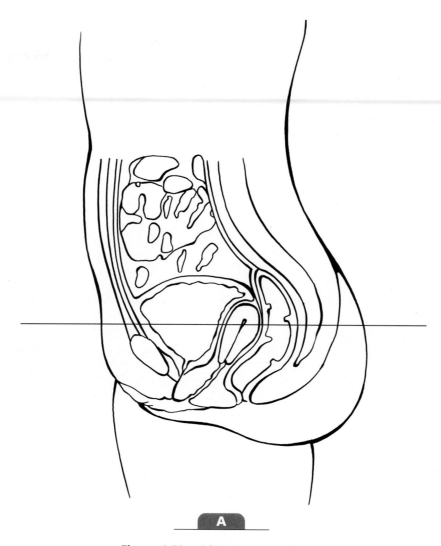

A

Figure 4-50 Axial CT image 19—female.

Figure 4-50 (A,B,C). Although small, the tip of the coccyx is cut in cross-section and provides attachment for the posterior pelvic diaphragm. On either side, the heads of the femurs are shown in the lower parts of the acetabula formed by the ischial and pubic bones. Within the bony pelvis, the bladder is somewhat smaller than in previous images but is still completely filled with contrast-enhanced urine. Adjacent to the posterior wall of the bladder, the body of the uterus is sectioned between the bladder and the rectum. Similar to previous images, the femoral arteries and veins are anterior to the bony pelvis as they extend into the region of the anterior thigh.

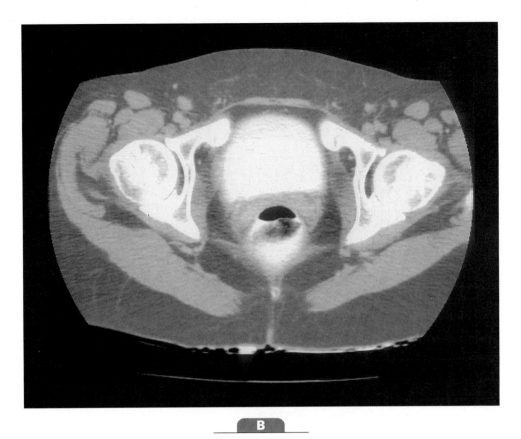

B

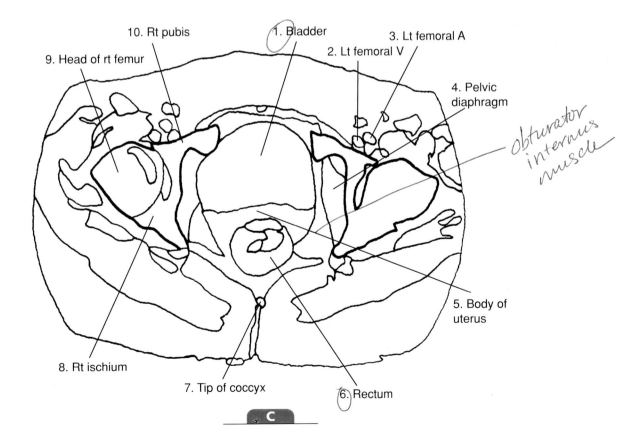

10. Rt pubis

1. Bladder

3. Lt femoral A

9. Head of rt femur

2. Lt femoral V

4. Pelvic diaphragm

obturator internus muscle

5. Body of uterus

8. Rt ischium

7. Tip of coccyx

6. Rectum

C

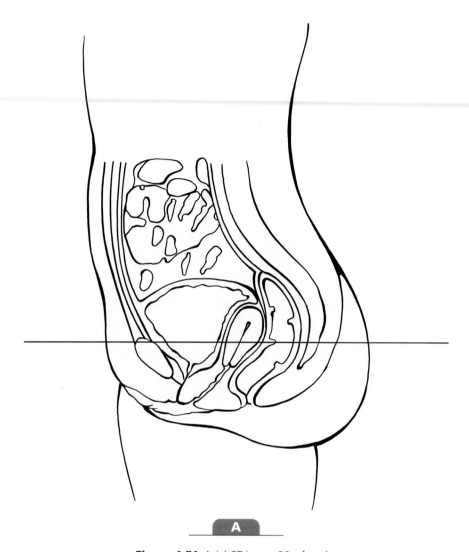

Figure 4-51 Axial CT image 20—female.

Figure 4-51 (A,B,C). This section below the level of the sacrum and the coccyx, demonstrates the symphysis pubis between the right and left pubic bones. On either side, the ischial bones are shown articulating with the proximal part of the femurs. The femurs appear irregularly shaped, demonstrating the heads, the necks, and the greater trochanters. Within the pelvic cavity, the contrast-enhanced bladder is seen anteriorly but is much smaller than in previous images, indicating that we are nearing the bottom of the bladder. Posteriorly, the rectum is sectioned and contains air and a small amount of contrast material, forming an air–fluid level. Between the rectum and the bladder, the cervix of the uterus has a density similar to that of the musculature of the pelvic diaphragm. Previously, this position was occupied by the body of the uterus, which was wider and appeared to wrap around the rectum. At this level, the cross-section through the pelvic diaphragm is V-shaped; it appears to be forming a sling around the rectum and is attached anteriorly to the pubic bones. Between the pelvic diaphragm and the ischial bones, deposits of fat can be found in the ischiorectal fossae. On the anterior pelvis, the femoral artery is again found lateral to the femoral vein, as they continue to extend into the anterior thigh.

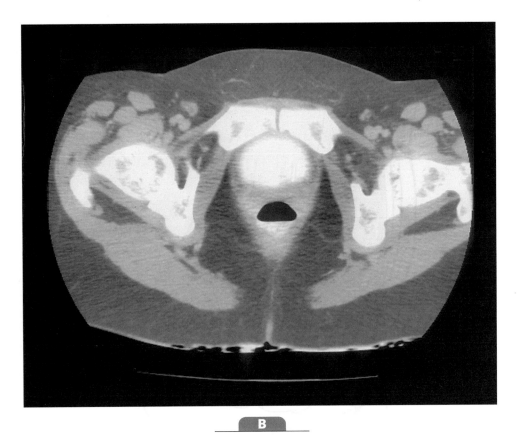

B

10. Rt femoral A

11. Rt femoral V

12. Rt pubis

1. Symphysis pubis

2. Bottom of bladder

3. Cervix of uterus

4. Neck of lt femur

5. Rectum

6. Lt ischiorectal fossa

7. Pelvic diaphragm

8. Rt ischium

9. Greater trochanter of rt femur

C

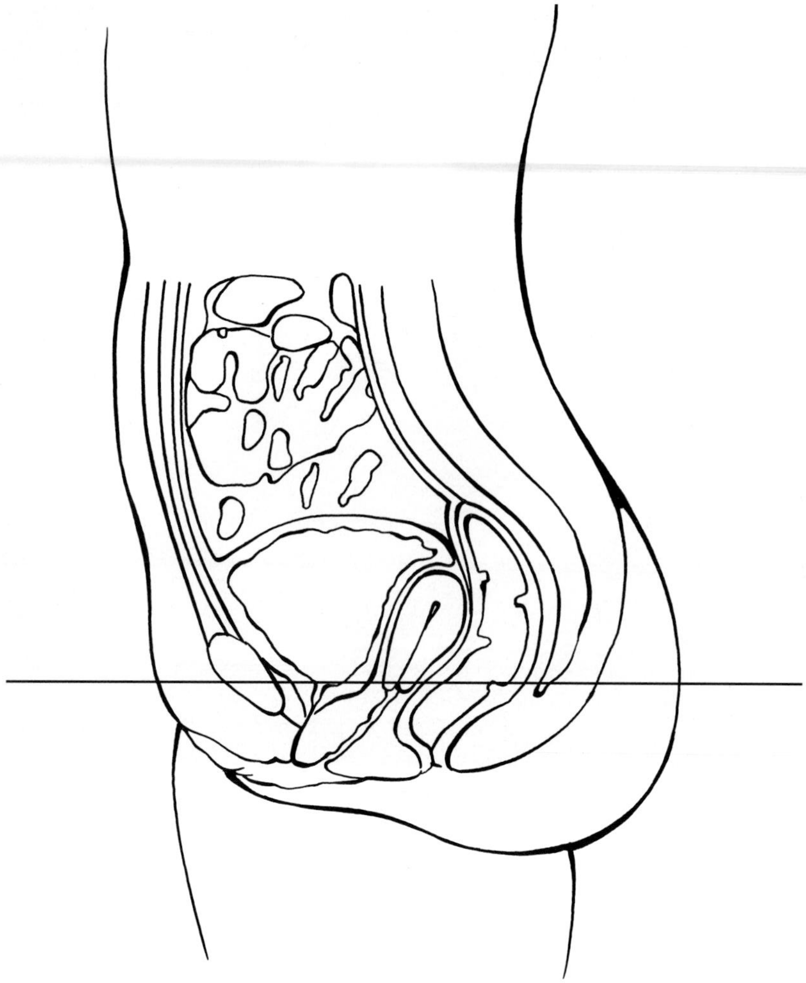

Figure 4-53 Axial CT image 22—female.

Figure 4-!
image betv
from the is
ischial bon
the level of
greater tro
pelvis, the
level of the
enhanceme
readily iden
V-shaped r
rectum, the
distinguish
tum and th
ischiorectal
anterior sur
section and
the femora

Figure 4-53 (A,B,C). Taken through the lower part of the pelvis, this image demonstrates the lower part of the symphysis pubis between the right and left pubic bones. On the left side, the ischial ramus can be seen to join the pubic ramus, forming continuous bone below the level of the obturator foramen. On the right side, only the ischial tuberosity is demonstrated in this section and is separated from the pubic bone by the obturator foramen. On either side of the bony pelvis, the femurs are demonstrated in cross-section posterior to the femoral vessels in the anterior region of the thigh. Within the pelvis, the air-filled rectum is centrally located and is surrounded by a wedge-shaped muscular structure. Similar to previous images, the pelvic diaphragm is V-shaped and forms a sling around the rectum attaching anteriorly to the pubic bones. Although a boundary cannot clearly be distinguished between the pelvic diaphragm and the cervix of the uterus, the air within the posterior vaginal fornix marks the site where the cervix joins the vagina. Between the cervix and the symphysis pubis, the urethra is shown in cross-section as a small, round structure near the same density as muscle. Between the pelvic diaphragm and the ischial bones, large triangular-shaped areas of fat are found within the ischiorectal fossae and are continuous with the fat on the posterior surface of the buttocks.

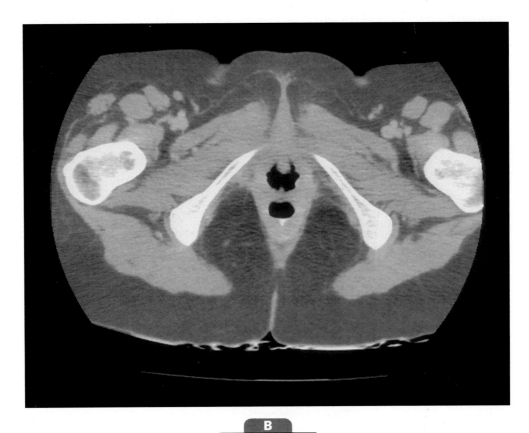

B

9. Shaft of the rt femur

10. Rt pubic ramus

1. Contents of femoral sheath

2. Urethra (not seen)

3. Vagina

8. Rt ischial ramus

4. Lt ischiorectal fossa

7. Rt ischial tuberosity

6. Pelvic diaphragm

5. Rectum

C

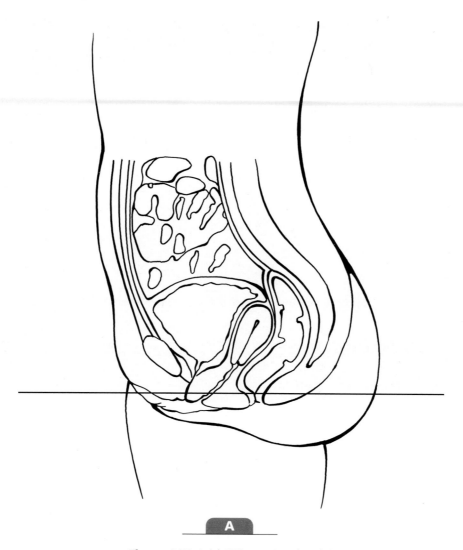

Figure 4-55 Axial CT image 24—female.

Figure 4-55 (A,B,C). The shafts of the femurs can be seen on either side of the image surrounding the pair of ischial bones centrally located in the lower pelvis. At this low level, the expanded portion of the ischial bone represents the ischial tuberosity, and the thin projection of bone is the ischial ramus. Within the pelvic cavity, air can be seen within the vagina, which appears less oval in shape than in the previous image. The air-filled rectum of the previous image has been replaced by the musculature of the pelvic diaphragm, which includes the external anal sphincter muscle. Between the pelvic diaphragm and the ischial bones, the ischiorectal fossae are again shown filled with fat. Within the musculature of the anterior thigh, a group of femoral vessels can be identified on either side.

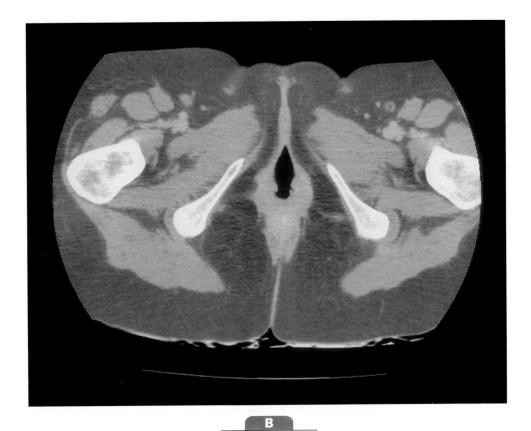

B

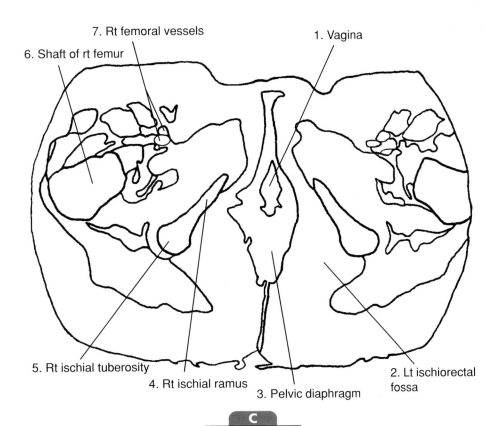

7. Rt femoral vessels

1. Vagina

6. Shaft of rt femur

5. Rt ischial tuberosity

4. Rt ischial ramus

3. Pelvic diaphragm

2. Lt ischiorectal fossa

C

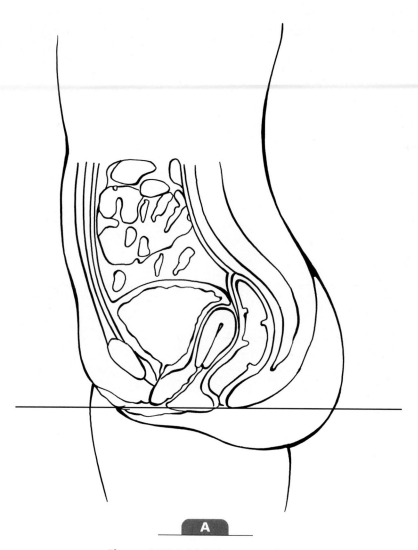

A

Figure 4-56 Axial CT image 25—female.

Figure 4-56 (A,B,C). This section, taken through the very lowest part of the pelvis, demonstrates the ischial bones on either side surrounded by the shafts of the femurs, which are thick, irregularly shaped bones. Within the pelvis, an air-filled opening can be seen extending from the region previously occupied by the vagina and the urethra, forming the vestibule posterior to the clitoris between the labia minora. Anterior to the vestibule, the labia majora are found on either side of the midline between the thighs. Similar to previous images, the femoral vessels are sectioned within the musculature of the anterior thigh.

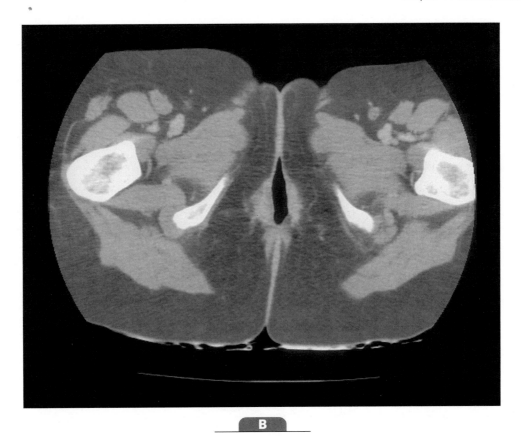

B

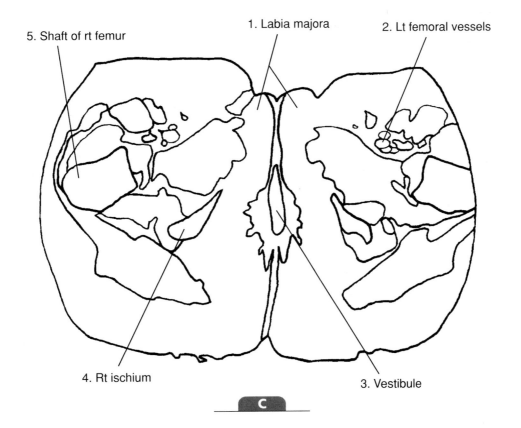

5. Shaft of rt femur

1. Labia majora

2. Lt femoral vessels

4. Rt ischium

3. Vestibule

C

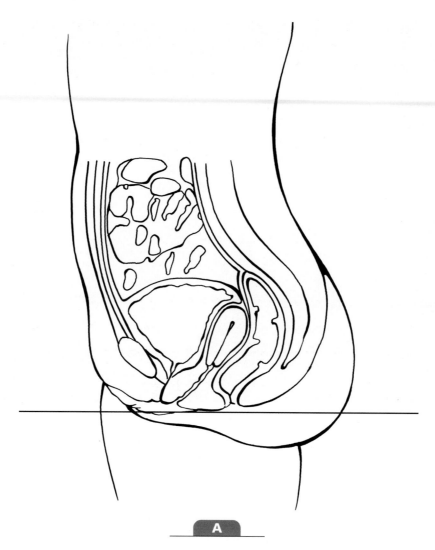

Figure 4-57 Axial CT image 26—female.

Figure 4-57 (A,B,C). This section is below the level of the pelvis and indicates completion of an axial examination of the pelvis. Because no pelvic bones can be seen in this image, the only bones are those of the femurs. In cross-section, the shafts of the femurs appear to be large, irregularly shaped bones surrounded by the musculature of the thigh. Within the anterior musculature, a group of femoral vessels can be identified on either side. Between the thighs, the fat-filled labia majora can be identified on either side and are separated by the opening between the thighs.

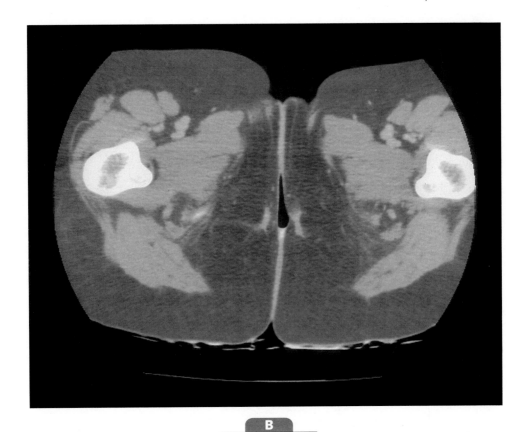

B

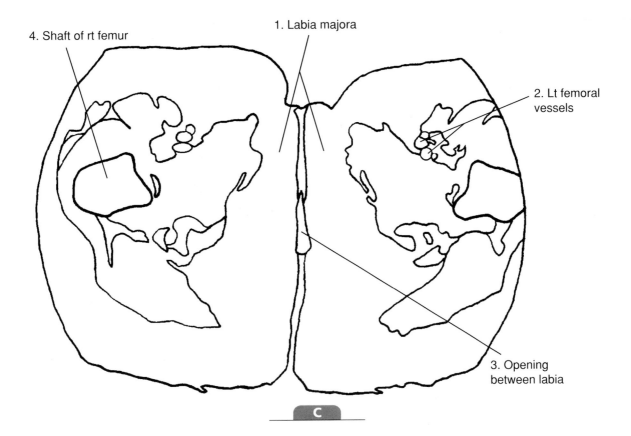

4. Shaft of rt femur

1. Labia majora

2. Lt femoral vessels

3. Opening between labia

C

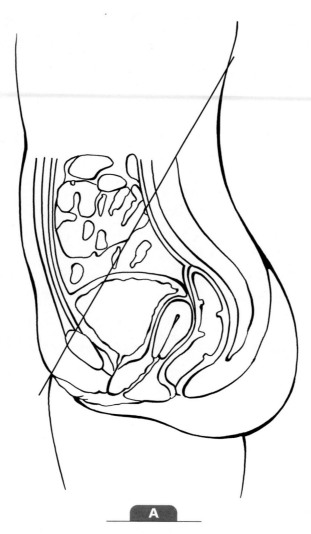

A

Figure 4-58 Coronal MR image 1—female.

Coronal MR Images: Female

In a typical scan of the pelvis, images are generated throughout the entire bony pelvis. However, the following descriptions will be limited to 11 selected images described at 5 mm intervals from anterior to posterior through the central region of the female pelvis. The images were generated at the following technical factors: TR = 500, TE = 20, FOV = 41 cm, TH = 10 mm (5 mm cuts). Abbreviations: TR = repetition time, TE = echo-time, FOV = field of view, TH = slice thickness.

Figure 4-58 (A,B,C). This section is through the anterior pelvis, because the symphysis pubis can be seen between the right and left pubic bones. Outside of the pubic bones, the only other bony structures apparent within this image are the right and left iliac bones forming the lateral borders for the greater or false pelvis. In regard to soft tissue structures, a distinct area of low signal can be seen above the pubic bones representing the anterior part of the urinary bladder. Above the bladder, parts of bowel are sectioned within the greater pelvis or lower abdominal cavity. On the left side, the sigmoid colon is longitudinally sectioned as it extends upward to join with the descending colon. On the opposite side of the lower abdomen, the outline of the cecum can be identified, representing the lowest part of the large intestine found on the right side of the body. Between the segments of large intestine just described, loops of small bowel and mesentery are loosely organized centrally.

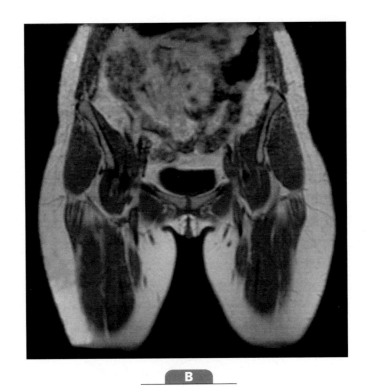

B

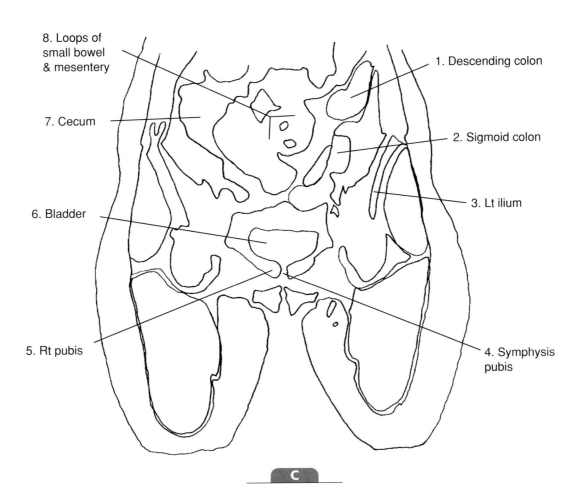

8. Loops of
small bowel
& mesentery

7. Cecum

6. Bladder

5. Rt pubis

1. Descending colon

2. Sigmoid colon

3. Lt ilium

4. Symphysis
pubis

C

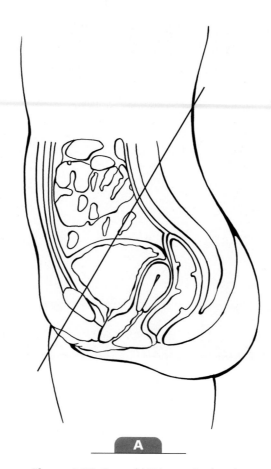

A

Figure 4-59 Coronal MR image 2—female.

Figure 4-59 (A,B,C). The symphysis pubis can again be seen separating the right and left pubic bones, indicating this plane of section lies within the anterior pelvis. Compared to the previous view, the iliac bones are slightly longer and appear almost continuous with the pubic bones. On the medial aspect of the iliac bones, the flat iliacus muscles are shown near their origin and extend downward through the pelvis to insert on the lesser trochanters of the femurs. Adjoining the iliac muscles, the psoas muscles can be seen on either side extending from their origin on the transverse process of L1 through L5 to join with the iliacus muscles and insert on the lesser trochanters of the femurs. As in the previous image, the urinary bladder is full and appears as a distinct region of low signal intensity directly above the pubic bones. Because this image demonstrates anatomy within the anterior pelvis, the vessels shown on the left side between the urinary bladder and left psoas muscle represent the left external iliac artery and vein. Although the vessels are also seen on the right side in a similar location, they are difficult to discern from surrounding structures. Above the structures just described, various parts of the bowel are sectioned within the greater pelvis. Medial to the left external iliac artery and vein, the sigmoid colon is shown in cross-section as it extends between the rectum in the posterior pelvis to the descending colon in the lower left abdominal cavity. Similar to the previous image, the cecum can be identified on the lower right side of the abdominal cavity and is separated from the descending colon by loops of small bowel and mesentery.

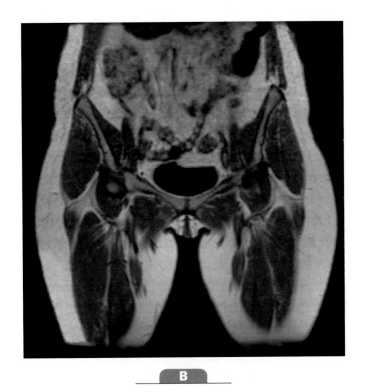

B

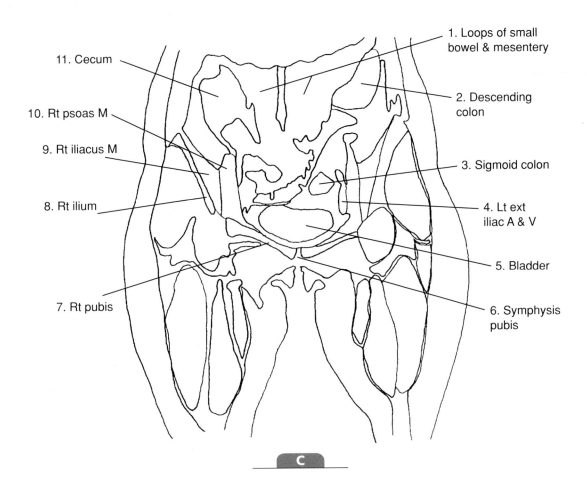

11. Cecum

10. Rt psoas M

9. Rt iliacus M

8. Rt ilium

7. Rt pubis

1. Loops of small bowel & mesentery

2. Descending colon

3. Sigmoid colon

4. Lt ext iliac A & V

5. Bladder

6. Symphysis pubis

C

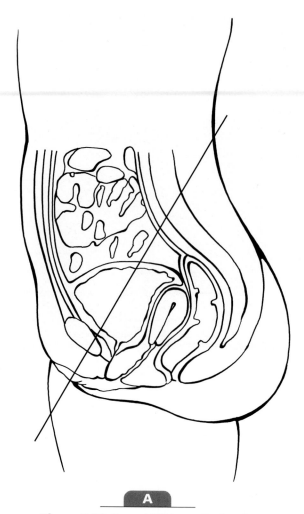

Figure 4-60 Coronal MR image 3—female.

Figure 4-60 (A,B,C). The heads of the femurs are on either side within the acetabula, which separate the iliac and pubic bones. Similar to previous images, the symphysis pubis can be seen between the right and left pubic bones and indicates that this section is within the anterior part of the pelvis. Directly below the symphysis pubis, two irregularly shaped regions of high signal intensity represent the fat-filled labia majora. Within the greater pelvis, the right external iliac artery and vein are more clearly discernible lying near the medial side of the right psoas muscle. Although they are not labeled, the left external iliac artery and vein are also shown medial to the left psoas muscle. Similar to previous images, several bowel structures can be identified within the greater pelvis. The sigmoid colon is again shown in cross-section directly above the bladder as it extends between the rectum and the descending colon. In the lower right abdominal cavity, the cecum is again shown lateral to randomly organized loops of small bowel and mesentery, which appear to lie on the roof of the bladder. Despite the loose organization, all of the bowel structures shown within this image are surrounded by sheets of connective tissue, the peritoneum, that suspend the bowel structures from the posterior abdominal wall and form a variety of mesenteric structures. In addition, the peritoneum forms the lining of the abdominal cavity and separates the structures found within the greater or false pelvis from those in the lesser or true pelvis.

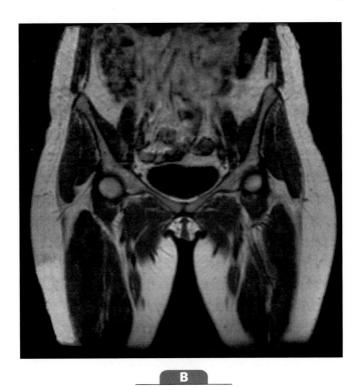

B

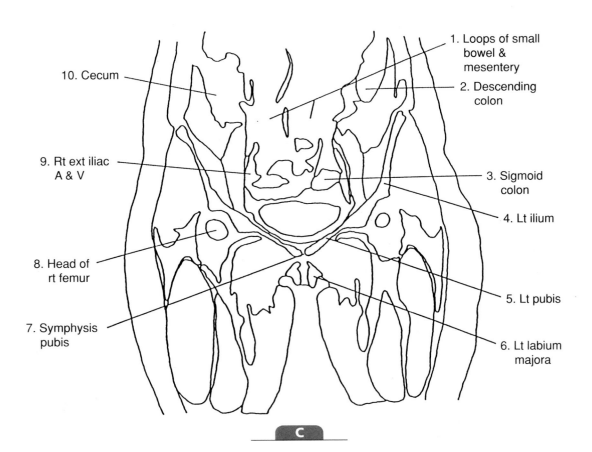

1. Loops of small bowel & mesentery

2. Descending colon

3. Sigmoid colon

4. Lt ilium

5. Lt pubis

6. Lt labium majora

7. Symphysis pubis

8. Head of rt femur

9. Rt ext iliac A & V

10. Cecum

C

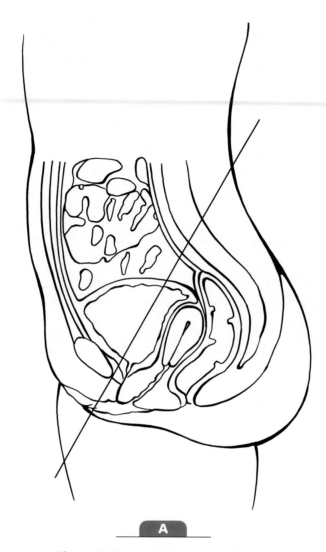

Figure 4-61 Coronal MR image 4—female.

Figure 4-61 (A,B,C). The heads of the femurs appear larger and the iliac bones appear thicker in this image than in the previous image, indicating we are nearing the mid-region of the bony pelvis. Although the pubic bones can again be seen on either side between the urinary bladder and the labia majora, they are thinner than in previous views, indicating we are nearing the region of the pelvic opening. Within the pelvis, the iliacus and psoas muscles are clearly shown on either side and appear to be joining together as they extend downward to insert on the lesser trochanters of the femurs. Because the psoas muscles originate from the transverse processes of the lumbar vertebrae, they form part of the posterior abdominal wall. Between the psoas muscles, the abdominal aorta is shown longitudinally sectioned, giving rise to the right and left common iliac arteries. A shadow slightly to the left of the abdominal aorta represents the inferior vena cava, which also bifurcates near this region to give rise to the right and left common iliac veins. Similar to previous images, the external iliac artery and vein are found on either side just medial to the psoas muscles. Above the urinary bladder, loops of small bowel and sigmoid colon are sectioned within the lower peritoneal cavity.

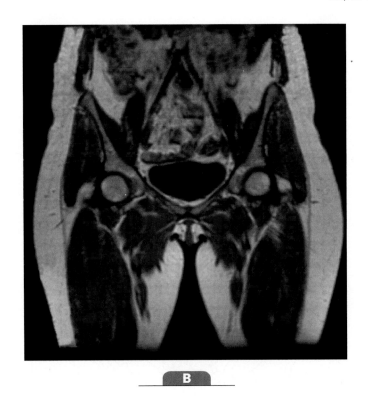

B

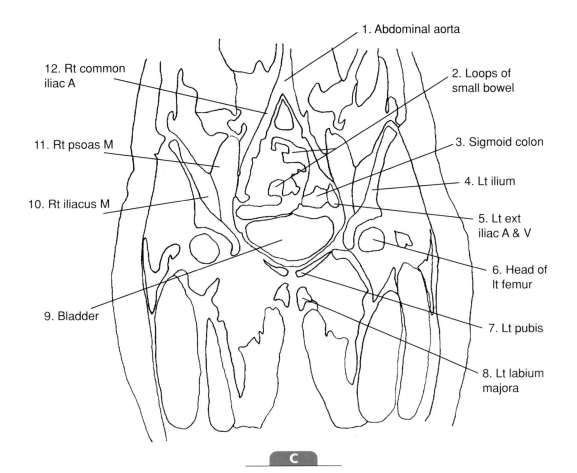

1. Abdominal aorta

12. Rt common
iliac A

2. Loops of
small bowel

11. Rt psoas M

3. Sigmoid colon

10. Rt iliacus M

4. Lt ilium

5. Lt ext
iliac A & V

6. Head of
lt femur

9. Bladder

7. Lt pubis

8. Lt labium
majora

C

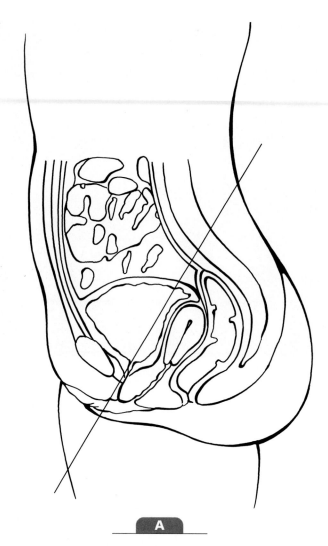

A

Figure 4-62 Coronal MR image 5—female.

Figure 4-62 (A,B,C). On either side, the proximal end of the femur is readily apparent and demonstrates the shaft in longitudinal section. On the upper part of the femur, the greater trochanter projects upward and provides a sight of attachment for musculature around the hip joint. The head of the femur is found within the acetabulum, which is formed in this image predominantly by the ilium. On the right side, an indention within the rounded portion of the head of the femur represents the fovea capitis femoris. The ligamentum teres originating within the acetabular fossa attaches to the head of the humerus at the fovea capitis femoris. Within the pelvis, the urinary bladder appears as a distinct region of low signal intensity. Similar to previous images, loops of small bowel and the sigmoid colon within the lower peritoneal cavity lie just above the bladder. In contrast to previous views, the anterior cortical margins of L4 and L5 are now seen between the proximal ends of the psoas muscles. As mentioned, the psoas muscles originate from the transverse processes of the lumbar vertebrae and extend downward to join with the iliacus muscles to insert on the lesser trochanters of the femurs.

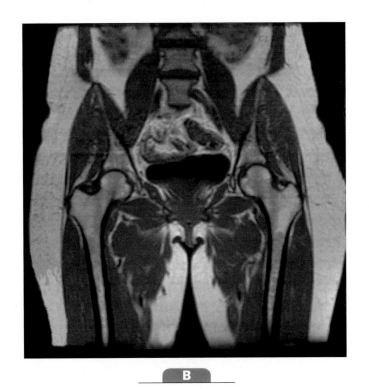

B

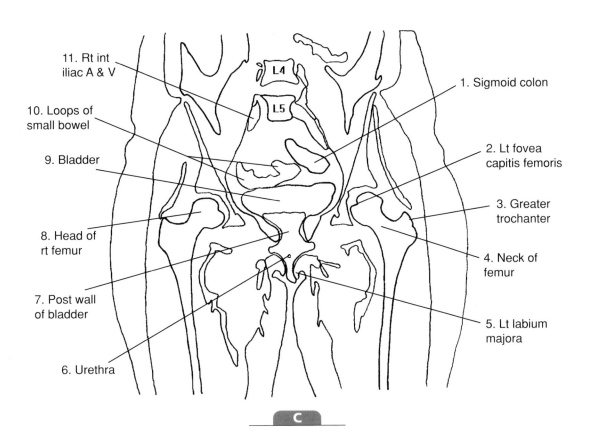

11. Rt int iliac A & V

10. Loops of small bowel

9. Bladder

8. Head of rt femur

7. Post wall of bladder

6. Urethra

L4

L5

1. Sigmoid colon

2. Lt fovea capitis femoris

3. Greater trochanter

4. Neck of femur

5. Lt labium majora

C

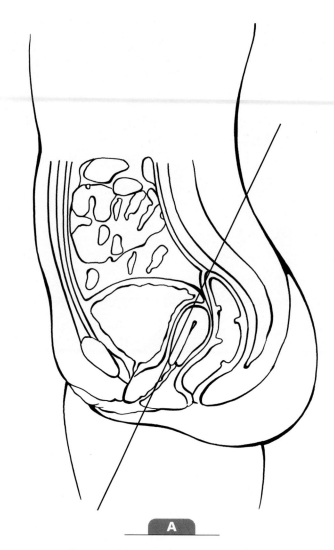

Figure 4-64 Coronal MR image 7—female.

Figure 4-64 (A,B,C). The proximal femurs are readily apparent on either side, indicating this section is through the mid-pelvic region. Within the pelvis, the posterior part of the bladder appears to lay over the uterus. The upper part of the uterus, the fundus, lies near the midline slightly above the right and left adnexal areas. As described earlier, the adnexal area includes the uterine appendages such as the ovaries, oviducts, and other structures found within the broad ligaments on either side of the uterus. Below the body of the uterus, the cervix or narrowed part is adjacent to the opening of the vagina. Shown in cross-section, the vagina lies between the cervix of the uterus and the labia majora. Above the urinary bladder, loops of small bowel and sigmoid colon are within the lower peritoneal cavity and appear to rest on the roof of the bladder. Above the bowel structures, the posterior branches of the common iliac vessels (the internal iliac artery and vein) are obliquely sectioned on either side of the vertebral body of L5.

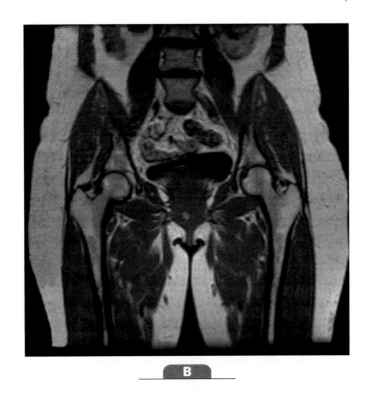

B

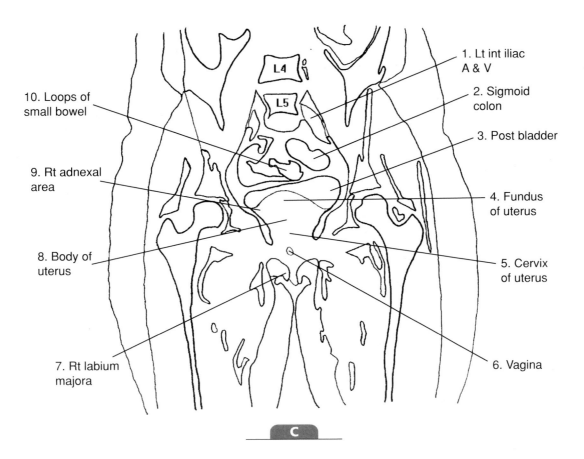

10. Loops of
small bowel

9. Rt adnexal
area

8. Body of
uterus

7. Rt labium
majora

1. Lt int iliac
A & V

2. Sigmoid
colon

3. Post bladder

4. Fundus
of uterus

5. Cervix
of uterus

6. Vagina

C

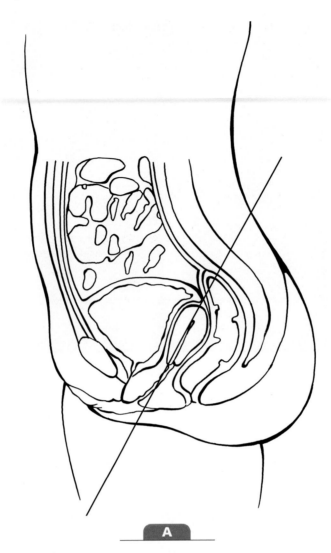

A

Figure 4-65 Coronal MR image 8—female.

Figure 4-65 (A,B,C). In this section, only the posterior part of the proximal femurs are shown on either side of the pelvis. Similar to the previous view, a small part of the posterior bladder appears to be draping over the fundus of the uterus and its appendages. In this patient, the posterior bladder is predominantly seen on the left side above the left adnexal area. The narrowed region representing the cervix of the uterus lies adjacent to the vagina, which is a muscular tube lined with mucous membrane connecting the uterine cavity to the exterior between the labia majora. Similar to previous images, the small bowel and sigmoid colon are within the lower peritoneal cavity above the posterior bladder. On either side of the vertebral body of L5, the internal iliac vessels are obliquely sectioned as they extend from their origin on the common iliac vessels to extend through the pelvis to become continuous with terminal branches in the gluteal region.

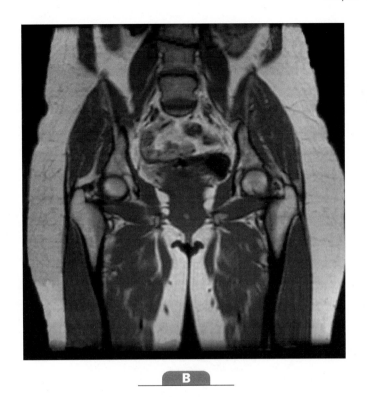

B

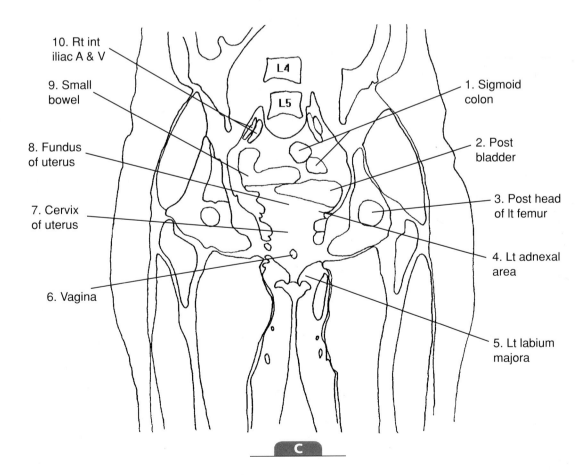

10. Rt int iliac A & V

9. Small bowel

8. Fundus of uterus

7. Cervix of uterus

6. Vagina

L4

L5

1. Sigmoid colon

2. Post bladder

3. Post head of lt femur

4. Lt adnexal area

5. Lt labium majora

C

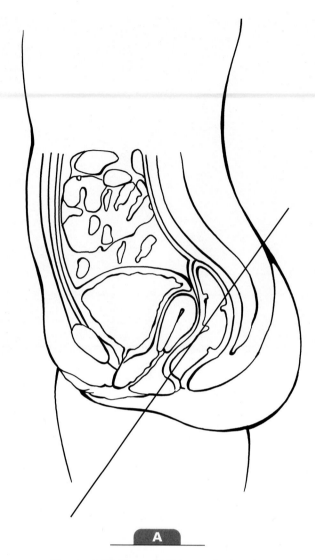

Figure 4-66 Coronal MR image 9—female.

Figure 4-66 (A,B,C). The proximal part of the femur can be seen on either side even though it appears to be in two parts. The rounded region representing the posterior head of the femur is still shown within the acetabulum, whereas the lesser trochanter and the intertrochanteric crest appear within the musculature of the upper thigh. Following the bladder from the previous section, only a small part of the posterior bladder is seen within this section on the left side. In the position previously occupied by the uterus, a region of low signal intensity represents the anterior part of the rectum. Found behind the bladder, the rectum extends between the distal part of the sigmoid colon and the anal canal. Directly below the rectum, the musculature of the anal sphincter is shown between the fat-filled ischiorectal fossae and the thin, flat muscular sheet representing the pelvic diaphragm. Similar to previous images, segments of the small bowel and sigmoid colon are sectioned within the lower peritoneal cavity and are found above the bladder and the rectum. On either side of the vertebral column, the internal iliac vessels are sectioned as they extend through the pelvis to enter the gluteal region. In the midline, the vertebral body of L5 is sectioned directly above the upper part of S1.

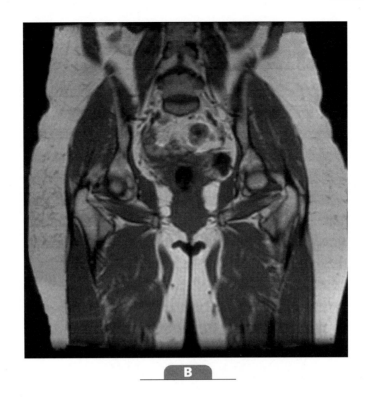

B

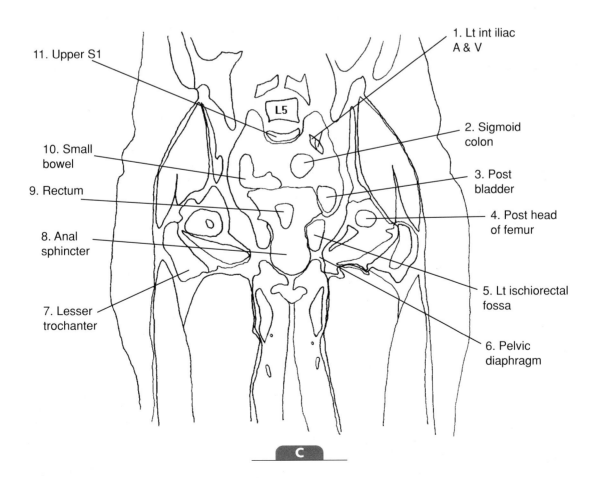

11. Upper S1

1. Lt int iliac
A & V

L5

10. Small
bowel

2. Sigmoid
colon

9. Rectum

3. Post
bladder

8. Anal
sphincter

4. Post head
of femur

7. Lesser
trochanter

5. Lt ischiorectal
fossa

6. Pelvic
diaphragm

C

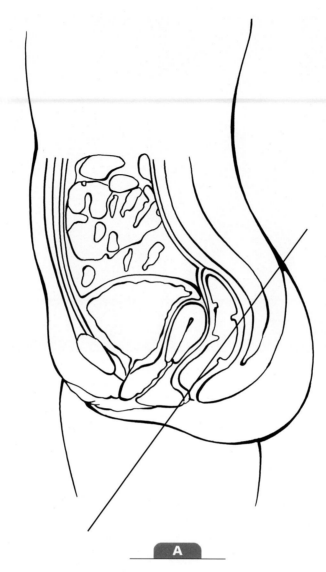

Figure 4-67 Coronal MR image 10—female.

Figure 4-67 (A,B,C). In the region previously occupied by the vertebral bodies of L4 and L5, the vertebral foramen now appears as a region of low signal intensity containing the dural sac and the cauda equina. In this coronal section, the vertebral body of S1 appears larger and is found between the iliac bones, which appear nearly vertical. On the lower part of the bony pelvis, the ischial tuberosities are found on either side and appear as enlarged or thickened regions of the ischial bones. Within the pelvis, the end of the sigmoid colon is sectioned just above the rectum, which appears larger than it did in the previous image. Below the rectum, the musculature of the anal sphincter is again surrounded by the fat-filled ischiorectal fossae and the thin, flat musculature of the pelvic diaphragm, shown in cross-section. As described earlier, the pelvic diaphragm is a group of flat muscles that form a sling across the pelvic cavity and support the pelvic viscera.

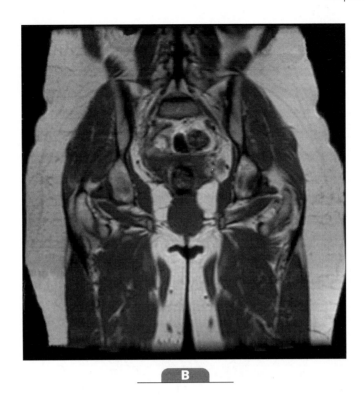

B

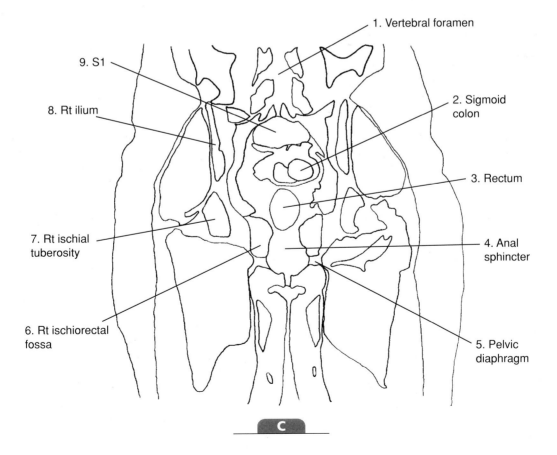

1. Vertebral foramen

9. S1

8. Rt ilium

2. Sigmoid colon

3. Rectum

7. Rt ischial tuberosity

4. Anal sphincter

6. Rt ischiorectal fossa

5. Pelvic diaphragm

C

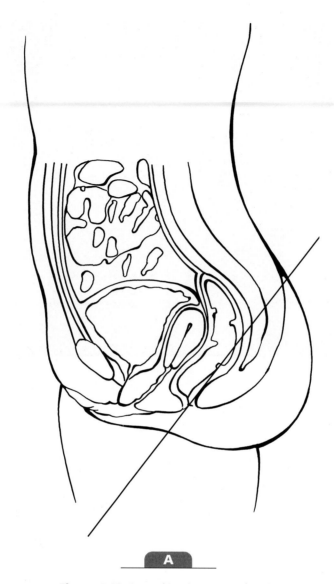

Figure 4-68 Coronal MR image 11—female.

Figure 4-68 (A,B,C). In this plane of section, the lateral parts of the sacrum are shown extending toward either side to articulate with the iliac bones to form the sacroiliac joints. In the position previously occupied by the vertebral bodies of L4 and L5, the vertebral foramen is longitudinally sectioned as it extends downward to the sacrum. Similar to the previous image, the iliac bones appear nearly vertical and are located above the thickened regions of bone found on either side of the pelvis that represent the ischial tuberosities. Within the pelvis, the rectum is centrally located, is larger than in previous views, and is nearing its juncture with the sigmoid colon. Below the rectum, the musculature of the anal sphincter is surrounded by the fat-filled ischiorectal fossae and the cross-section of flat muscles representing the pelvic diaphragm.

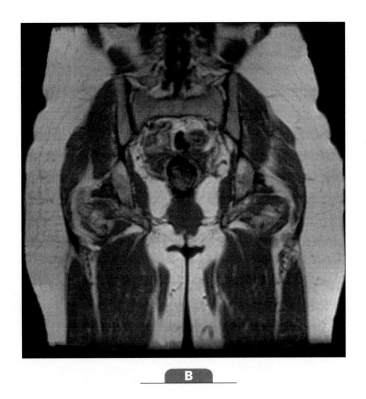

B

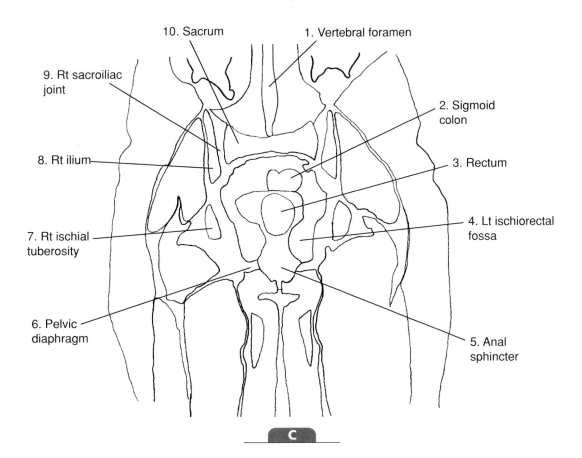

10. Sacrum   1. Vertebral foramen

9. Rt sacroiliac
joint

2. Sigmoid
colon

8. Rt ilium

3. Rectum

7. Rt ischial
tuberosity

4. Lt ischiorectal
fossa

6. Pelvic
diaphragm

5. Anal
sphincter

C

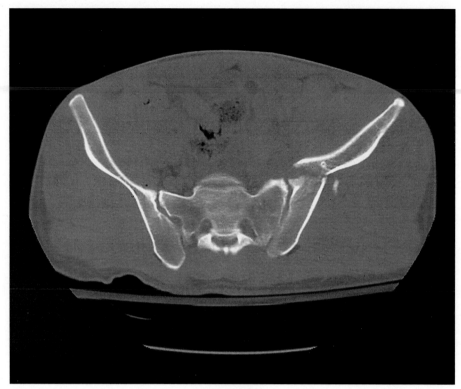

Figure 4-69

Supplement 4-1. *Figure 4-69 shows a 37-year-old man who was injured when he was struck in the pelvis by a forklift. The emergency room physician ordered a CT examination of the pelvis; it revealed a comminuted fracture of the left ilium. In a selected CT image generated at window settings for bone, several fragments can be seen within the left ilium. Somewhat surprisingly, the right ilium is normal, and the sacroiliac joints are intact on both sides. Even though there was little displacement of the bone fragments, the comminuted fracture required surgical repair.*

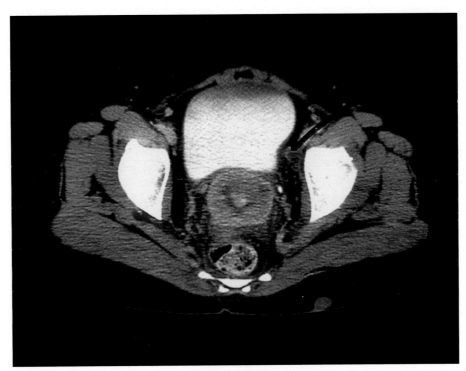

Figure 4-70

Supplement 4-2. *Figure 4-70 is a CT scan of the pelvis of a 42-year-old woman that was ordered to evaluate a palpable pelvic mass found the previous day. The results of the biopsy obtained on the same day indicated the mass was a carcinoma of the cervix. The large abnormal structure between the rectum and the contrast-enhanced bladder is readily apparent. The image shows an enlarged cervix measuring 6 cm in diameter. In the central part of the cervix, some low attenuation material is seen and is likely from postbiopsy changes. Metastatic disease was found in subsequent scans of the abdomen and chest (not shown), and the prognosis for this patient was poor.*

REVIEW QUESTIONS

1. The_____supplies most of the structures within the lesser pelvic cavity with arterial blood.

2. Which of the following is considered retroperitoneal in location?
   A. Ileum
   B. Transverse colon
   C. Jejunum
   D. Ascending colon

3. The acetabulum is formed by the following bones: _____forms the upper part,_____ forms the lower anterior part, and_____the forms the lower posterior part.

4. The femoral vein is located lateral to the femoral artery. True or false.

5. Which of the following is the erectile tissue forming the anterior part of the penis?
   A. Cavernosum spongiosum
   B. Corpus cavernosum
   C. Corpus spongiosum
   D. Cavernosum spongiosum

6. Which sacral segment corresponds with the origin of the rectum from the sigmoid colon?
   A. S1
   B. S2
   C. S3
   D. S4

7. Which of the following structures would be considered most posterior in the pelvis?
   A. Lower bladder
   B. Urethra
   C. Prostate
   D. Seminal vesicles

8. Which of the following would not be considered part of the adnexal area?
   A. Uterus
   B. Ovaries
   C. Broad ligament
   D. Oviduct

9. To enter the abdominal cavity, the spermatic cord passes_____ the pubic bones. Above or below.

10. All of the following muscles form the pelvic diaphragm except
    A. Iliacus
    B. Levator ani
    C. Coccygeus
    D. All of the above from the pelvic diaphragm

11. The ovaries are located on which side of the broad ligament? Anterior or posterior.

12. The femoral artery originates from the
    A. Common iliac artery
    B. Gluteal artery
    C. External iliac artery
    D. Internal iliac artery

13. In an axial section through the pelvis, which alimentary structure would be most inferior?
    A. Ascending colon
    B. Descending colon
    C. Sigmoid colon
    D. Rectum

14. Which of the following spaces forms the lowest part of the abdominal cavity?
    A. Ischiorectal fossa
    B. Adnexal area
    C. Area above bladder
    D. Rectouterine pouch

15. Describe the parts of the uterus.

16. Which of the following is located most inferiorly?
    A. Acetabulum
    B. Coccyx
    C. Symphysis pubis
    D. Obturator foramen

17. Which of the following best describes the position of the greater trochanter of the femur?
    A. Anterior and medial
    B. Posterior and medial
    C. Anterior and lateral
    D. Posterior and lateral

18. The most distinctive difference between the lower segments of the sacrum and the coccyx is the absence of the_____.

19. What space surrounds the cervix of the uterus extending into the vagina?

20. If you were asked to perform a CT examination of the pelvis, what bony structures would need to be included within the first and last axial images to ensure that all the pelvic structures would be visualized?

Chapter 5

Head

OBJECTIVES

Upon completion of this chapter, the student should be able to:

1. Describe the inferior boundary of the head.
2. Identify and describe the bones making up the skull.
3. Identify and describe the location of the central nervous system structures within the head.
4. Describe the structures separating the skull cavity.
5. Describe the dural venous system and the major arteries in the head.
6. List the general functions of the cerebrum, cerebellum, basal ganglia, and brainstem and each structure's locations on sagittal, coronal, and axial images.
7. Follow the course of the cerebrospinal fluid (CSF) as it passes through the central nervous system.
8. Describe the cranial nerves.
9. Explain the relationships among structures located within the skull.
10. Correctly identify anatomical structures on patient CT and MR images of the head.

ANATOMICAL OVERVIEW

Most students consider the head to be one of the more difficult regions of the body to study, owing to the large number of structures in a relatively small area. The major bony structure, the skull, houses the brain and the organs of the special senses. When imaging the head, the base of the skull is the inferior boundary of the head. The bones making up the skull will be reviewed first to provide a framework for learning the soft tissue structures.

Skeletal

Ethmoid (*ETH-moyd*). The bone between the orbits (Fig. 5-1); generally described as spongy, because it has thin layers of bone separated by air pockets and numerous channels.

Cribriform (KRIB-ri-fōrm) plate. The section of the ethmoid that forms part of the floor midline in the anterior cranial cavity (the term means "like a sieve"). It is filled with perforations that transmit the olfactory nerves originating from the mucous membrane within the nasal cavity to the first pair of cranial nerves.

Crista galli (KRIS-tă GAL-li). A triangular process projecting upward from the cribriform plate that provides attachment for the falx cerebri.

Perpendicular plate. Also called the vertical plate. Part of the ethmoid that is found below the cribriform plate that joins with the vomer and septal cartilage to separate the nasal cavity into right and left parts.

Sinuses. Also called *air cells*. Their number and arrangement within the ethmoid are highly variable; there are generally 3 to 18 cells. Collectively, they form the two ethmoidal sinuses on the right and left sides of the nasal cavity. The mucous membrane–lined cells drain into the nasal cavity in the superior and middle meatus and have interconnections with the sphenoid sinus.

Nasal conchae (KON-kă). Two thin, seashell-shaped bones on either side of the ethmoid that project into the nasal cavity, forming the superior and middle conchae. Their unique scroll shape provides efficient circulation and filtration of inhaled air before it passes on to the trachea and lungs.

Frontal. The bone forming the forehead, the anterior part of the skull, and the roofs of the orbital cavities (Fig. 5-1 and 5-2).

Sinuses. Compartments of air centrally located within the frontal bone that are usually separated by a septum and drain into the nasal cavity in the middle meatus (opening below middle concha).

Orbital plate. The part of the frontal bone that forms the roof of the orbital cavities. The frontal sinuses extend over the orbits in some individuals (Fig. 5-1).

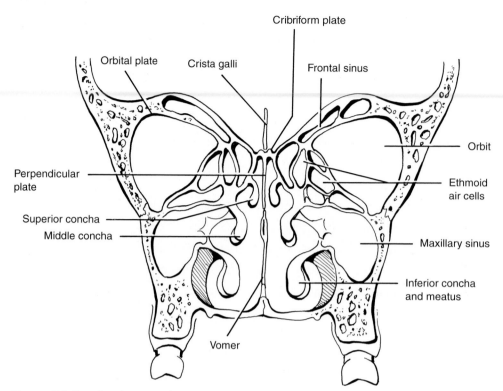

Figure 5-1 Drawing demonstrating a posterior coronal view of the nasal cavity.

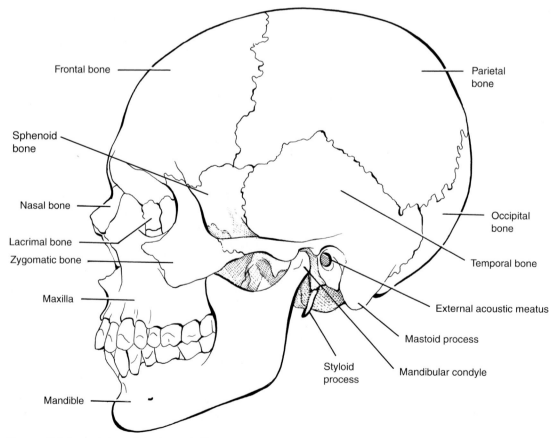

Figure 5-2 Lateral view of the bony skull.

Lacrimal (*LAK-ri-măl*). The small bone forming the floor of the nasolacrimal duct on the anteromedial wall of the orbit (Fig. 5-2).

Maxilla (*mak-SIL-ă*). Made up of the two maxillary (*MAK-si-lār-ē*) bones, which unite to form the upper part of the mouth and the anterior three-quarters of the hard palate. Every bone in the face articulates with the maxilla except the mandible.

Sinuses. Each maxillary bone contains a pocket of air that empties into the nasal cavity through the middle meatus (Fig. 5-1).

Nasals. Two fused bones that form the upper bridge of the nose. Cartilage and skin extend inferiorly, forming the lower nose (Fig. 5-2).

Zygomatics (*ZĪ-gō-MAT-iks*). Commonly called the cheek bones, because they form a prominence on either side of the face. The bones form much of the inferior and lateral walls of the orbit and have a process that articulates with the temporal bone to form the zygomatic arch.

Mandible. Commonly called the jaw bone. The only movable bone in the skull and the largest and strongest facial bone. It is frequently divided into two major parts: the ramus (*RĀ-mŭs*), the vertical projection of bone on either side, and the body, the horizontal projection containing the teeth.

Condyles (*KON-dīlz*). The rounded processes above the mandibular rami (*RĀ-mi*) that articulate with the temporal bones to form the temporomandibular (*TEM-pŏ-rō-man-DIB-yū-lăr*) joints.

Vomer (*VŌ-mer*). Forms the posterior part of the nasal septum. A thin, flat bone extending from the hard palate and articulating with the perpendicular plate of the ethmoid (Figs. 5-1 and 5-3).

Palatines (*PAL-ă-tīnz*). Pair of bones forming the posterior part of the hard palate (Fig. 5-3). Because they are L-shaped, they also form part of the lateral walls and floor of the nasal cavity.

Parietals (*pă-RĪ-ĕ-tălz*). Pair of flat bones that form much of the lateral walls and roof of the cranial cavity (Fig. 5-2).

Sphenoid (*SFĒ-noyd*). Found within the floor of the cranial cavity. Called the keystone of the cranium, because it articulates with all the other cranial bones (Figs. 5-2 to 5-4).

Clivus (*KLĪ-vŭs*). The bony structure within the posterior cranial fossa (*FOS-ă*) between the dorsum sellae and the foramen magnum (Fig. 5-3). The upper part lies just posterior to the dorsum sellae and is formed by the body of the sphenoid bone. On the other end, the lower part extends to the foramen magnum and is formed by the basilar part of the occipital bone.

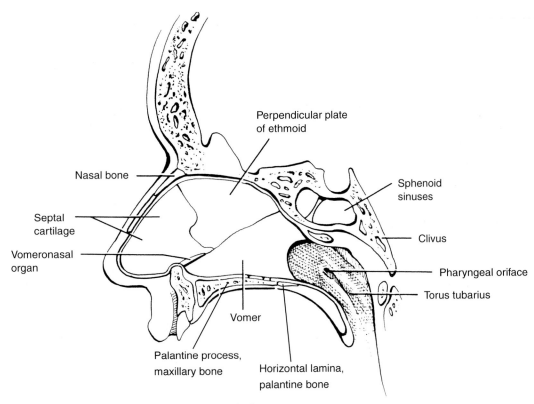

Figure 5-3 Median sagittal view of the bony skull.

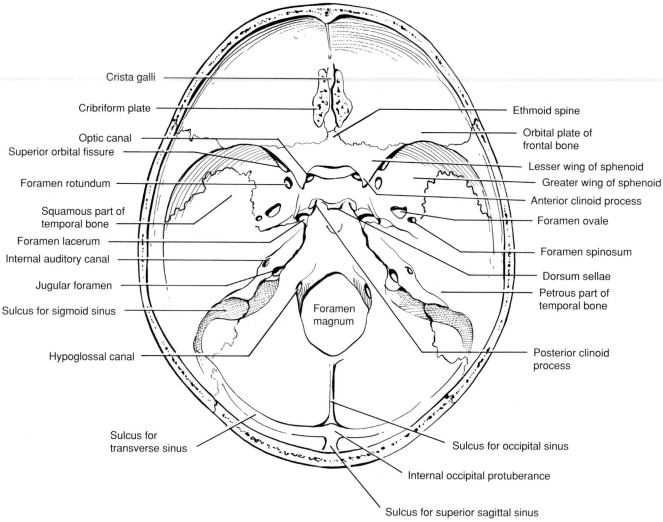

Figure 5-4 Superior axial view of the base of the skull.

Sinuses. The central portion of the sphenoid bone, located inferior to the sella turcica (*SEL-ă TUR-sĭ-kă*), usually contains two air cells asymmetrically divided by a septum and continuous with the posterior nasal cavity.

Greater and lesser wings. Within the cranial floor, the wings of the sphenoid bone are lateral to the sella turcica (Fig. 5-4). The lesser wings are anterior and superior to the sella turcica and form part of the posterior part of the bony orbit. The greater wings are larger and more inferior; they form part of the floor of the cranial cavity and part of the lateral cranial walls (Fig. 5-2).

Anterior and posterior clinoid (KLĪ-noyd) processes. They surround the sella turcica and provide a site of attachment for the dura mater, anchoring the pituitary gland within the sella turcica (Fig. 5-4).

Dorsum sellae (DŌR-sŭm SEL-ē). The posterior boundary of the sella turcica, containing the posterior clinoid processes and forming the upper part of the clivus.

Temporals (*TEM-pŏ-rălz*). Pair of irregularly shaped bones that form the inferior part of the lateral wall of the cranial cavity and much of the middle cranial floor (Figs. 5-2 and 5-4). Its petrous (*PET-rŭs*) portion, within the floor of the cranial cavity, contains the internal ear.

External auditory meatus (mē-Ā-tŭs). Found on the lateral side of the skull (Fig. 5-2). The opening within the temporal bone that forms a canal to reach the middle ear.

Mastoid (MAS-toyd) sinuses. Found within the mastoid processes of the temporal bones (posterior and inferior to the external auditory meatus). They are continuous with the inner ear.

Occipital (*ok-SIP-i-tăl*). Forms the posterior part of the cranium and contains the largest opening of the skull, the foramen magnum (Fig. 5-4).

Foramina (*fō-RAM-i-nă*)

All are bilateral, except the foramen (*fō-RĀ-men*) magnum.

Carotid (ka-ROT-id). Located within the petrous portion of the temporal bone. Transmits the internal carotid artery into the cranial cavity.

Cribriform (KRIB-ri-fōrm). Found in the ethmoid bone (Fig. 5-4). Transmits bundles of nerve fibers originating from mucous membranes lining the nasal cavity to the olfactory (I) nerves.

Hypoglossal (hī-pō-GLOS-ăl) canal. Transmits the hypoglossal (XII) nerve out of the skull through the occipital bone just above the occipital condyles.

Internal auditory canal. Also called the internal acoustic meatus. Located within the petrous part of the temporal bone, it transmits the facial (VII) and the acoustic (VIII) nerves.

Jugular (JŬG-yū-lar). Located just posterior to the carotid foramen between the petrous part of the temporal bone and the occipital bone. Contains the internal jugular vein, glossopharyngeal (IX) nerve, vagus (X) nerve, and spinal accessory (XI) nerve.

Lacerum (LAS-er-ŭm). Found between the occipital, temporal, and sphenoid bones. Transmits small vessels, nerves, and lymphatics.

Magnum (MAG-nŭm). Found at the base of the occipital bone. Transmits the spinal cord.

Optic. Located within the lesser wing of the sphenoid bone. Transmits the optic (II) nerve and the ophthalmic (of-THAL-mik) artery into the orbital cavity (Fig. 5-4).

Ovale (Ō-vă-lē). The opening through the greater wing of the sphenoid bone. Transmits the mandibular branch of the trigeminal (V) nerve to the lower face (Figs. 5-4 and 5-5).

Superior orbital fissure. Found between the lesser and greater wings of the sphenoid bone. Transmits the oculomotor (III), trochlear (IV), ophthalmic branch of the trigeminal (V), and the abducens (VI) nerves.

Cranial Nerves

All are paired. The mnemonic for remembering the cranial nerves is "*On old Olympus towering tops a Finn and Greek viewed some hops.*"

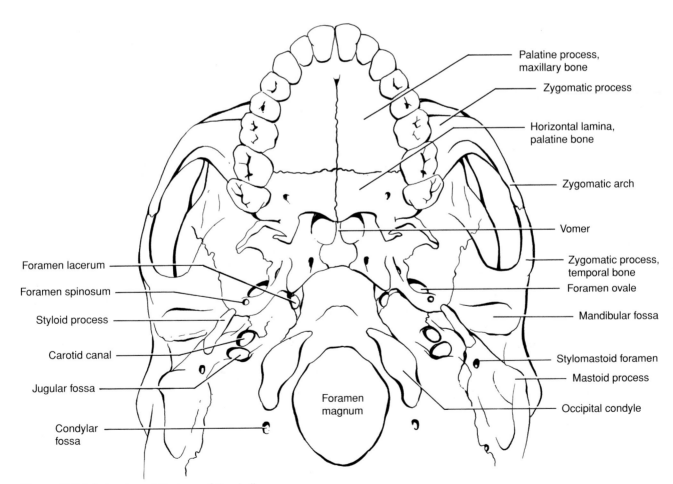

Figure 5-5 Inferior view of the base of the skull.

Labels (clockwise from top right):
- Palatine process, maxillary bone
- Zygomatic process
- Horizontal lamina, palatine bone
- Zygomatic arch
- Vomer
- Zygomatic process, temporal bone
- Foramen ovale
- Mandibular fossa
- Stylomastoid foramen
- Mastoid process
- Occipital condyle
- Foramen magnum
- Condylar fossa
- Jugular fossa
- Carotid canal
- Styloid process
- Foramen spinosum
- Foramen lacerum

I: *olfactory* (*ol-FAK-tŏ-rē*). Originate from the olfactory bulb and terminate within the nasal cavity in the mucous membranes. Transmit the sense of smell.

II: *optic.* Originates from the retina. Transmit the sense of sight.

III: *oculomotor* (*OK-yū-MŌ-tŏr*). Originate from the interpeduncular fossa. Innervate the external muscles of the eyes, except the superior oblique and lateral rectus muscles.

IV: *trochlear* (*TROK-lē-ar*). Originate lateral to the cerebral peduncles. Innervate the superior oblique muscles of the eyes.

V: *trigeminal* (*tri-JEM-i-năl*). Emerge from the lateral side of the pons and have both sensory and motor functions. The three branches provide sensory fibers to most of the head and the motor fibers innervate the muscles of mastication.

VI: *abducens* (*ab-DŪ-senz*). Emerge from the groove between the pons and medulla. Innervates the lateral rectus muscles of the eyes.

VII: *facial.* Attach to the brainstem at the cerebellopontine (*ser-e-BEL-ō-PON-tēn*) angle and have both sensory and motor functions. The sensory fibers carry the sense of taste from the anterior two-thirds of the tongue, and the motor fibers innervate the muscles of facial expression.

VIII: *acoustic.* Extend from the brainstem beside the facial nerve. Transmit the senses of equilibrium and hearing.

IX: *glossopharyngeal* (*GLOS-ō-fă-RIN-je-ăl*). Emerge from the medulla and have both sensory and motor functions. The sensory fibers transmit the sense of taste from the posterior third of the tongue, and the motor fibers innervate the muscles of the pharynx.

X: *vagus* (*VĀ-gŭs*). Emerge from the medulla. Carry both sensory and motor fibers from the pharynx, larynx, thorax, and abdomen.

XI: *spinal accessory.* Emerge from the medulla. Innervate the trapezius (*tra-PĒ-zē-ŭs*) and sternocleidomastoid (*STER-nō-KLĪ-dō-MAS-toyd*) muscles.

XII: *hypoglossal* (*hī-pō-GLOS-ă*). Emerge from the medulla. Innervate the muscles of the tongue.

Brain

Cerebellum (*ser-e-BEL-ŭm*). The second largest part of the brain. Located behind the face and brainstem in the posterior cranial fossa (Fig. 5-6). Its outer layer, containing a concentration of cell bodies, is called gray matter; its deeper layers, containing mostly cell processes and supportive cells, is called white matter. Coordinates movements and maintains posture and balance.

Vermis (*VER-mis*). The constricted region joining the two cerebellar hemispheres.

Pedunculi (*pe-DŬNG-kyū-li*). Bundles of nerves traveling between the cerebellum and the brainstem. The superior joins the midbrain; the middle connects with the pons; and the inferior extends to the medulla and spinal cord.

Cerebellar tonsils. Located on the lower and medial part of the cerebellar hemispheres, next to the foramen magnum.

Cerebrum (*SER-ĕ-bŭm*). The largest part of the brain, it consists of two hemispheres. The cortex contains mostly nerve cell bodies and appears as gray matter in unstained specimens. Below the cortex, nerve fibers traveling toward and away from the cortex form the white matter. Most regions function as association areas related to memory, reasoning, judgment, intelligence, and personality.

Sylvian (*SIL-vē-an*) **fissure.** Also called the lateral cerebral sulcus (*SUL-kŭs*). Located on the lateral side of the cerebrum (Fig. 5-7), where many grooves or sulci are found between rounded protrusions or gyri (*JĪ-ri*). It is deeper than the sulci and divides the lateral cerebrum into the temporal and frontal lobes.

Central sulcus. A centrally located sulcus found on the top of the cerebrum, extending around the upper hemispheres dividing the parietal and temporal lobes.

Frontal lobe. Part of the cerebral hemispheres, located anterior to the central sulcus and above the Sylvian fissure. The motor, or muscle, control areas are found just in front of the central sulcus; and the association areas are found in the anterior frontal lobe.

Parietal (*păRĪ-ĕ-tăl*) **lobe.** Located between the central sulcus and the parieto-occipital fissure and found above the Sylvian fissure. The general sensory, or somesthetic, areas that represent specific parts of the body are found directly posterior to the central sulcus. The remaining section functions as part of the association areas.

Temporal lobe. Located inferior to the Sylvian fissure and anterior to an extension of the parieto-occipital fissure. The upper part contains the primary auditory area, and the rest is thought to be part of the association areas.

Hippocampal (*hip-ō-KAM-păl*) *formation.* Deep within the temporal lobe, this curved sheet of gray matter extends upward into the floor of the lateral ventricle (*VEN-tri-kl*). It is considered part of the limbic system and is involved in the emotional aspects of behavior.

Occipital lobe. The posterior part of the cerebral hemisphere, located behind the parieto-occipital fissure. Considered the primary visual area of the brain.

Corpus callosum (*KOR-pŭs ka-LO-sŭm*). Large bundles of transverse or commissural fibers of white matter connecting the right and left cerebral hemispheres. The commissural fibers transmit impulses from a gyrus on one cerebral hemisphere to the corresponding gyrus on the opposite side (Fig. 5-8).

Genu (*JE-nū*). Describes the anterior part of the corpus callosum, which transmits commissural fibers between the frontal lobes (Latin for "bend" or "kneel").

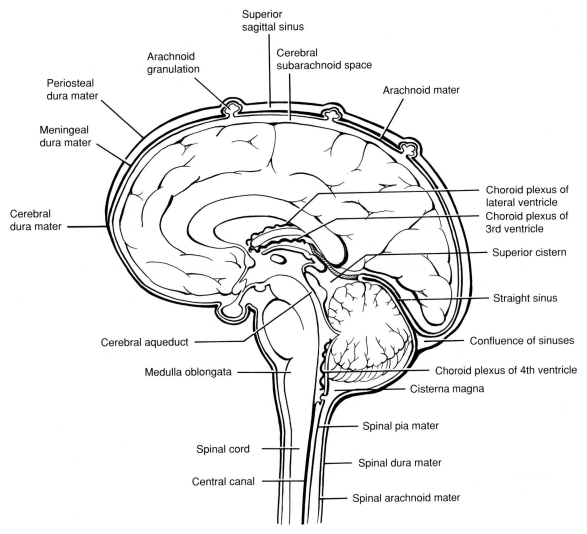

Figure 5-6 Median sagittal drawing of the central narvous system.

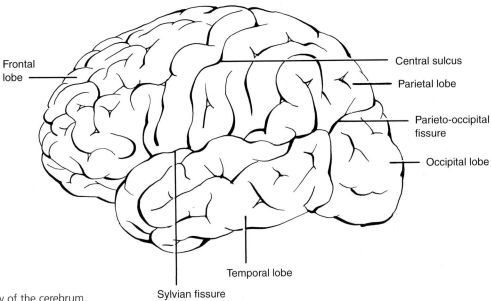

Figure 5-7 Lateral view of the cerebrum.

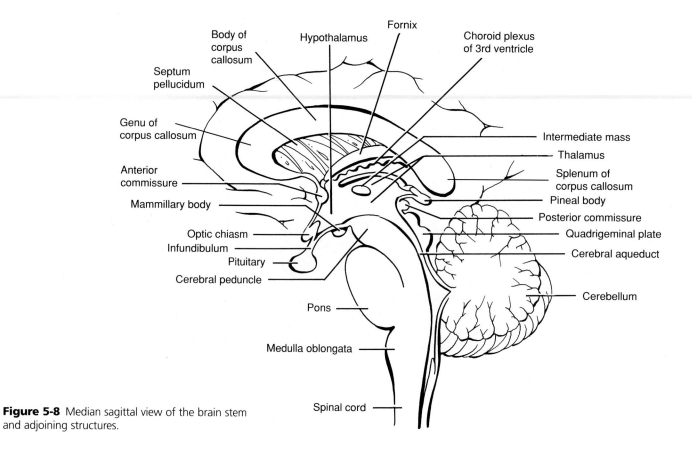

Figure 5-8 Median sagittal view of the brain stem and adjoining structures.

Body. The middle part of the corpus callosum, formed by commissural fibers from the parietal and temporal lobes extending to the opposite hemisphere.

Splenium (SPLE-nē-ŭm). The posterior and thicker part of the corpus callosum formed by fibers extending from the posterior parietal and occipital lobes to the corresponding lobe on the opposite side.

Fornix (*FŌR-niks*). On either side, the arched columns formed by tracts of fibers joining together posteriorly under the splenium of the corpus callosum. Together, they form the roof of the third ventricle.

Septum pellucidum (*SEO-tŭm pe-LŪ-sid-ŭm*). A thin, double-layered membrane between the columns of the fornix and the corpus callosum that separates the anterior horns of the lateral ventricles.

Anterior commissure. An oval-shaped bundle of fibers traveling between the temporal and frontal lobes of the right and left cerebral hemispheres. Found below the inferior end of the fornix, it forms part of the anterior wall of the third ventricle.

Posterior commissure. A complex bundle of fibers traveling between hemispheres from a variety of nuclei. Forms part of the posterior wall of the third ventricle.

Pineal (*PIN-ē-ăl*) **body.** Pinecone-shaped endocrine gland attached to the roof of the third ventricle; found below the

splenium of the corpus callosum. At about the time of puberty, it starts to calcify or collect what is commonly called brain sand.

Intermediate mass. Also called the interthalamic adhesion. A bundle of gray matter that serves as a bridge through the third ventricle, joining the right and left thalamic nuclei.

Thalamus (*THAL-ă-mŭs*). Oval-shaped nucleus that forms the lateral walls of the third ventricle; usually about 2.5 cm (1 in.) long. Although the nucleus is mostly gray matter, it does contain small areas of white matter, subdividing the structure into smaller groups. Primarily serves as the "switching center" for directing sensory impulses to the appropriate region of the cerebral cortex.

Hypothalamus (*HĪ-pō-THAL-ă-mŭs*). Forms the floor and part of the lateral walls of the third ventricle. The nucleus includes the mammillary body and is protected by the upper part of the sphenoid bone. Although relatively small, it controls many bodily functions related to maintaining homeostasis, or stability, within the body.

Pituitary (*pi-TŪ-i-tār-ē*). Also called the hypophysis (*hi-POF-i-sis*). Located within the sella turcica of the sphenoid bone. An endocrine gland that regulates so many of the body's activities it is often called the "master gland"; the hormones are absorbed by a capillary plexus surrounding the gland.

Infundibulum (*in-fŭn-DIB-yū-lŭm*). The stalk connecting the pituitary to the hypothalamus.

Midbrain. The bundle of nervous tissue connecting the cerebrum with the cerebellum and spinal cord. Although the majority of the area consists of nerve fibers, a variety of nuclei are found embedded within the white matter.

Cerebral peduncles (*pe-DŬNG-klz*). Found on the anterior portion of the midbrain. A pair of large fiber bundles that carry motor impulses from the cerebral cortex to the pons and spinal cord.

Red nucleus. Found below the thalamus in the superior part of the cerebral peduncles. An oval-shaped region of gray matter considered to be a motor nucleus. Fibers from the cerebral cortex and cerebellum terminate here and give rise to fibers traveling downward in the spinal cord.

Substantia nigra (*sŭb-STAN-shē-ă NI-gră*). The layer of deeply pigmented gray matter lining much of the posterior surface of the cerebral peduncles. Fibers from the cell bodies within the nucleus project to the cerebral cortex, basal nuclei, thalamus, hypothalamus, and other regions of the brain.

Quadrigeminal (*KWAH-dri-JEM-i-năl*) *plate.* Also called the corpora quadrigemina. The posterior portion of the midbrain, behind the cerebral aqueduct. Consists of four rounded eminences containing small nuclei. Responsible for reflex movements in response to auditory and visual stimuli.

Pons (*ponz*). Located anterior to the cerebellum. The enlarged portion of the brainstem where fibers from the cerebellum join those from the cerebrum and spinal cord. Like the midbrain, it consists of mostly white matter but also contains a number of nuclei.

Medulla oblongata (*me-DŪL-ă ob-long-GAH-tă*). Forms the lower brainstem directly below the pons and contains all the ascending and descending tracts that communicate between the spinal cord and the brain. Despite having a large amount of white matter formed by the nerve fibers, it contains a variety of nuclei. Many motor nerve fibers decussate (*DĒ-kŭ-sāt*), or cross over, to the opposite side, causing one side of the brain to control motor function on the opposite side of the body.

Spinal cord. Found within the spinal foramina. It connects the brain with the body. Like the cerebrum and cerebellum, it consists of both gray and white matter; however, unlike the cerebrum and cerebellum, its outer layer is white matter.

Caudate (*KAW-dāt*) **nucleus.** C-shaped area of gray matter found following the curve of the lateral ventricle. Involved in muscle control (Fig. 5-9).

Head. The enlarged part of the caudate nucleus bulges into the floor of the anterior horn of the lateral ventricle.

Body. The central portion of the caudate nucleus anterior to the collateral trigone (*TRI-gōn*) of the lateral ventricle.

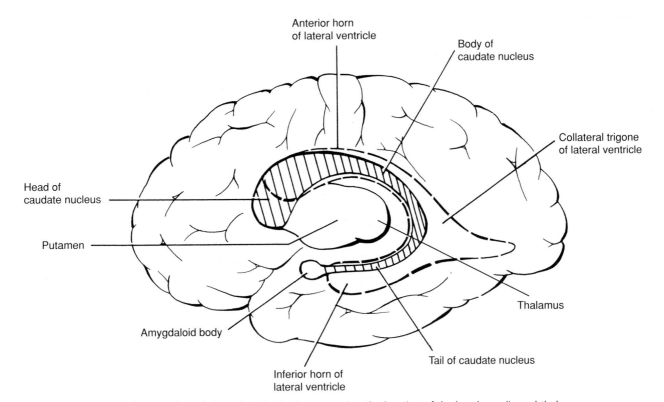

Figure 5-9 Drawing from the lateral view of the brain demonstrating the location of the basal ganglia and thalamus.

Tail. The tapered part of the caudate nucleus in the roof of the inferior horn of the lateral ventricle.

Internal capsule. The group of sensory and motor nerves connecting the cerebral cortex with the brainstem and spinal cord (Fig. 5-10). Because the tracts separate the thalamus from the basal ganglia (globus pallidus, putamen, and caudate), they form what appears as a "capsule" for the thalamus.

Lenticular (*len-TIK-YŪ-lăr*) **nuclei.** Found lateral to the internal capsule and the thalamus. Shaped like an acorn, with the pointed end surrounded by internal capsule. Consist of the globus pallidus and the putamen.

Globus pallidus (*GLŌ-bŭs PAL-i-dŭs*). The medial lenticular nucleus located next to the internal capsule. Laterally, it is separated from the putamen by a small lamina of fibers. Considered primarily a motor nucleus. Cellular extensions from the structure connect with most of the nuclei within the brain and the cerebral cortex.

Putamen (*pyū-TA-men*). The lateral lenticular nucleus found next to the globus pallidus and medial to the external capsule. Has numerous connections and is generally considered a motor nucleus. Generally thought to inhibit function of cortical-induced motor activity.

External capsule. A thin layer of white matter between the putamen and the claustrum. Its fibers are derived from the insula; the subthalamic connections are unknown.

Claustrum (*KLAWS-trŭm*). A sheet of gray matter bounded by laminae of white matter on either side, the external capsule medially, and the extreme capsule laterally. The connections and function of the nucleus are not yet clearly understood.

Extreme capsule. The thin layer of white matter between the claustrum and insula. Contains fibers from both areas.

Insula (*IN-sū-lă*). Commonly called the inner lobe. The region of the cerebral cortex located deep within the Sylvian or lateral cerebral fissure. Medially, it is separated from the claustrum by the extreme capsule, which carries its fibers to other parts of the brain and spinal cord. Although the function is not clearly understood, stimulation results in visceral sensations and autonomic responses.

Corona radiata (*kō-RŌ-nă RA-dē-ă-tă*). Found above the thalamus and basal ganglia. Fibers radiating between the

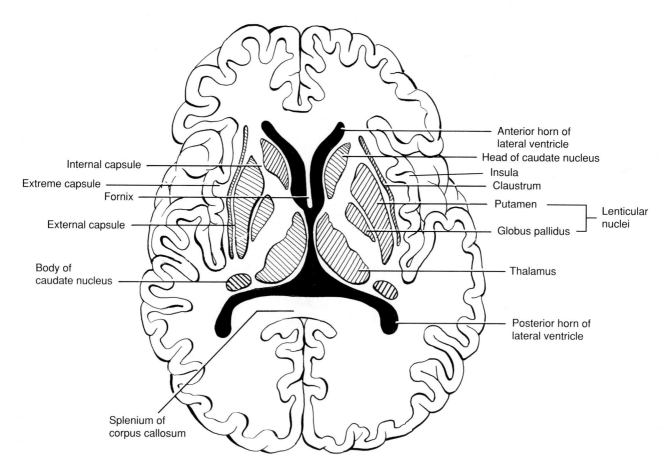

Figure 5-10 Axial section through the head demonstrating the basal ganglia and thalamic nuclei.

internal capsule and the cerebral cortex form sheets, creating a crown of white matter above the nuclei (Fig. 5-11).

Enclosing Structures

Dura mater (*DŪ-ră MA-ter*). The outermost and toughest of the three membranes covering the brain and spinal cord (Latin for "hard mother"). The meningeal layer located closest to the bone surrounding the CNS (Fig. 5-12). Although not shown in Figure 5-12, meningeal arteries are frequently found between the dura mater and calvarial bone in the epidural space. The arachnoid mater is deep to the dura mater, and the two membranes can be separated, creating a subdural space.

Arachnoid (*ă-RAK-noyd*) **mater.** The middle, delicate meningeal membrane covering the brain and spinal cord. Connected to the underlying pia mater by trabeculae (*tră-BEK-yū-lă*), or thin fibrous threads, much like spiderwebs. Between the trabeculae, the subarachnoid space is filled with CSF and contains most of the major arteries supplying blood to the brain.

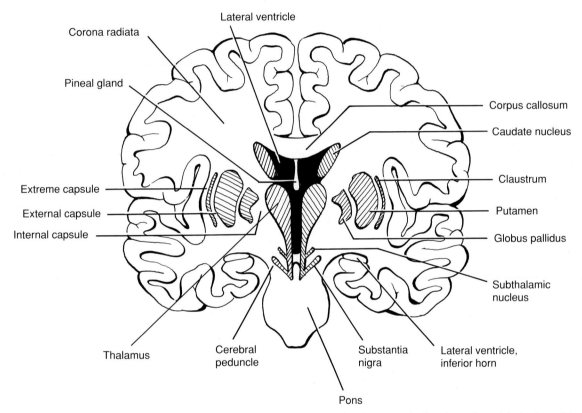

Corona radiata — Lateral ventricle — Pineal gland

Corpus callosum
Caudate nucleus
Claustrum
Putamen
Globus pallidus
Subthalamic nucleus

Extreme capsule
External capsule
Internal capsule

Thalamus — Cerebral peduncle — Substantia nigra — Lateral ventricle, inferior horn — Pons

Figure 5-11 Coronal section through the brain demonstrating relationships between the basal ganglia and thalamic nuclei.

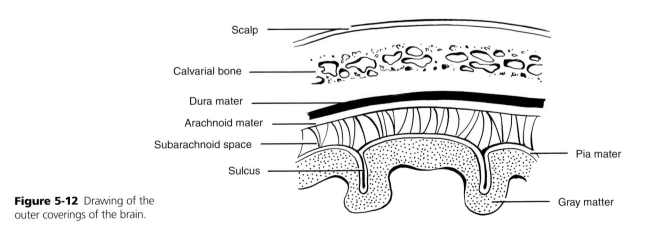

Scalp
Calvarial bone
Dura mater
Arachnoid mater
Subarachnoid space
Sulcus
Pia mater
Gray matter

Figure 5-12 Drawing of the outer coverings of the brain.

Pia (*PĪ-ă*) **mater.** The innermost membrane surrounding the brain and spinal cord. In a cadaver specimen, it is difficult to separate from the nervous system structures, because it is tightly adhered and intimately related to the surface of the brain and spinal cord.

Falx cerebri (*falks se-RĒ-bri*). Separates the cerebral hemispheres. A reflection of dura mater that extends caudally from the upper calvarium and ends just above the corpus callosum (Fig. 5-13). Its anterior end attaches to the crista galli of the ethmoid bone, and the posterior end joins other dural reflections in the posterior cranial fossa.

Falx cerebelli (*ser-ĕ-BEL-i*). The reflection of dura mater separating the cerebellar hemispheres in the posterior cranial cavity.

Tentorium (*ten-TŌ-rē-ŭm*) **cerebelli.** The dural reflection extending horizontally between the cerebrum and cerebellum. Laterally, it is attached to the petrous ridge on either side; it extends posteriorly to the juncture of the falx cerebri and falx cerebelli.

Dural Sinuses and Veins

Superior sagittal (*SAJ-i-tăl*) **sinus.** Within the upper margin of the falx cerebri, the layers of dura form a sinus for venous blood draining from the upper cerebral hemispheres. Following the superior margin of the falx cerebri, it lies near the inner surface of the calvarium.

Inferior sagittal sinus. Within the lower margin of the falx cerebri, venous blood from the medial part of the cerebral hemispheres is collected in a space between the layers of dura. In a coronal section, it is demonstrated between the cerebral hemispheres just above the corpus callosum.

Vein of Galen. Located below the splenium of the corpus callosum, it drains the internal cerebral hemispheres into the straight sinus.

Straight sinus. The space for venous blood between the layers of the dura mater at the juncture of the falx cerebri, falx cerebelli, and tentorium cerebelli. Receiving blood from the inferior sagittal sinus and the vein of Galen, it extends posteriorly to empty into the confluence of sinuses.

Confluence of sinuses. The opening formed between the layers of dura mater where the superior sagittal, straight, occipital, and transverse sinuses meet.

Transverse sinuses. Within the posterior margin of the tentorium cerebelli, they extend laterally on either side (Fig. 5-14). Within the layers of dura, each one drains venous blood from the confluence of sinuses to the petrous part of the temporal bone where it bends caudally to join the sigmoid sinus.

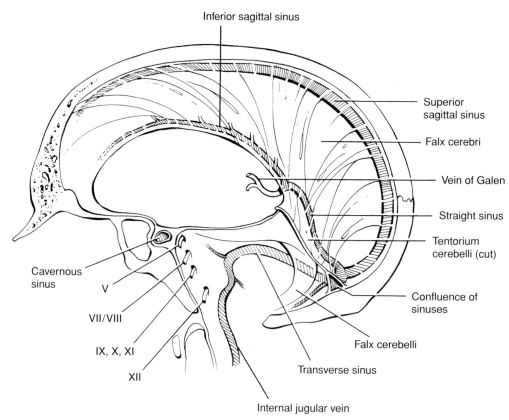

Figure 5-13 Dural reflections and associated venous sinuses within the head.

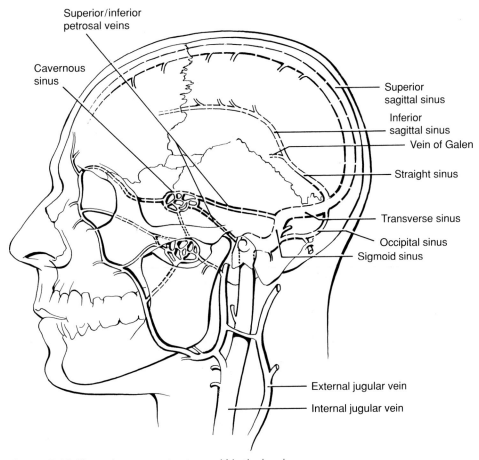

Figure 5-14 The major venous structures within the head.

Sigmoid (*SIG-moyd*) **sinuses.** Drain venous blood from the transverse and petrosal sinuses into the internal jugular veins. They curve through the petrous parts of the temporal bones.

Internal jugular veins. Originating from the sigmoid sinuses, they are the major route for drainage of venous blood from the head. Each one exits the base of the skull through the jugular foramen on the inferior surface of the petrous part of the temporal bone and extends through the neck to join the brachiocephalic vein in the chest.

Arteries

To help you learn the location of the major arteries, think of a stick man named Willis. Willis's legs are formed by the vertebral arteries, his trunk is formed by the basilar artery, his arms are the posterior cerebral arteries, and his head is formed by the circle of Willis (Fig. 5-15).

Vertebral (*VER-tĕ-brăl*). Originating from the subclavian arteries in the thorax, these bilateral arteries ascend through the transverse foramina of C6 through C1.

Superior to C1, they pass through the foramen magnum and the dura mater to enter the subarachnoid space. Found on either side of the medulla oblongata, the right and left arteries merge to give rise to the basilar artery at the level of the lower pons.

Basilar (*BAS-i-lăr*). Found near the midline on the anterior surface of the pons, this artery is within the subarachnoid space and originates from the juncture of the right and left vertebral arteries. Extending to the upper border of the pons, it divides and gives rise to the right and left posterior cerebral arteries.

Circle of Willis. A ring of vessels located within the subarachnoid space below the hypothalamus and midbrain that supplies arterial blood to the cerebrum.

Posterior cerebral. Located along the upper border of the pons, these bilateral arteries originate from the basilar artery and extend above the tentorium cerebelli to supply the occipital lobes with arterial blood. The right and left arteries are separated by the falx cerebri and appear to wrap around the splenium of the corpus callosum joining the right and left cerebral hemispheres.

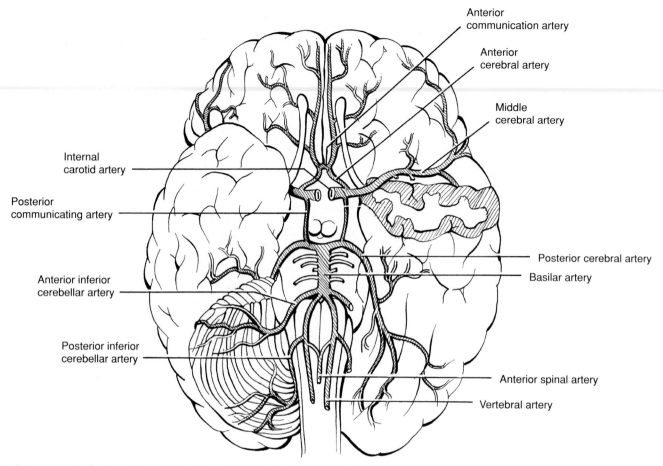

Figure 5-15 Inferior view of the major arteries of the brain.

Posterior communicating. Shortly after the posterior cerebral artery originates from the basilar artery, a small branch connects with the internal carotid artery. Although small, these arteries provide a collateral route for blood flow between the major arteries (vertebrals and internal carotids) that supply arterial blood to the brain.

Internal carotid. Beginning at the bifurcation of the common carotids in the neck, these arteries ascend next to the internal jugular veins to enter the skull through the carotid canals. As they pass along the S-shaped groove on the lateral surface of the sella turcica, they extend through the dural layers of the cavernous sinus to enter the subarachnoid space. Within the subarachnoid space, they branch to form the posterior communicating, middle cerebral, and anterior cerebral arteries.

Middle cerebral. The major branches from the internal carotid arteries, these arteries extend laterally through the Sylvian fissures to supply blood to the temporal and parietal lobes.

Anterior cerebral. Slightly smaller than the middle cerebral artery, these branches of the internal carotid arteries travel anteriorly in the interhemispheric fissure. The right and left arteries are found on either side of the falx cerebri and appear to wrap around the genu of the corpus callosum to supply blood to the frontal and medial part of the parietal lobes.

Anterior communicating. The anterior cerebral arteries are joined by a small vessel that provides a collateral route for blood flow between the right and left sides.

Ventricles and Cisterns

Lateral ventricles. Within each cerebral hemisphere, there is a C-shaped cavity with a horn radiating from the posterior part of the curve (Fig. 5-16). The cavities are lined by ependyma (*ep-EN-di-mă*), which in certain regions is highly vascularized, forming the choroid plexus (*KO-royd PLEK-sŭs*). The choroid plexus produces CSF from the blood to fill the ventricles.

Anterior horn. The part of the lateral ventricles found within the frontal lobe. The roof is formed by the corpus cal-

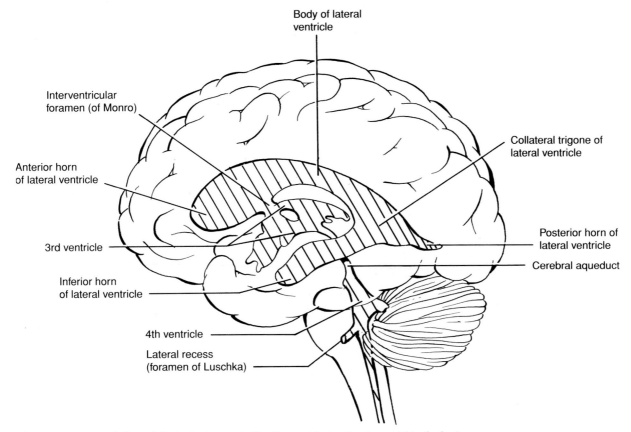

Figure 5-16 Lateral view of the brain demonstrating the ventricular structures within the brain.

losum, the floor and lateral wall are formed by the head of the caudate nucleus, and the medial wall is formed by the septum pellucidum.

Body. The anterior horn continues posteriorly to join with the body of the lateral ventricle within the parietal lobe. Like the anterior horn, the roof is formed by the corpus callosum and the medial wall is formed by the septum pellucidum. In this region, however, the floor is formed by the body of the caudate and the thalamus.

Collateral trigone. The triangular-shaped regions of the lateral ventricles that join the body, posterior horn, and inferior horn.

Posterior horn. The posterior part of the lateral ventricle. Found within the occipital lobe of the cerebrum. The roof and lateral walls are formed by groups of myelinated fibers extending to the splenium of the corpus callosum. In coronal section, it is found near the center of the cerebral hemisphere and is roughly triangular in shape. In all other planes of section, it is continuous with the collateral trigones.

Inferior or lateral horn. Located within the temporal lobe. Part of the lateral ventricle that extends forward and inferiorly from the collateral trigone. It is near the center of the temporal lobe and is lateral to all the other ventricular structures.

Interventricular foramen. Also called the foramen of Monro. Small openings that join the lateral ventricles with the third ventricle.

Third ventricle. A small, narrow opening found near the median sagittal plane between the thalamic and hypothalamic nuclei. CSF, produced by the choroid plexuses of the lateral ventricles, travels through the interventricular foramina to drain into this structure (Fig 5-17).

Cerebral aqueduct. The opening transmitting CSF from the lateral and third ventricles to the fourth ventricle. Located within the posterior part of the midbrain, this small opening is found in the midline between the cerebral peduncles and the quadrigeminal plate.

Fourth ventricle. The base of this pyramidal-shaped structure rests on the pons and medulla oblongata; the apex extends toward the cerebellum. This opening receives CSF through the cerebral aqueduct. Like the other ventricles, its choroid plexus produces CSF that travels either down through the spinal cord or empties out into the subarachnoid space.

Lateral recess. Although a large section of the fourth ventricle can be found at the midline, it has an opening extending laterally on each side. CSF in the lateral recess drains

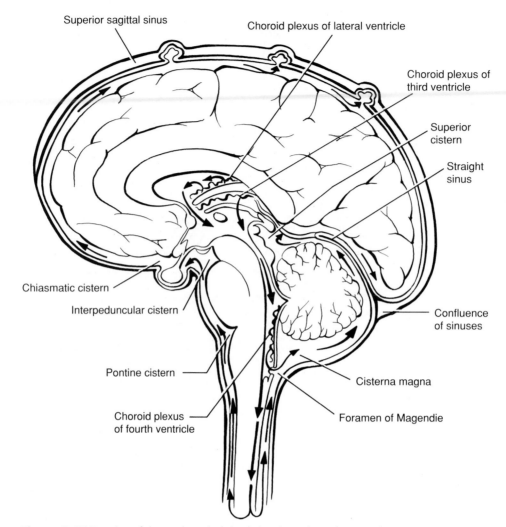

Figure 5-17 Drawing of the cerebrospinal circulation throughout the central nervous system.

through the lateral aperture, the foramen of Luschka, and into the subarachnoid space (Fig. 5-16).

Superior cistern. Also called superior cerebellar cistern. An enlarged region of subarachnoid space above the cerebellum below the tentorium cerebelli (Fig. 5-17). Located posterior to the midbrain, the opening is near the cerebral

aqueduct; and in axial sections, they are frequently demonstrated together.

Cisterna magna. Also called the cerebellomedullaris cistern. An enlarged region of subarachnoid space located posterior to the medulla oblongata between the cerebellum and the occipital bone.

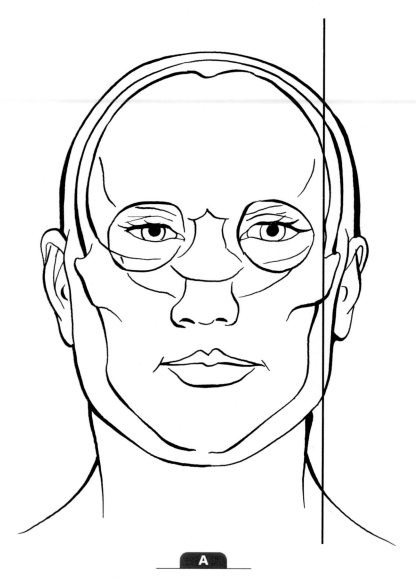

Figure 5-18 Sagittal MR image 1.

SAGITTAL MR IMAGES

The following 8 sagittal MR images of the head will be described at 8.0 mm intervals from the left side to the midsagittal plane. The right side will not be described, because the structures are generally the same as those on the left side. The images were generated at the following technical factors: TR = 650, TE = 20, RF = 90°, FOV = 25 cm, TH = 7.5 mm. Abbreviations: TR = repetition time, TE = echo-time, RF = radiofrequency, FOV = field of view, TH = slice thickness.

Figure 5-18 (A,B,C). The image generated on the left side of the head is the first sagittal section demonstrating brain anatomy and would be the first in a series of sagittal images throughout the brain (Fig. 5-18). At first glance, the sulci can be seen separating the gyri of the temporal lobe. The darkened area surrounding the temporal lobe represents the bones of the skull. Inferior to the temporal lobe within the region of the bones of the skull, the oblong structure represents the external auditory meatus. To the left of the meatus, the lateral edge of the face is demonstrated as a bright area, owing to the amount of fat and glandular material found just anterior to the ear.

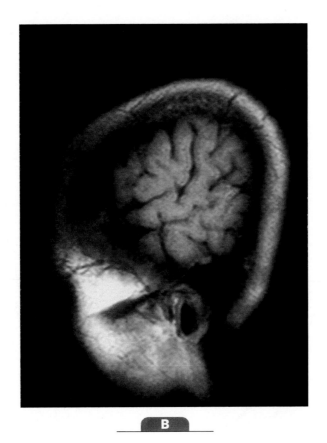

B

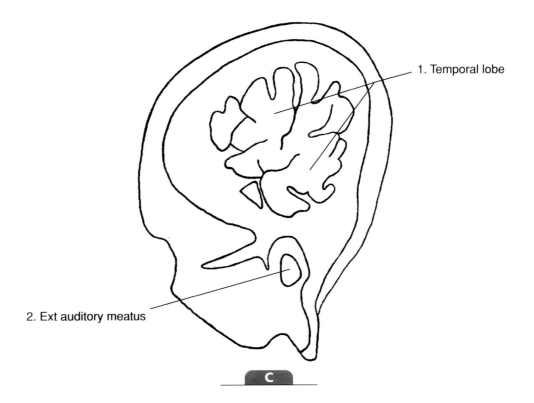

1. Temporal lobe

2. Ext auditory meatus

C

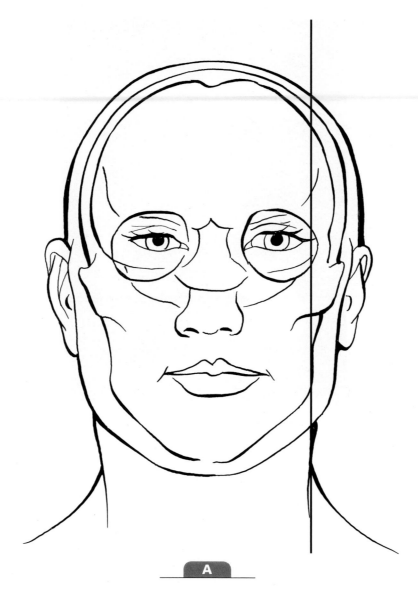

Figure 5-19 Sagittal MR image 2.

Figure 5-19 (A,B,C). Compared to the previous image, more of the cerebral hemisphere is shown in this sagittal section which also demonstrates the sulci dividing the gyri of the temporal lobe. Surrounding the temporal lobe, the darkened area representing the bones of the skull contain the opening of the external auditory meatus below the cerebrum. Within this darkened region, an enlarged, low-density area is found immediately posterior to the external auditory meatus and represents the mastoid air cells. Anterior to the meatus, the muscles of the cheek are now sectioned below the fat and glandular material, as described in the previous section.

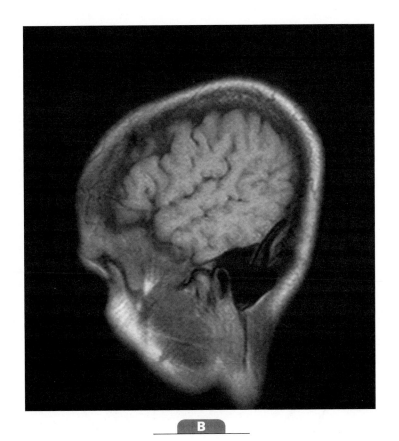

B

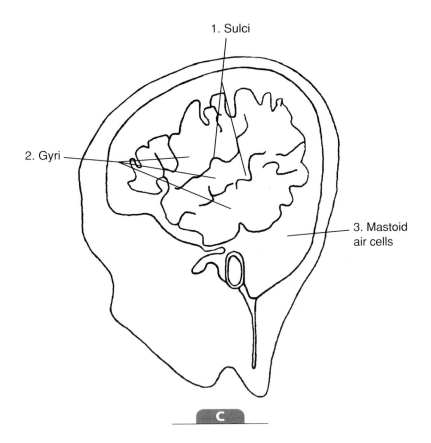

1. Sulci

2. Gyri

3. Mastoid
air cells

C

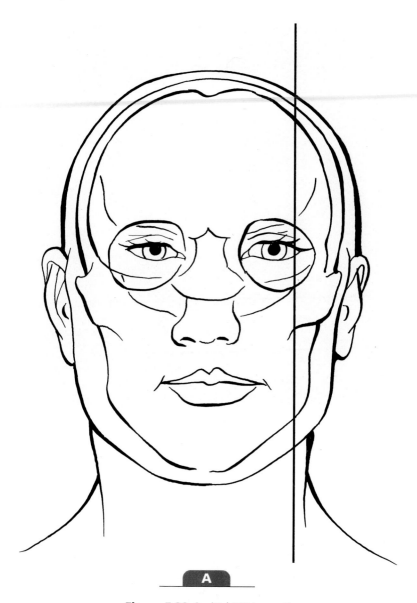

Figure 5-20 Sagittal MR image 3.

Figure 5-20 (A,B,C). This section is distinctly different from the two previous images because the brain can now be distinguished as having three identifiable parts. The temporal lobe is separated from the parietal lobe by the darkened region of the Sylvian fissure. Below the temporal lobe, the mastoid air cells are again found as an enlarged region of the skull, shown as a darkened area. In contrast to previous images, part of the brain can now be seen adjacent to the mastoid air cells with a more linear pattern than the convoluted pattern of the cerebrum. Located within the posterior cranial fossa, the posterior part of the brain is the cerebellum.

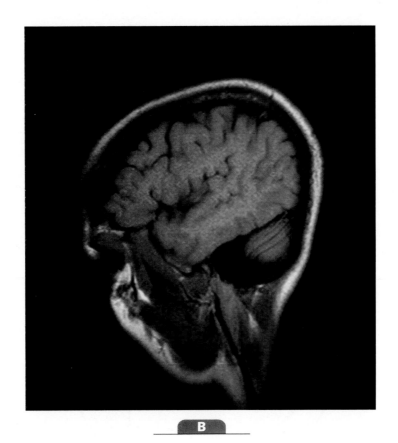

B

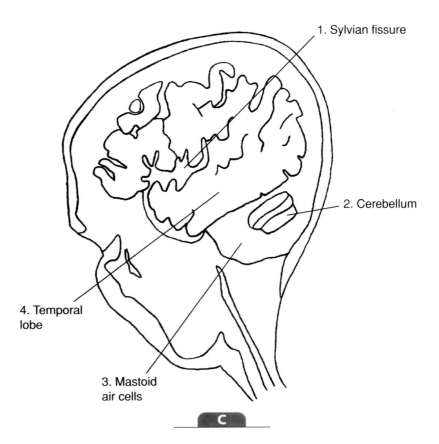

1. Sylvian fissure

2. Cerebellum

4. Temporal
lobe

3. Mastoid
air cells

C

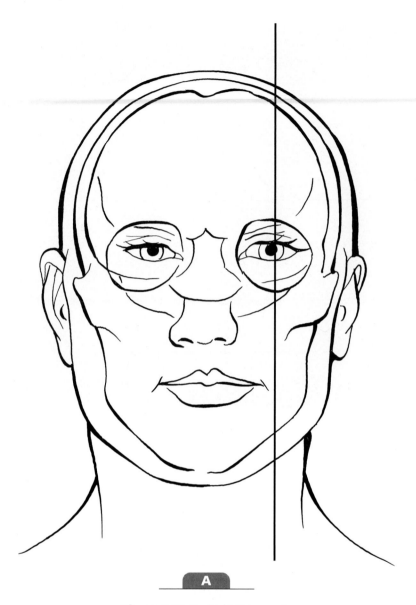

Figure 5-21 Sagittal MR image 4.

Figure 5-21 (A,B,C). At first glance, the most readily identifiable structure on this image is the globe of the eye, which is surrounded by a layer of fat within the bony orbital cavity. The area of high signal intensity represents the fat between the dark area of the globe of the eye and the more inferiorly located maxillary sinus. Posterior to the eye, the medial border of the Sylvian fissure is now seen extending toward the insula, or the inner lobe of the cerebrum. Similar to the previous image, the parietal lobe is found above the insula and the temporal lobe is below the insula. These lobes are not labeled here, because the borders cannot clearly be seen at this level. Below the temporal lobe, a larger portion of the cerebellum is shown. Because most of the section is below the surface of the cerebellum, the linear striations are less evident than in the previous image.

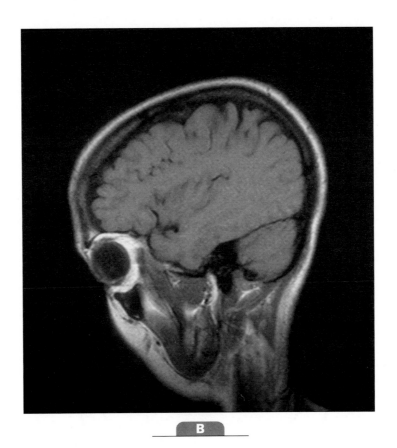

B

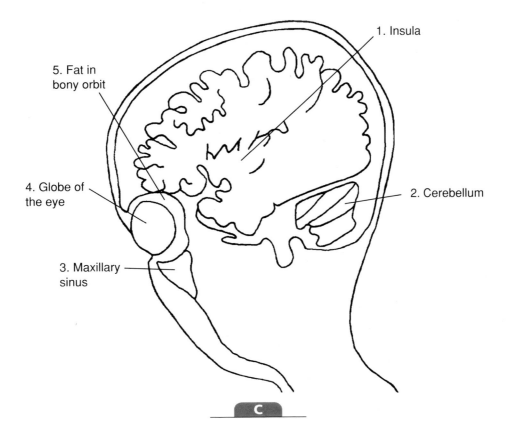

1. Insula

5. Fat in
bony orbit

2. Cerebellum

4. Globe of
the eye

3. Maxillary
sinus

C

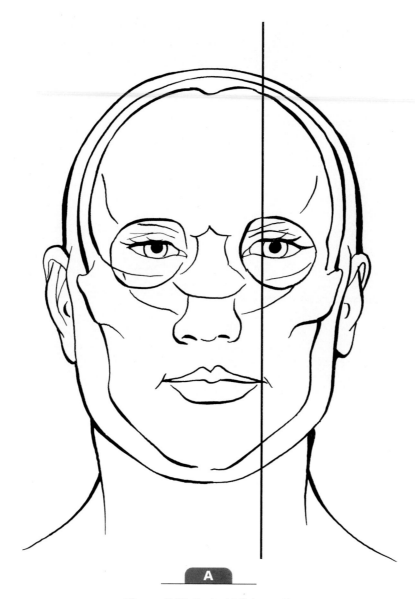

Figure 5-22 Sagittal MR image 5.

Figure 5-22 (A,B,C). The anatomy within this section lies near the midline of the left eye. Similar to the previous image, the globe of the eye can be readily identified. In addition, the optic nerve is longitudinally sectioned, extending off the posterior aspect of the globe through the layer of orbital fat. Attached to the upper pole of the globe of the eye, the superior rectus muscle is extending through the orbital fat back to attach to the skull. On the inferior pole of the globe, the inferior rectus muscle can also be seen extending through the orbital fat back to attach to the skull. As in the previous image, the maxillary sinus appears as a dark area immediately below the region of the eye. Inside the cranial cavity, the central lobe of the brain, the insula, is found above the temporal lobe. In the deep temporal lobe, the inferior horn of the lateral ventricle is shown along with the body of the caudate nucleus. In this section, the inferior horn appears separate from the triangular-shaped area of the posterior horn located deep within the occipital lobe. Inferior to the occipital lobe, the cerebellum is shown in the posterior cranial fossa.

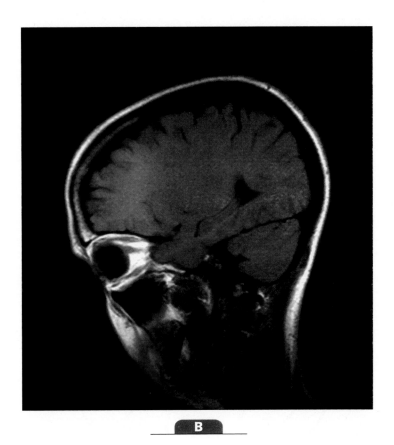

B

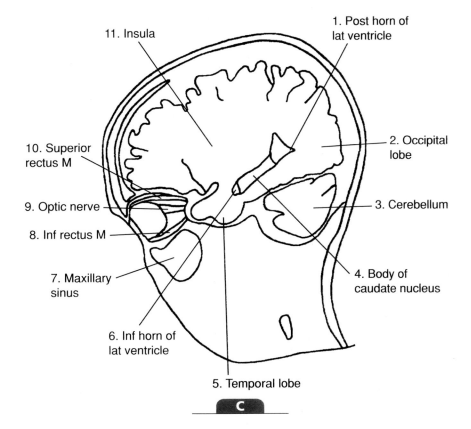

11. Insula

1. Post horn of
lat ventricle

10. Superior
rectus M

2. Occipital
lobe

9. Optic nerve

3. Cerebellum

8. Inf rectus M

7. Maxillary
sinus

4. Body of
caudate nucleus

6. Inf horn of
lat ventricle

5. Temporal lobe

C

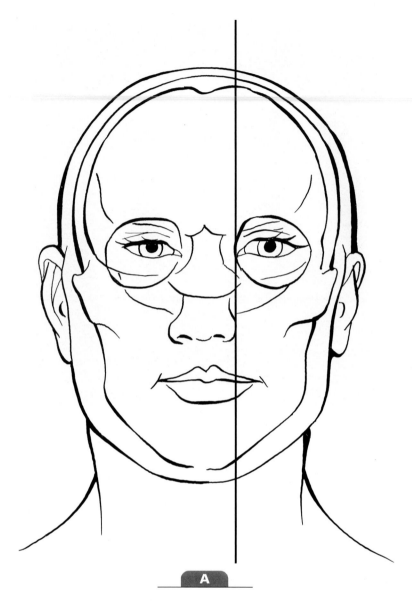

Figure 5-23 Sagittal MR image 6.

Figure 5-23 (A,B,C). This image shows the largest part of the maxillary sinus. Within the cranial cavity, the nuclei sectioned deep to the insula are the lenticular nuclei, the putamen and globus pallidus. The lenticular nuclei are separated from the thalamus by a collection of nerve processes collectively referred to as the internal capsule. Because the previous section included the inferior and posterior horns of the lateral ventricles, the enlarged region of the lateral ventricle now sectioned is labeled as the collateral trigone. As in previous images, the cerebellum is shown below the occipital lobes of the cerebrum.

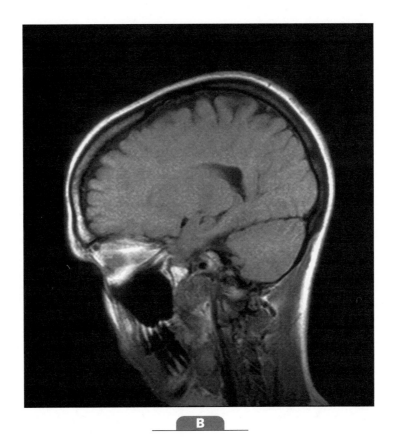

B

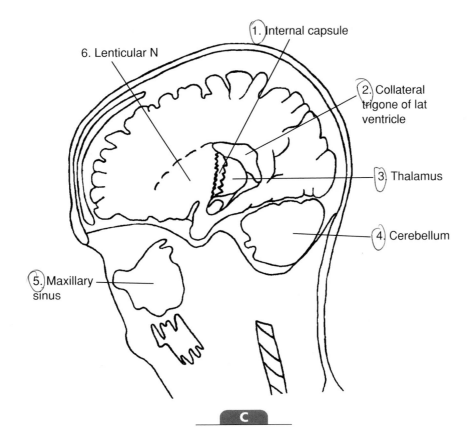

6. Lenticular N

1. Internal capsule

2. Collateral trigone of lat ventricle

3. Thalamus

4. Cerebellum

5. Maxillary sinus

C

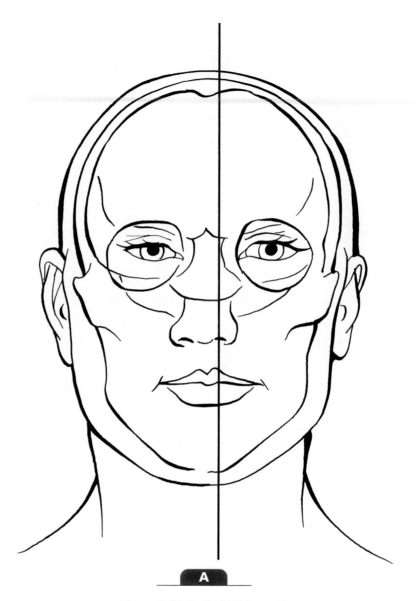

Figure 5-24 Sagittal MR image 7.

Figure 5-24 (A,B,C). This image is nearing the midline, as evidenced by the surface outline, which demonstrates a small part of the lateral aspect of the nose. In this section, the maxillary sinus is no longer seen and has been replaced by the ethmoid air cells. Above the ethmoid air cells, an enlarged region of the skull represents the frontal sinus in the position formerly occupied by the upper bony orbit. Within the cranial cavity, the body of the lateral ventricle is longitudinally sectioned continuous with the anterior horn in the frontal lobe of the cerebrum. Forming the roof of the lateral ventricle, the corpus callosum is a band of white matter formed by commissural fibers projecting between the right and left cerebral hemispheres. Below the lateral ventricles, the head of the caudate nucleus is protruding into the anterior horn of the lateral ventricle, and the thalamus is protruding into the body of the lateral ventricle. Below the thalamus, the pons can be seen as an enlarged region of the brainstem anterior to the cerebellum.

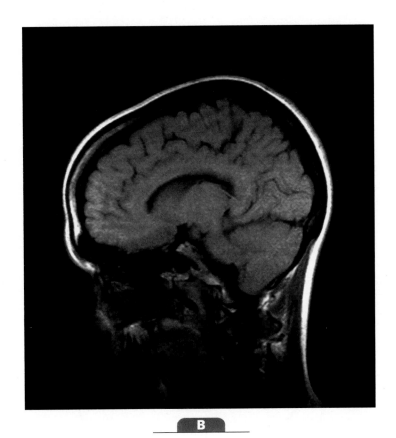

B

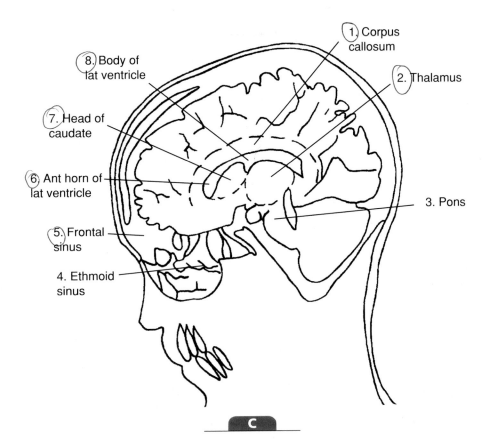

1. Corpus callosum

8. Body of lat ventricle

2. Thalamus

7. Head of caudate

6. Ant horn of lat ventricle

3. Pons

5. Frontal sinus

4. Ethmoid sinus

C

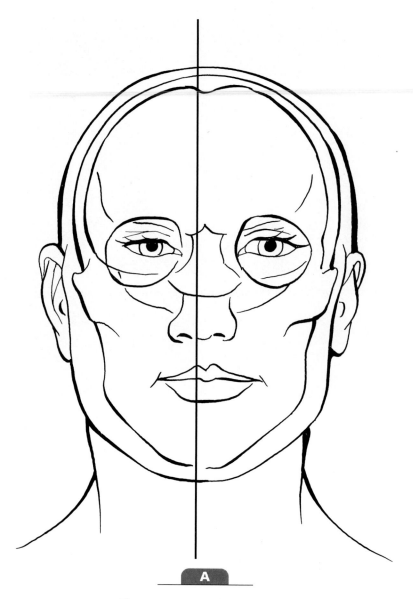

Figure 5-25 Sagittal MR image 8.

Figure 5-25 (A,B,C). On the surface outline of this image, the nose is shown in full profile, indicating this section is near the mid-sagittal plane. Below the nasal cavity, the muscles of the tongue are shown in front of the vertebral column. Similar to the previous image, the frontal sinus appears as an enlarged area of the skull just above the nasal cavity. Because this image is near the midline, the ethmoid air cells are no longer visualized; and an enlarged region of the skull, the sphenoid sinus, is forming the posterior border of the nasal cavity. Immediately posterior to the sphenoid sinus, a dense area formed by the sphenoid bone and basilar part of the occipital bone is labeled the clivus. In the upper part of the sphenoid sinus, the pituitary gland is demonstrated on the base of the brain centrally situated between the cerebral hemispheres. The commissural fibers of the corpus callosum are now found anteriorly forming a bend, or genu, that gives rise to the anterior commissure at its most inferior point. Posteriorly, the enlarged part of the corpus callosum forms the splenium. In the region previously occupied by the thalamus, a round commissural bundle called the intermediate mass is shown in cross-section as it extends through the third ventricle between the right and left thalamic nuclei. In this section, the fibers connecting with the cerebrum are shown forming the most superior part of the brainstem, the cerebral peduncles. Below the cerebral peduncles, the fibers from the cerebellum join those from the cerebrum, forming an enlarged region (the pons) that makes up the anterior border of the fourth ventricle. The lower part of the brainstem, the medulla oblongata, gradually narrows as it travels toward the foramen magnum, where it continues as the spinal cord as it exits the cranial cavity.

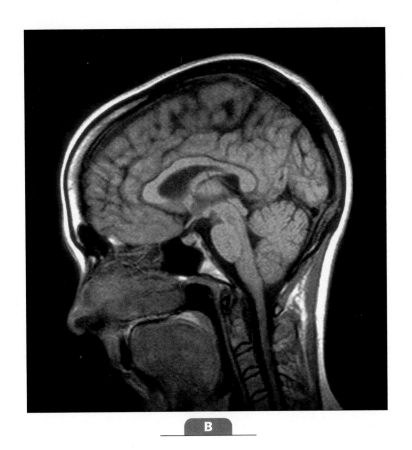

B

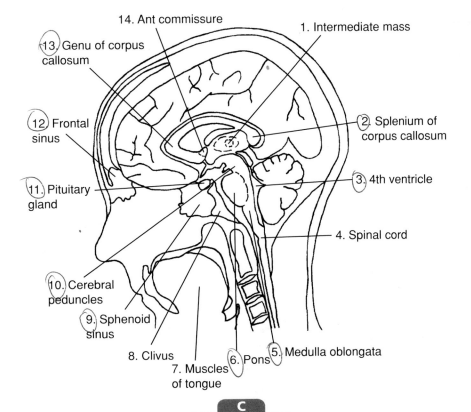

C

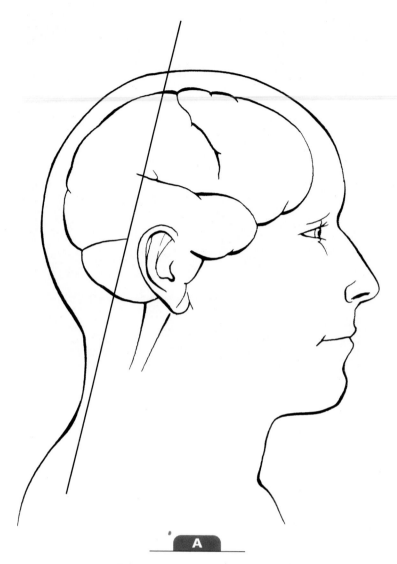

Figure 5-26 Coronal MR image 1.

CORONAL MR IMAGES

The following 16 images of the head will be described at 5.5 mm intervals from posterior to anterior. The images were generated at the following technical factors: TR = 2000, TE = 80, RF = 90°, FOV = 25 cm, TH = 5.0 mm. Abbreviations: TR = repetition time, TE = echo-time, RF = radiofrequency, FOV = field of view, TH = slice thickness.

Figure 5-26 (A,B,C). Generated through the posterior part of the brain, this section demonstrates the occipital lobes and the underlying cerebellum in the posterior cranial fossa. The right and left cerebral hemispheres are separated by the falx cerebri, and the cerebrum is separated from the underlying cerebellum by the tentorium cerebelli. Unlike the cerebral hemispheres, the cerebellar hemispheres are not clearly separable, except on the lower border where the indentation creates the enlarged subarachnoid space just above the foramen magnum known as the cisterna magna. On either side of the cisterna magna, the cerebellar tonsils are labeled as the lower and medial segments of the cerebellar hemispheres.

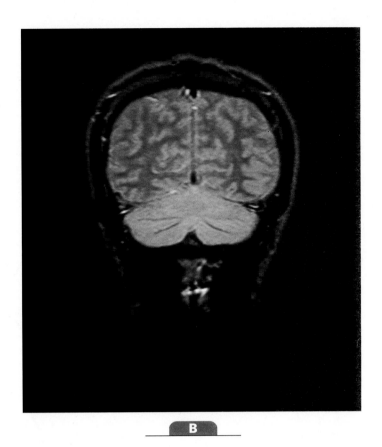

B

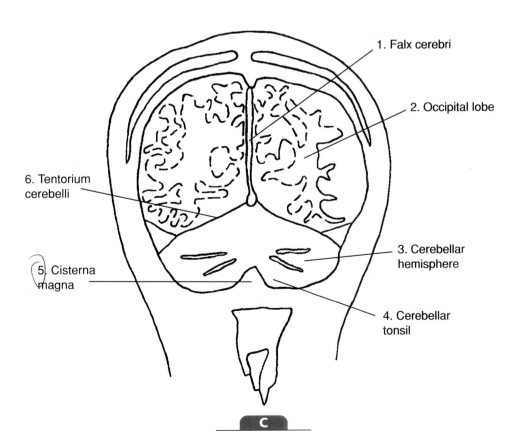

1. Falx cerebri

2. Occipital lobe

6. Tentorium cerebelli

3. Cerebellar hemisphere

5. Cisterna magna

4. Cerebellar tonsil

C

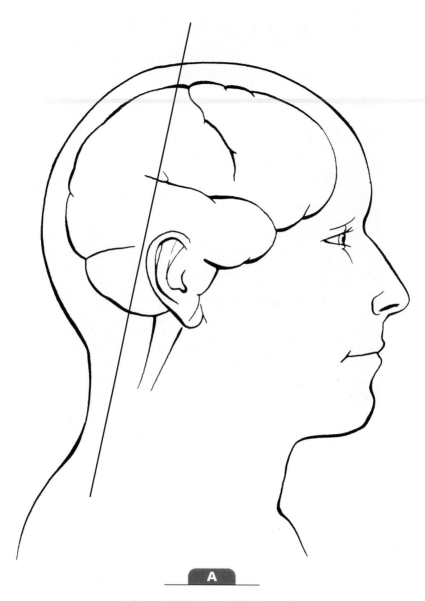

Figure 5-27 Coronal MR image 2.

Figure 5-27 (A,B,C). Compared to the previous image, the more anterior location of this section better demonstrates the white matter within the occipital lobe surrounded by the gray matter of the cortex. The falx cerebri separates the right and left cerebral lobes and creates a lumen along its boundary, forming parts of the dural venous sinuses, the straight sinus, and superior sagittal sinus. Similar to the cerebral hemispheres, the white matter within the cerebellar hemispheres is now better visualized within the central part of the cerebellum. Although the cerebellar tonsils are no longer seen on the lower cerebellum, the superior cerebellar vermis is sectioned as it joins the two cerebellar hemispheres. As described in the previous image, the tentorium cerebelli separates the cerebrum and cerebellum. The lateral borders of the tentorium cerebelli and the endosteal dura lining the inside of the skull form the transverse sinuses. In the midline, the tentorium cerebelli and the falx cerebri join together to form the straight sinus.

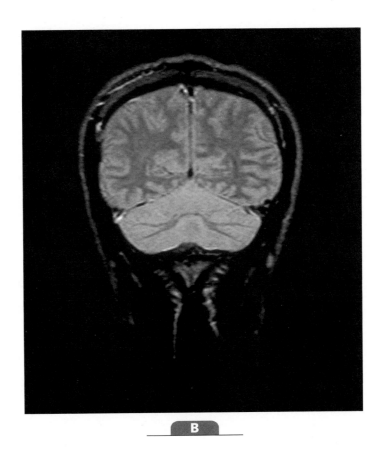

B

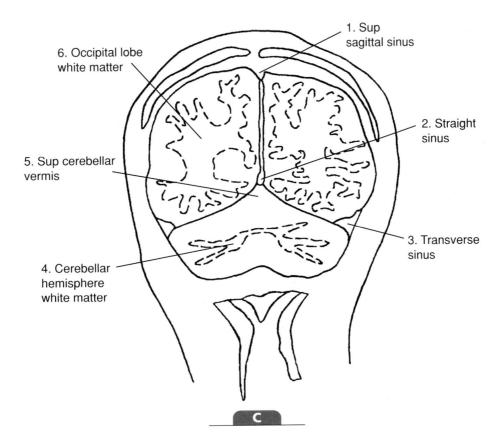

6. Occipital lobe
white matter

1. Sup
sagittal sinus

2. Straight
sinus

5. Sup cerebellar
vermis

3. Transverse
sinus

4. Cerebellar
hemisphere
white matter

C

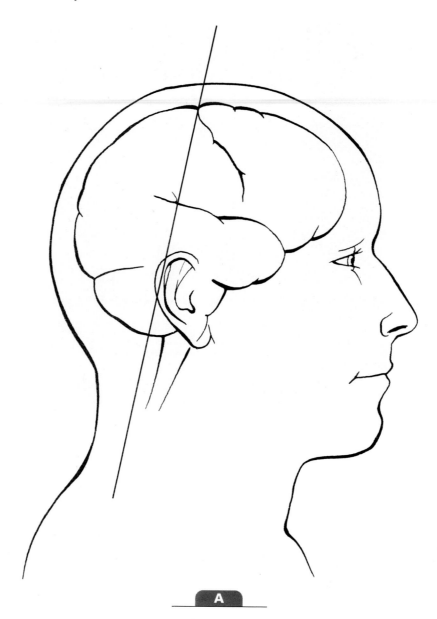

Figure 5-28 Coronal MR image 3.

Figure 5-28 (A,B,C). As in the previous images, the falx cerebri separates the right and left cerebral hemispheres. Below the cerebrum, the cerebellum appears more triangular in shape and the superior cerebellar vermis lies directly below the tentorium cerebelli. The cerebellar vermis is a median strip joining the right and left cerebellar hemispheres. Below the cerebellum, the occipital bone is seen as a dark area extending around the neural structures just described. Outside of the occipital bone, several layers of the scalp can be delineated on the top of the skull.

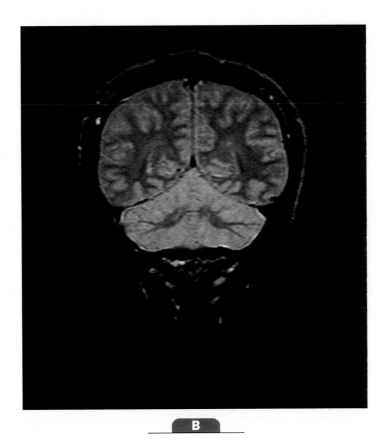

B

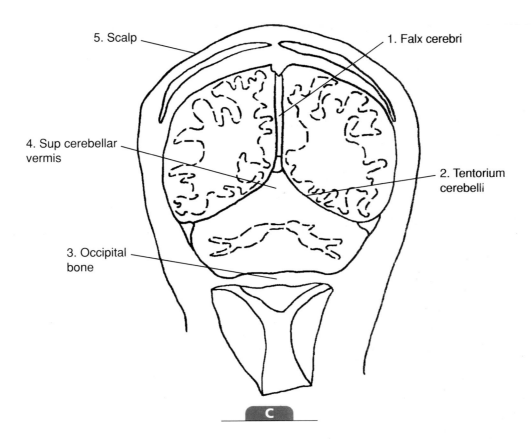

5. Scalp

1. Falx cerebri

4. Sup cerebellar vermis

2. Tentorium cerebelli

3. Occipital bone

C

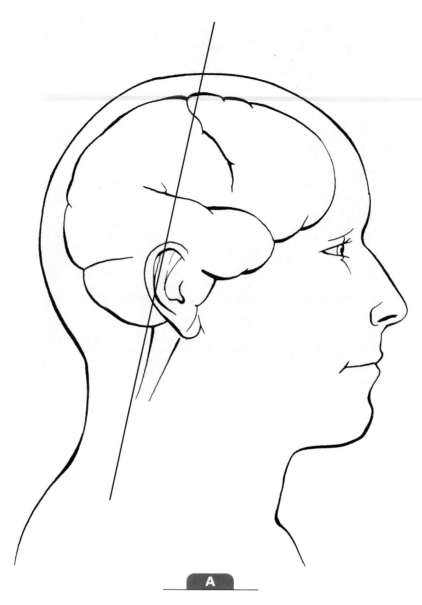

Figure 5-29 Coronal MR image 4.

Figure 5-29 (A,B,C). The unique shape of the cerebellum in this image demonstrates that the plane of section is near the anterior part of the cerebellum. Compared to the previous image, an inferior projection now appears continuous with the cerebellum, representing the posterior medulla oblongata. Although it cannot clearly be delineated here, the fourth ventricle is above the posterior medulla oblongata in the central region of the cerebellum. On either side of the cerebellar hemispheres, the transverse sinuses are within the lateral margin of the tentorium cerebelli. Above the cerebellum, the straight sinus is near the midline in the tentorium cerebelli and is connected via the falx cerebri to the superior sagittal sinus. Within the cerebral hemispheres, fluid-filled regions within the white matter are now discernible, representing the posterior horns of the lateral ventricles.

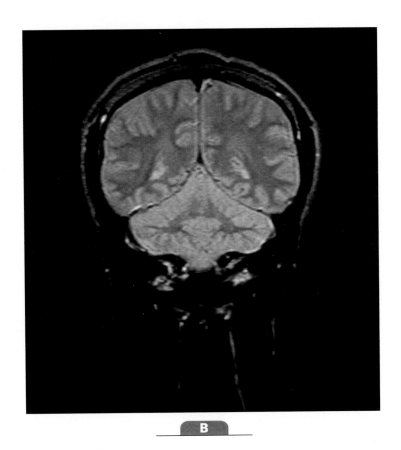

B

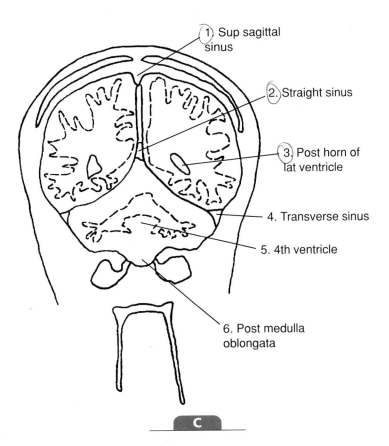

1. Sup sagittal sinus

2. Straight sinus

3. Post horn of lat ventricle

4. Transverse sinus

5. 4th ventricle

6. Post medulla oblongata

C

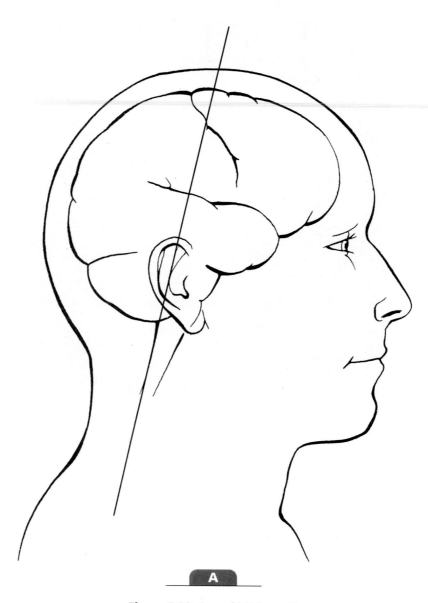

Figure 5-30 Coronal MR image 5.

Figure 5-30 (A,B,C). The diamond shape of the cerebellar region in this image indicates that this section includes the anterior cerebellum and the lower part of the brainstem, the medulla oblongata. Although not clearly discernible, the fourth ventricle is within the central cerebellum and the superior cerebellar vermis is just below the superior cistern. Together, these structures lie just below the tentorium cerebelli that joins with the falx cerebri to form the straight sinus. Within the cerebral hemispheres, the enlarged hyperdense regions within the white matter are labeled the posterior horns of the lateral ventricles within the occipital lobes.

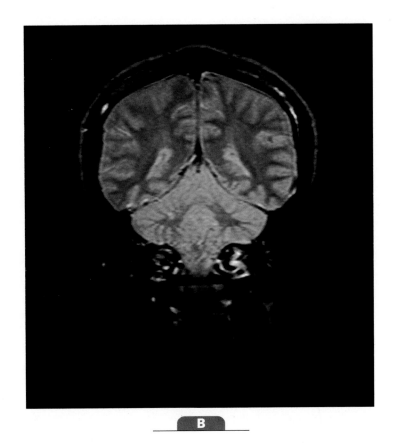

B

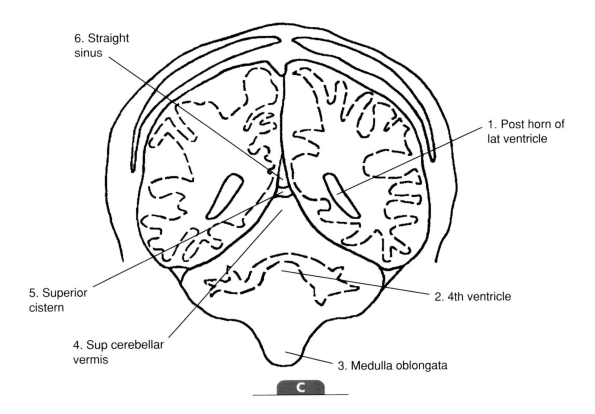

6. Straight
sinus

1. Post horn of
lat ventricle

5. Superior
cistern

2. 4th ventricle

4. Sup cerebellar
vermis

3. Medulla oblongata

C

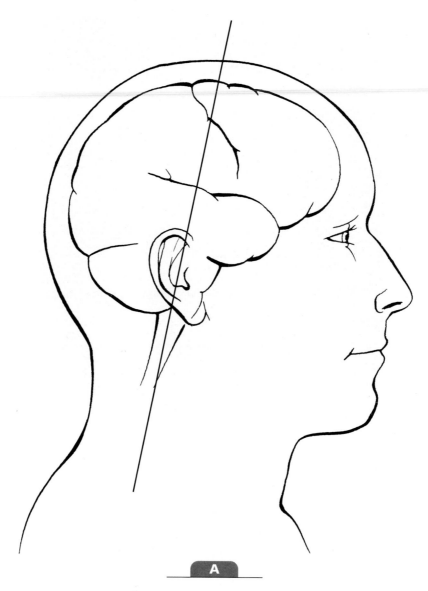

A

Figure 5-31 Coronal MR image 6.

Figure 5-31 (A,B,C). The cervical spinal cord on the lower part of this image indicates the plane of this section includes the contents of the foramen magnum. Forming the lower brainstem, the medulla oblongata and the posterior pons are surrounded on either side by the margins of the right and left cerebellar hemispheres. Although the lateral margins and transverse sinuses are still found between the cerebrum and cerebellum, the tentorium cerebelli and straight sinus are no longer seen centrally. Instead, a pair of internal cerebral veins are directly below the splenium of the corpus callosum. This pair of internal cerebral veins drain into the vein of Galen that extends only a short distance before emptying into the straight sinus. As described earlier, the splenium of the corpus callosum is continuous with the white matter of the cerebral hemispheres and acts as a commissural route for fibers to extend between the right and left cerebral hemispheres. Lateral to the splenium of the corpus callosum, the deep groove of the Sylvian fissure divides the parietal and temporal lobes of the cerebrum. Within the white matter of these lobes, the CSF-filled lateral ventricle appears enlarged, representing the region of the collateral trigone. Immediately below the collateral trigone of the lateral ventricle, a convoluted region of gray matter deep within the temporal lobe represents the hippocampal formation. As described previously, the hippocampal formation is considered part of the limbic system and serves a vital role in emotional behavior.

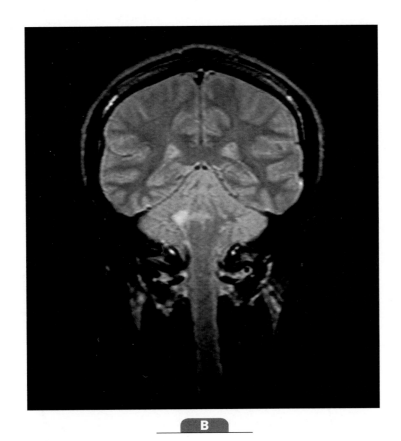

B

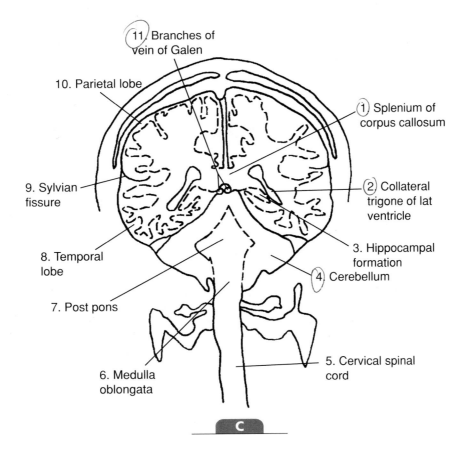

11. Branches of vein of Galen

10. Parietal lobe

1. Splenium of corpus callosum

9. Sylvian fissure

2. Collateral trigone of lat ventricle

8. Temporal lobe

3. Hippocampal formation

4. Cerebellum

7. Post pons

5. Cervical spinal cord

6. Medulla oblongata

C

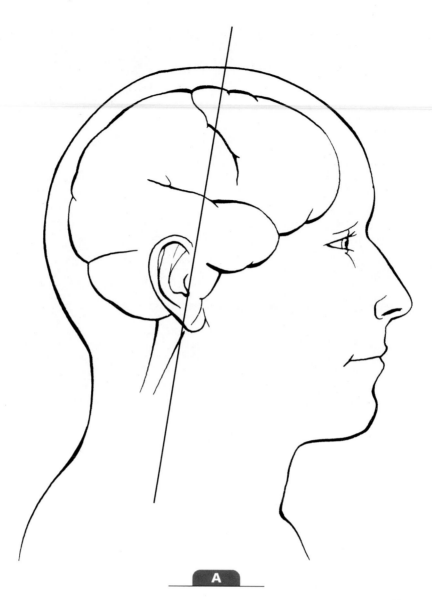

Figure 5-32 Coronal MR image 7.

Figure 5-32 (A,B,C). The absence of much of the cerebellar hemispheres in this image indicates the plane of the section to be near the midline of the head. The enlarged region of the brainstem (the pons) is centrally located in the region previously occupied by the cerebellum. Immediately below the pons, the medulla oblongata appears as the enlarged part of the brainstem that continues as the spinal cord below the occipital bone. Unlike previous images, this section demonstrates all three of the parts of the brainstem: the medulla oblongata, the pons, and the midbrain. Although not labeled the midbrain, the quadrigeminal plate and the cerebral aqueduct are within the midbrain region of the brainstem. The quadrigeminal plate is found in the region previously occupied by the cerebellar vermis. Below the quadrigeminal plate, the opening of the cerebral aqueduct is cross-sectioned, extending between the third and fourth ventricles. The pineal gland is found medially between the bodies of the lateral ventricles. In this more anterior section, the collateral trigone of the lateral ventricle has given rise to the body and inferior horns of the lateral ventricles separated by a region of gray matter, the thalamus. As in previous images, the white matter extending between the cerebral cortex and the basal ganglia are collectively called the corona radiata.

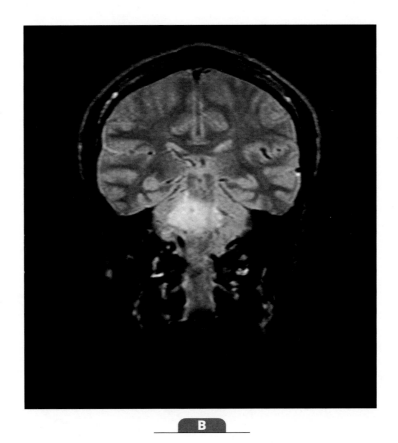

B

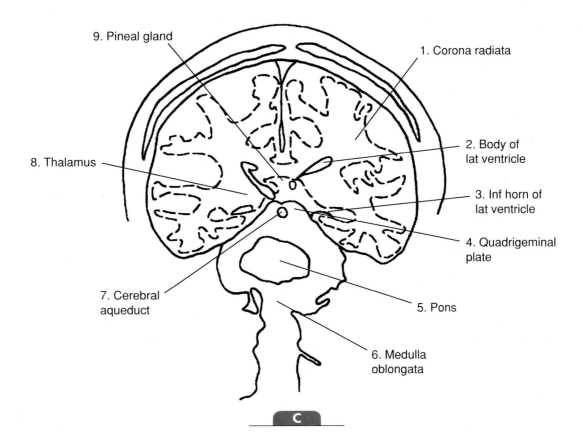

9. Pineal gland

1. Corona radiata

8. Thalamus

2. Body of lat ventricle

3. Inf horn of lat ventricle

4. Quadrigeminal plate

7. Cerebral aqueduct

5. Pons

6. Medulla oblongata

C

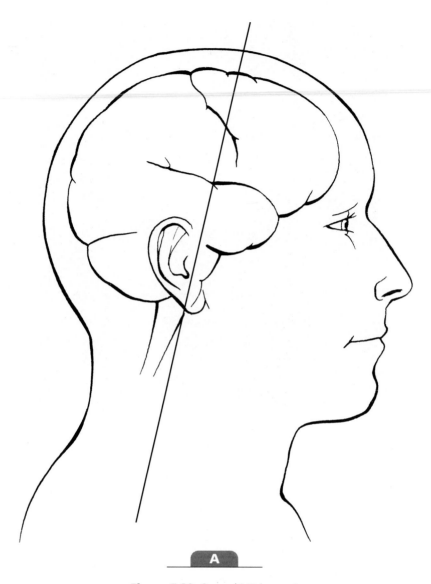

Figure 5-33 Coronal MR image 8.

Figure 5-33 (A,B,C). The pons is a hyperdense region near the center of this image, below the cerebral hemispheres. Directly above the pons, the cerebral peduncles are found below the opening of the third ventricle. On either side of the third ventricle, the thalamic nuclei are found between the body and inferior horns of the lateral ventricles. Directly below the inferior horn of the lateral ventricle, the convoluted regions of gray matter represent the hippocampal formations. Lateral to the thalamic nuclei, the deep groove or Sylvian fissure is found dividing the cerebral hemispheres. Surrounding the medial part of the Sylvian fissure, the insula is the region of gray matter forming what is also referred to as the inner lobe of the brain.

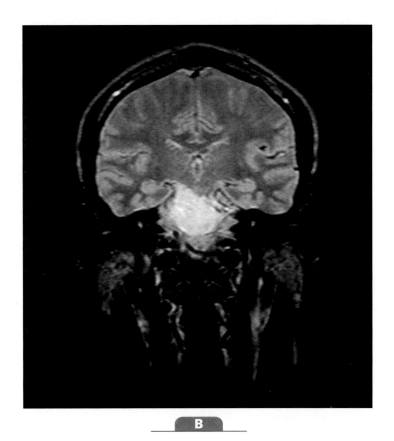

B

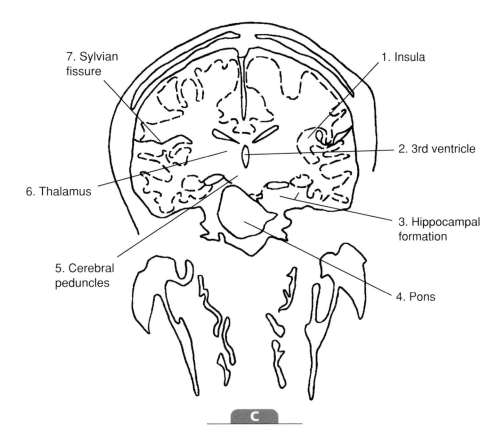

7. Sylvian fissure

1. Insula

2. 3rd ventricle

6. Thalamus

3. Hippocampal formation

5. Cerebral peduncles

4. Pons

C

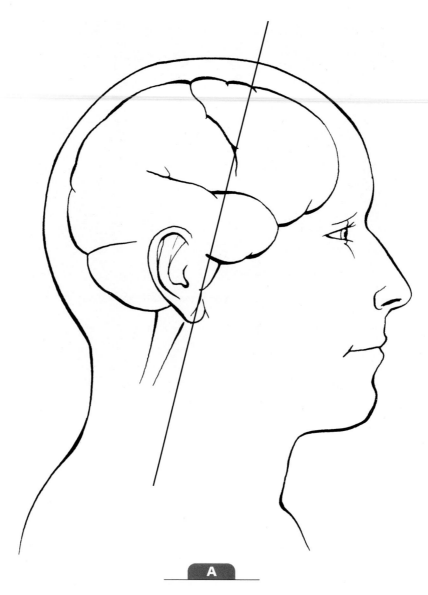

Figure 5-34 Coronal MR image 9.

Figure 5-34 (A,B,C). Similar to the previous image, the pons can be readily identified as a hyperdense region immediately below the cerebral hemispheres. Directly above the pons, the third ventricle is demonstrated in the midline and appears continuous with the lateral ventricles. On either side of the third ventricle, the oval-shaped thalamic nuclei occupy a medial location in the cerebral hemispheres. Below the thalamic nuclei, a small pair of round nuclei, the red nuclei, are demonstrated within the upper midbrain. Below the red nuclei, the substantia nigrae appear as thin striations of gray matter within the cerebral peduncles of the midbrain.

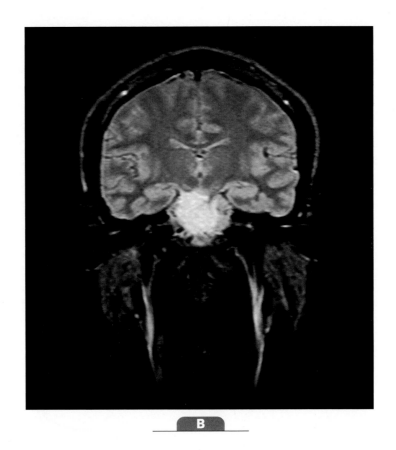

B

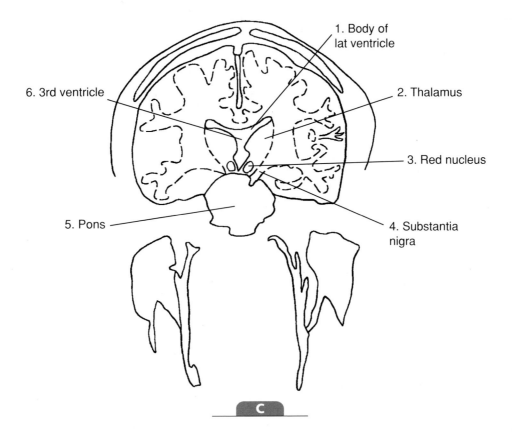

1. Body of
   lat ventricle

6. 3rd ventricle

2. Thalamus

3. Red nucleus

5. Pons

4. Substantia
   nigra

C

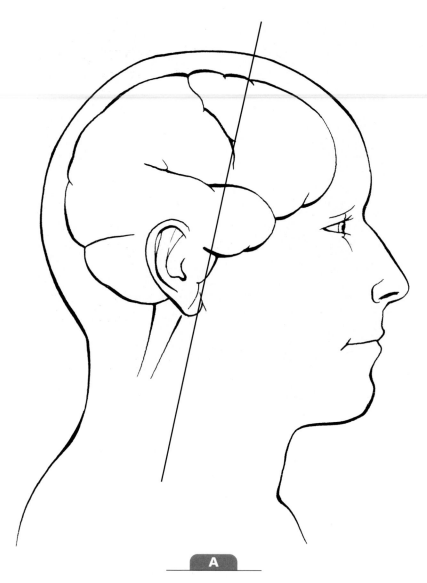

Figure 5-35 Coronal MR image 10.

Figure 5-35 (A,B,C). Although slightly smaller than in previous images, the pons appears as a hyperdense region just below the cerebral hemispheres The midbrain connects the pons with the cerebral hemispheres and is found just below the third ventricle. Within the lower part of the cerebral hemispheres, in the region previously occupied by the inferior horn of the lateral ventricle, the gray matter of the hippocampal formation lies deep within the temporal lobe. Above the lateral ventricles, the body of the corpus callosum extends between the right and left cerebral hemispheres. Immediately above the corpus callosum, the lower margin of the falx cerebri forms a dural venous sinus known as the inferior sagittal sinus. On the superior margin of the falx cerebri and directly below the parietal bones, the superior sagittal sinus is formed, which reabsorbs the majority of the CSF into the venous bloodstream.

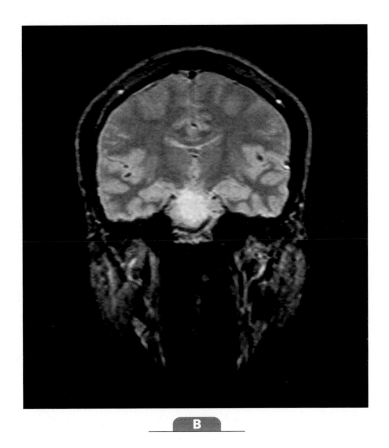

B

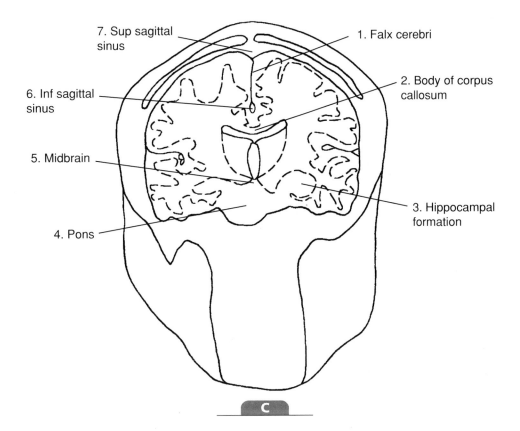

7. Sup sagittal
sinus

1. Falx cerebri

2. Body of corpus
callosum

6. Inf sagittal
sinus

5. Midbrain

3. Hippocampal
formation

4. Pons

C

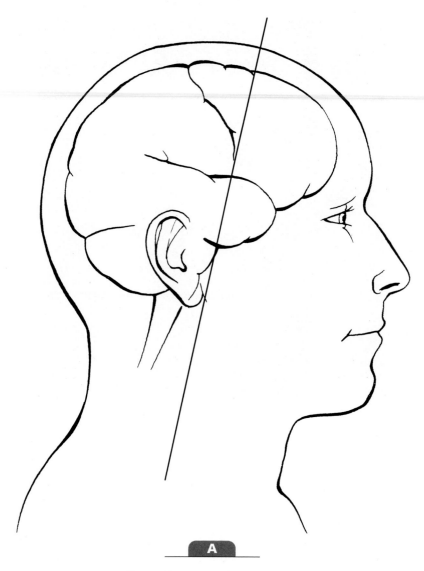

Figure 5-36 Coronal MR image 11.

Figure 5-36 (A,B,C). At this level, only the most anterior part of the pons is seen below the cerebral hemispheres. Similar to the previous images, the third ventricle is found medially located between the thalamic nuclei. In this section, a band of white matter forms what appears as a capsule surrounding the thalamus. The internal capsule separates the thalamus from the lenticular nuclei, the globus pallidus and the putamen.

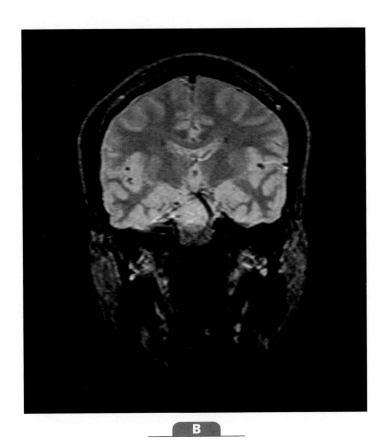

B

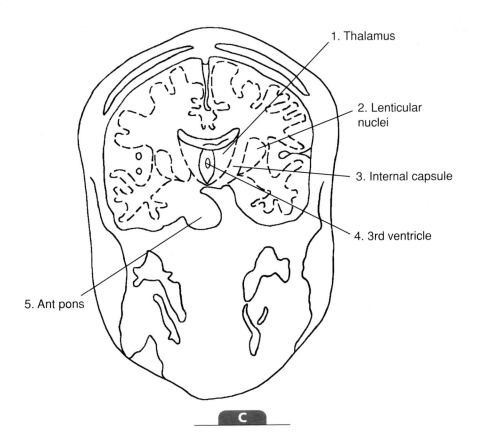

1. Thalamus

2. Lenticular nuclei

3. Internal capsule

4. 3rd ventricle

5. Ant pons

C

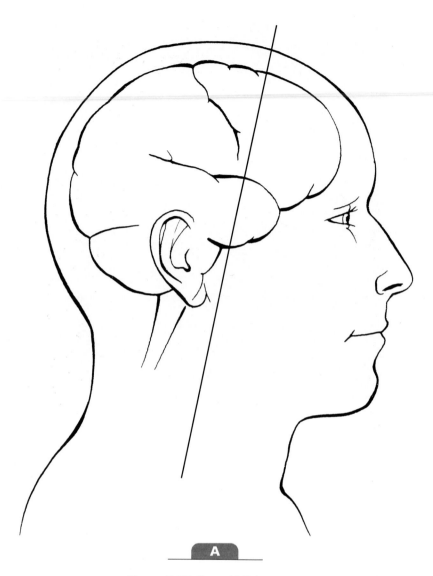

Figure 5-37 Coronal MR image 12.

Figure 5-37 (A,B,C). The right and left cerebral hemispheres are separated by the falx cerebri, which contains the superior sagittal sinus and inferior sagittal sinus. Directly below the falx cerebri, the body of the corpus callosum is found joining the right and left cerebral hemispheres. The Sylvian fissure divides each cerebral hemisphere into parietal and temporal lobes. Although not clearly seen here, the third ventricle would again occupy a medial position below the body of the corpus callosum separating the anterior part of the thalamic nuclei. Lateral to the thalamic nuclei, the lenticular nuclei are now separable into the globus pallidus and the putamen.

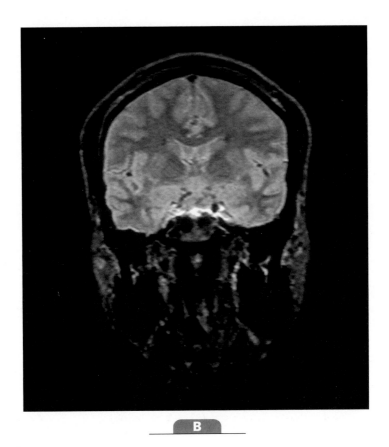

B

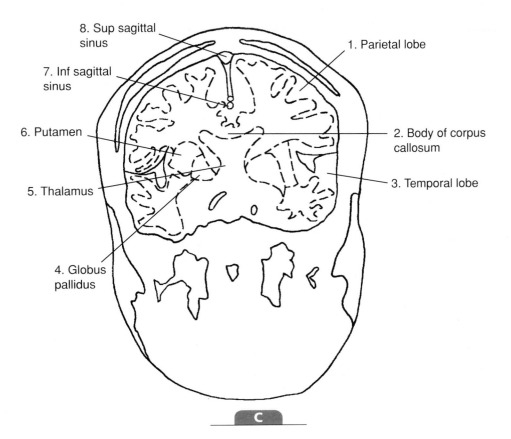

8. Sup sagittal
sinus

7. Inf sagittal
sinus

6. Putamen

5. Thalamus

4. Globus
pallidus

1. Parietal lobe

2. Body of corpus
callosum

3. Temporal lobe

C

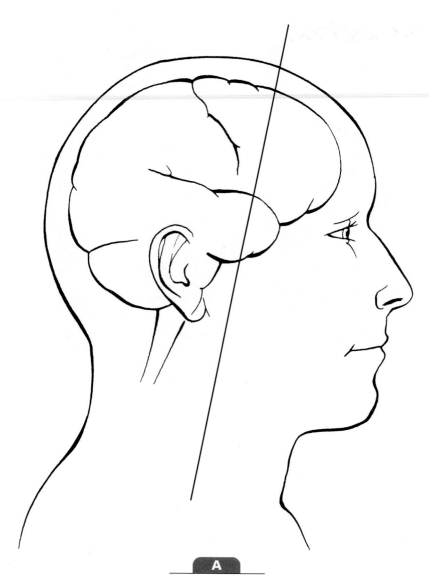

Figure 5-38 Coronal MR image 13.

Figure 5-38 (A,B,C). Directly below the cerebral hemispheres in the region previously occupied by the pons, an enlarged region of the skull can be seen representing the sphenoid sinus. Just above the sphenoid sinus in the region of the sella turcica, the oval-shaped pituitary gland can be identified below the cerebrum. Directly above the pituitary gland, the nerve fibers within the optic chiasma are sectioned as they extend from the cerebral hemispheres toward the globes of the eyes. On either side of the optic chiasma, the internal carotid arteries are sectioned as they ascend to bifurcate into the anterior and middle cerebral arteries. Although the lumina are not readily apparent, the anterior horns of the lateral ventricles are found directly below the body of the corpus callosum. Within the anterior horns of the lateral ventricles, the heads of the caudate nuclei are shown protruding into the opening on either side.

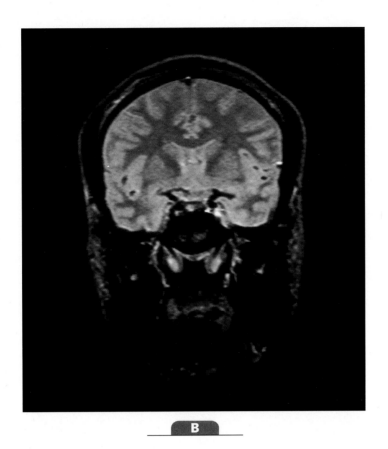

B

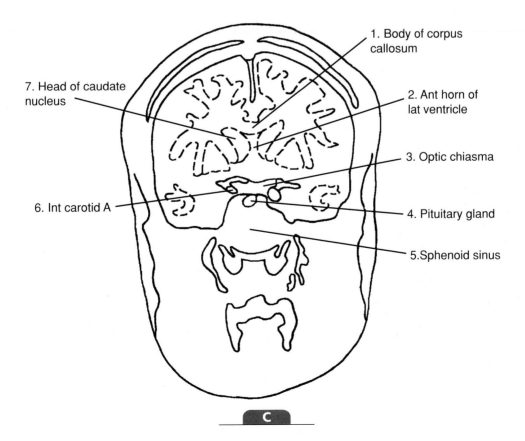

1. Body of corpus callosum

7. Head of caudate nucleus

2. Ant horn of lat ventricle

3. Optic chiasma

6. Int carotid A

4. Pituitary gland

5.Sphenoid sinus

C

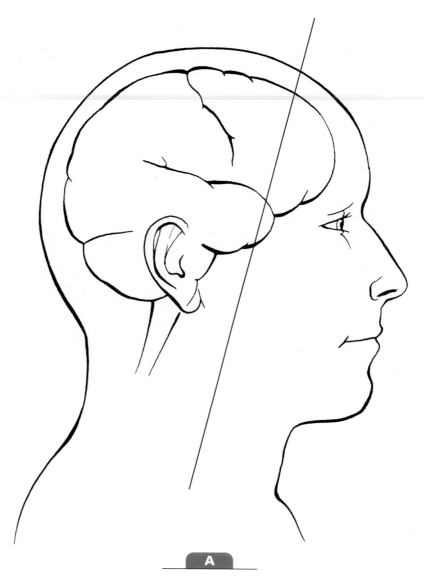

A

Figure 5-39 Coronal MR image 14.

Figure 5-39 (A,B,C). Sectioned through the anterior cerebrum, the frontal lobe is separated from the anterior part of the temporal lobe by the Sylvian fissure, which contains branches of the middle cerebral artery. As described earlier, the middle cerebral artery originates from the internal carotid artery just above the sphenoid sinus. Similar to the previous image, the anterior horns of the lateral ventricles are barely visible between the septum pellucidum and the heads of the caudate nuclei. The internal capsule is the band of white matter separating the gray matter of the caudate nucleus from that of the lenticular nuclei. On the lower part of the image, a distinct hypodense region can be identified below the sphenoid sinus as the region of the nasopharynx.

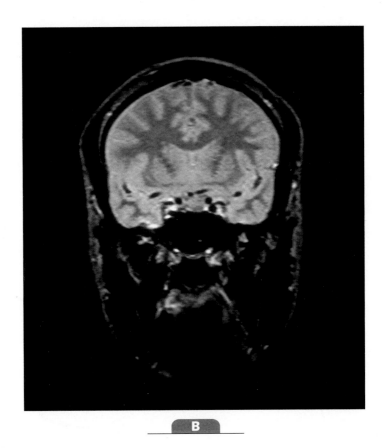

B

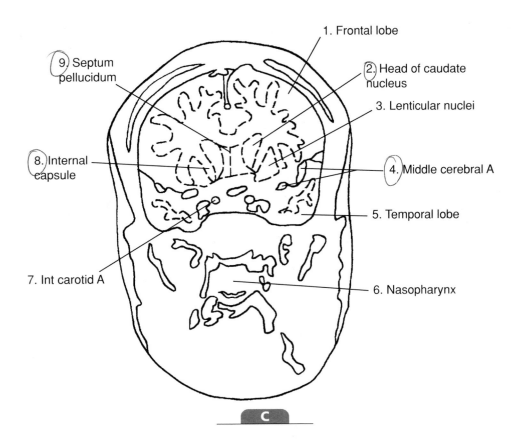

9. Septum pellucidum

1. Frontal lobe

2. Head of caudate nucleus

3. Lenticular nuclei

8. Internal capsule

4. Middle cerebral A

5. Temporal lobe

7. Int carotid A

6. Nasopharynx

C

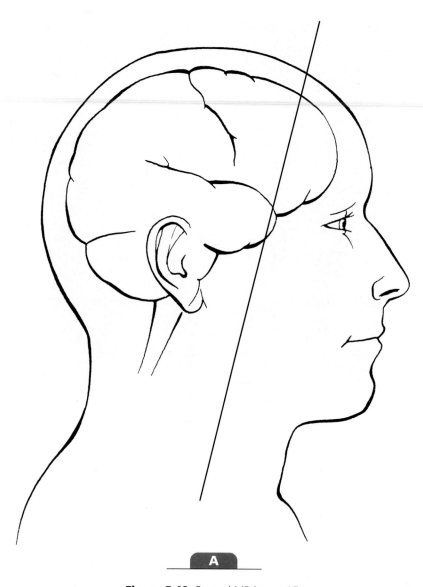

Figure 5-40 Coronal MR image 15.

Figure 5-40 (A,B,C). This image of the anterior head clearly demonstrates the relationship between the nasopharynx and the more superiorly located sphenoid sinus. Directly above the sphenoid sinus, the anterior cerebral arteries are cut in cross-section as they extend from their origin, the internal carotid arteries, to their destination in the anterior cerebrum. Within the cerebral hemispheres, the white matter is formed by a collection of nerve fibers, and the gray matter of the cerebral cortex is formed by a collection of nerve cell bodies.

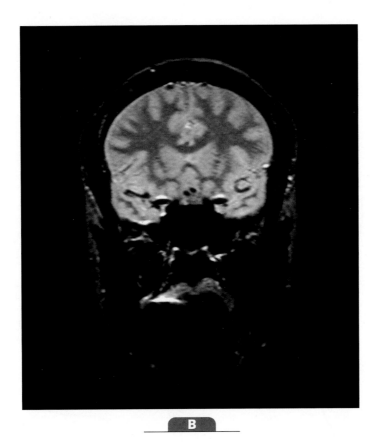

B

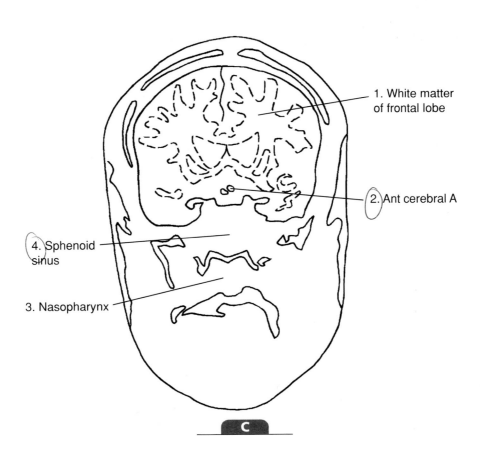

1. White matter of frontal lobe

2. Ant cerebral A

4. Sphenoid sinus

3. Nasopharynx

C

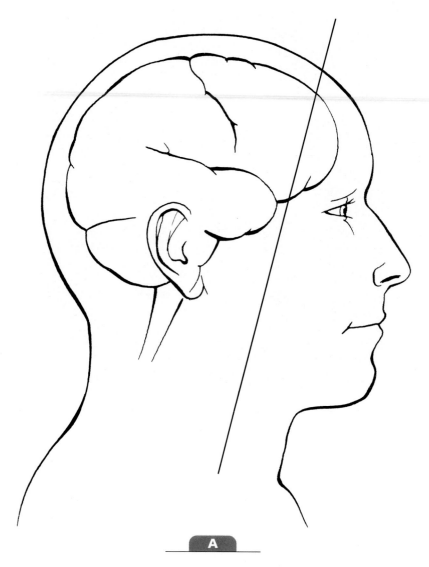

Figure 5-41 Coronal MR image 16.

Figure 5-41 (A,B,C). This image shows the anterior-most section through the cerebral hemispheres. The right and left frontal lobes are connected through the commissural fibers forming the genu of the corpus callosum located between the hemispheres. In the region previously occupied by the anterior horn of the lateral ventricle, the head of the caudate nucleus appears as an island of gray matter surrounded by white matter. Below the cerebrum, the right and left optic nerves are found in cross-section as they extend toward the globe of the eye. In the midline, the hypodense region of the sphenoid sinus is labeled between the optic nerves. Below the sphenoid sinus, in the location previously occupied by the nasopharynx, the inferior nasal conchae are sectioned on either side within the nasal cavity.

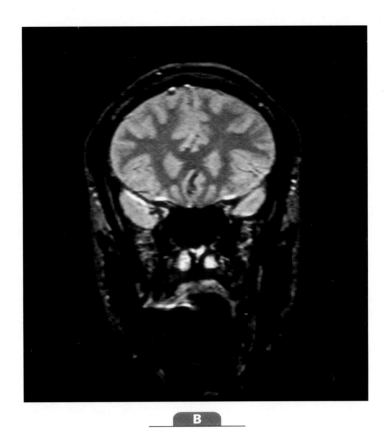

B

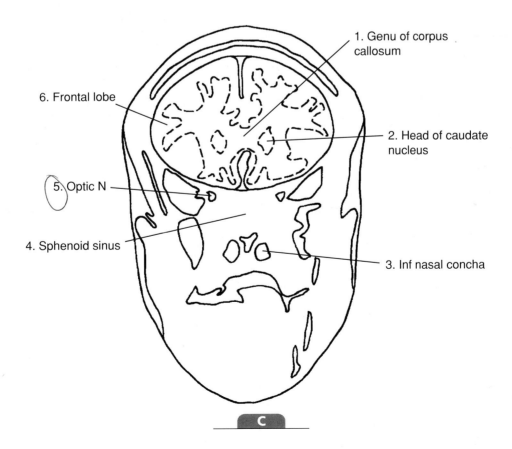

1. Genu of corpus callosum

6. Frontal lobe

2. Head of caudate nucleus

5. Optic N

4. Sphenoid sinus

3. Inf nasal concha

C

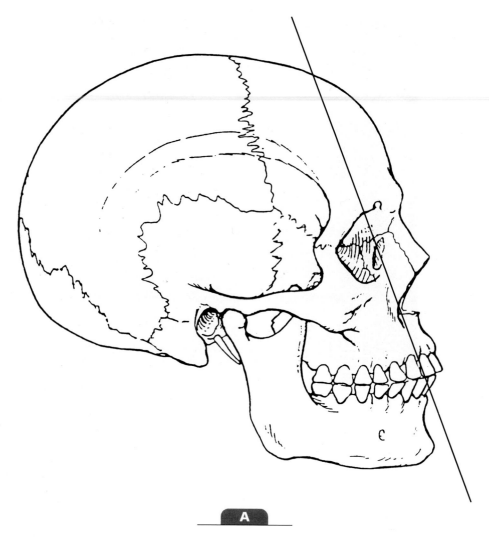

A

Figure 5-42 Axial CT image 1.

Coronal CT Images

The following 5 images of the face will be described at 4.0 mm intervals from anterior to posterior. The images were generated at the following technical factors: 120 kVp and 180 mA-s. Abbreviations: kVp = kilovolt peak, mA-s = milliampere-second.

Figure 5-42 (A,B,C). The frontal sinus is readily identified encased within the frontal bone at the upper part of this image and is found above the nasal cavity. Within the nasal cavity, the perpendicular plate of the ethmoid bone and septal cartilage divide the area into right and left parts. Below the nasal cavity, the maxillary bones extend to the upper teeth bordering the anterior oral cavity. On the right side, the anterior-most part of the right maxillary sinus is found between the nasal cavity and the region of the right eye. Because this plane of section runs through the anterior-most part of the eye, the right cornea is shown between the upper and lower eyelids.

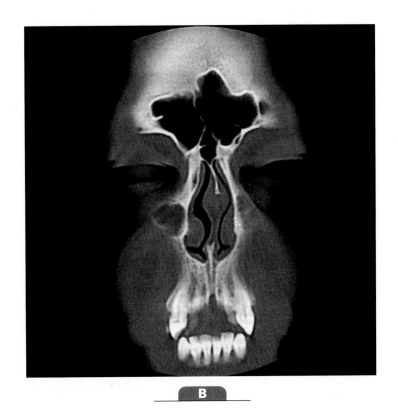

B

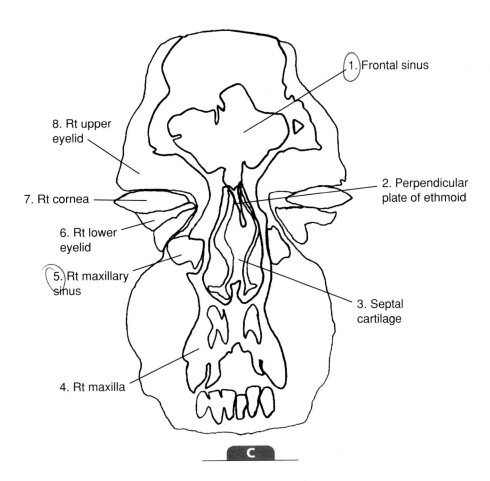

1. Frontal sinus

8. Rt upper eyelid

7. Rt cornea

6. Rt lower eyelid

5. Rt maxillary sinus

4. Rt maxilla

2. Perpendicular plate of ethmoid

3. Septal cartilage

C

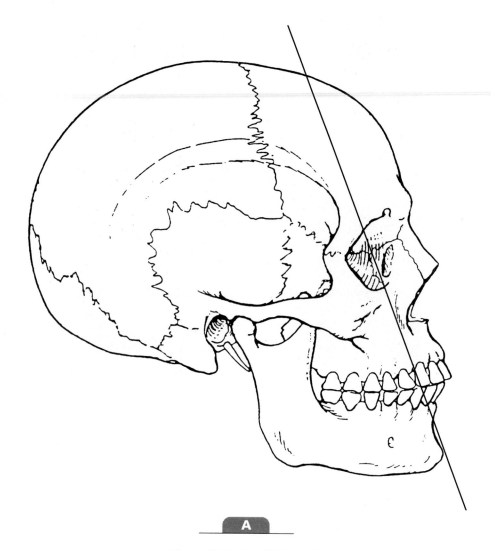

Figure 5-43 Axial CT image 2.

Figure 5-43 (A,B,C). The frontal bone is again shown to contain the frontal sinus, which is located above the contents of the nasal cavity. Within the nasal cavity, the nasal septum is formed by two bony projections on either end that are separated by septal cartilage. As described earlier and shown in Figure 5-3, the perpendicular plate of the ethmoid bone is the more superior part of the nasal septum, whereas the vomer forms the lower part. On either side of the nasal septum, the inferior conchae are found adjacent to the wall of the maxillary sinus. Below the nasal cavity, the maxillary bones are shown projecting downward to the teeth on either side and form the roof of the oral cavity.

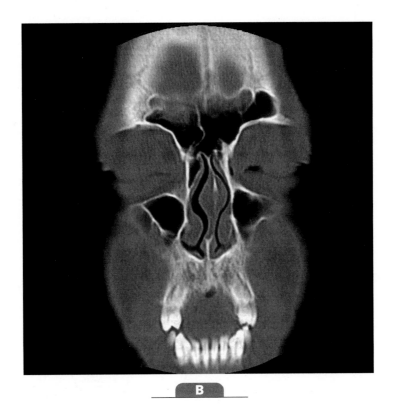

B

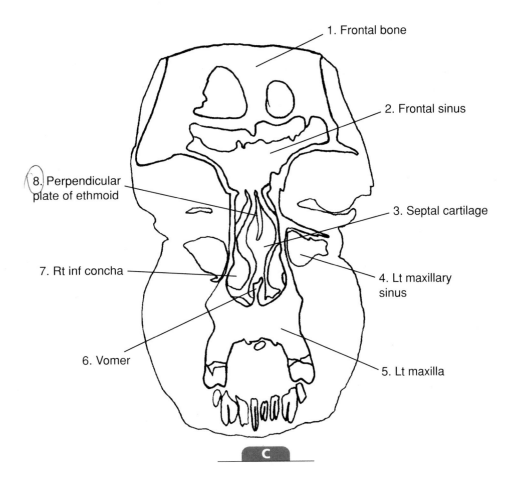

1. Frontal bone

2. Frontal sinus

8. Perpendicular plate of ethmoid

3. Septal cartilage

7. Rt inf concha

4. Lt maxillary sinus

6. Vomer

5. Lt maxilla

C

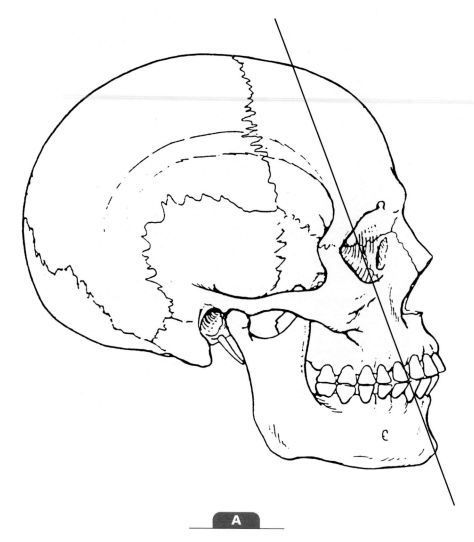

A

Figure 5-44 Axial CT image 3.

Figure 5-44 (A,B,C). Similar to the previous images, the frontal sinus is shown encased by the frontal bone, but it appears smaller in this image. Although the frontal sinus is still located above the nasal cavity, several air cells found directly between the eyes separate the frontal sinus from the lower nasal cavity. Similar to the previous image, the septum dividing the nasal cavity is formed by the perpendicular plate of the ethmoid, septal cartilage, and the vomer. Although one would expect this nasal septum to divide the nasal cavity into equal and symmetrical parts, the deviation of the septum to the left side seen in this patient is not an uncommon finding. On either side of the nasal septum, the inferior conchae span from superior to inferior through most of the nasal cavity. On either side of the nasal cavity, the maxillary sinuses are shown within the maxillary bones and are larger than in previous images. The maxillary bones extend downward on either side, forming the roof of the oral cavity, which is filled with the musculature of the upper tongue, the genioglossus muscle.

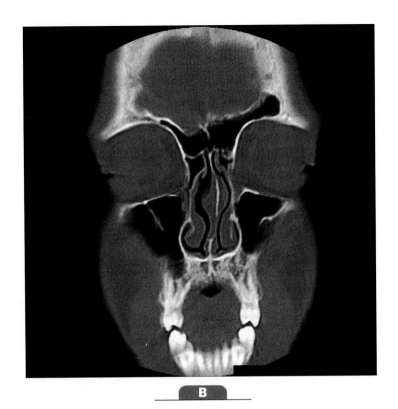

B

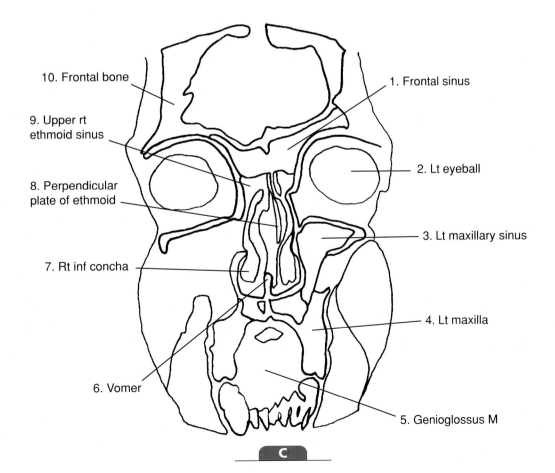

10. Frontal bone

9. Upper rt
ethmoid sinus

8. Perpendicular
plate of ethmoid

7. Rt inf concha

6. Vomer

1. Frontal sinus

2. Lt eyeball

3. Lt maxillary sinus

4. Lt maxilla

5. Genioglossus M

C

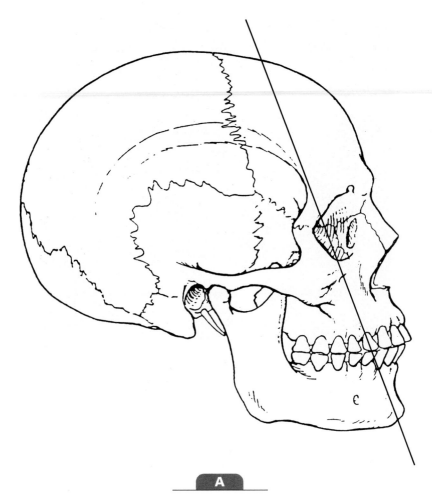

A

Figure 5-45 Axial CT image 4.

Figure 5-45 (A,B,C). At this level through the anterior face, the orbital plate of the frontal bone is shown forming the upper margin of the bony orbit. Between the right and left orbital cavities, several specific structures can now be identified within the ethmoid bone. Near the midline, a small projection of bone can be seen extending upward, representing the crista galli, which is surrounded on either side by the cribriform plate. As described earlier, perforations in the cribriform plate transmit the first pair of cranial nerves, the olfactory nerves, from the mucous membranes lining the nasal cavity. Below the cribriform plate, the air cells forming the ethmoid sinus are again shown between the orbits. In this more posterior plane, the inferior and middle conchae are shown in either side of the nasal cavity. By comparison, the middle conchae is shorter and more superior than the inferior concha. On either side of the nasal cavity, air is found within the large, triangular-shaped maxillary sinuses. On the lateral side of the face, the zygomatic bones are now shown, in section, forming the lower lateral boundary of the bony orbit. Below the nasal cavity, the palatine process of the maxilla is shown forming the roof of the oral cavity. Below the oral cavity, the tongue, or genioglossus muscle, is again shown and is bounded inferiorly by the mandible.

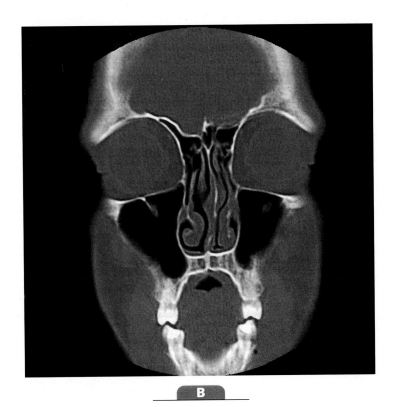

B

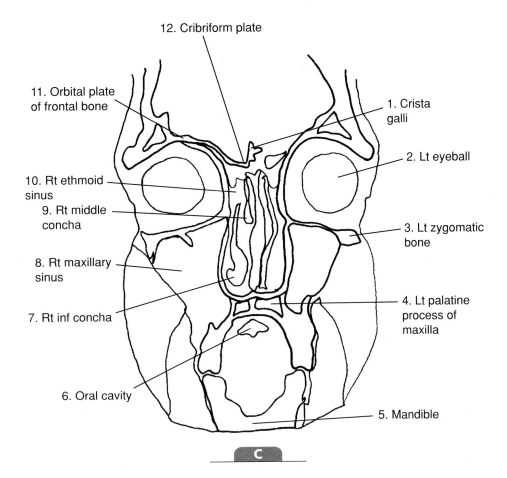

12. Cribriform plate

11. Orbital plate
of frontal bone

10. Rt ethmoid
sinus

9. Rt middle
concha

8. Rt maxillary
sinus

7. Rt inf concha

6. Oral cavity

1. Crista
galli

2. Lt eyeball

3. Lt zygomatic
bone

4. Lt palatine
process of
maxilla

5. Mandible

C

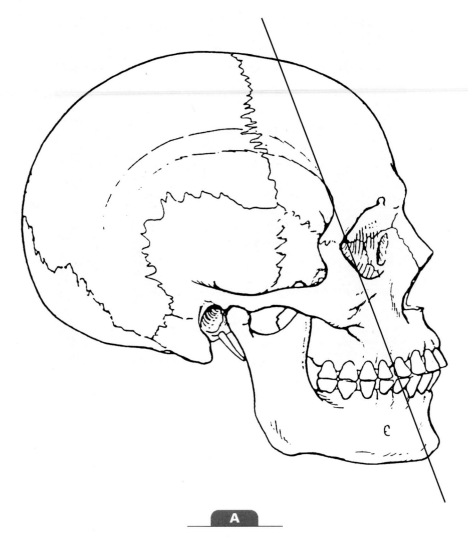

Figure 5-46 Axial CT image 5.

Figure 5-46 (A,B,C). The orbital plate of the frontal bone separates the contents of the orbital cavity from the frontal lobe of the cerebrum. Near the midline, the bony extension of the ethmoid bone projecting upward into the cranial cavity can again be labeled the crista galli, which is bounded on either side by the cribriform plate. Also within the ethmoid bone, the air cells forming the ethmoid sinuses are shown sectioned between the orbits; the middle and inferior conchae are shown on either side of the nasal septum. Similar to the previous image, the large triangular-shaped maxillary sinuses can be seen on either side of the nasal cavity. On the lateral aspect of the maxillary sinuses, the zygomatic bones form the lower outer margin of the bony orbits. Forming the lower margin of the maxillary sinuses, the palatine processes of the maxillae form the roof of the oral cavity, which is labeled above the musculature of the tongue (the genioglossus) and the mandible.

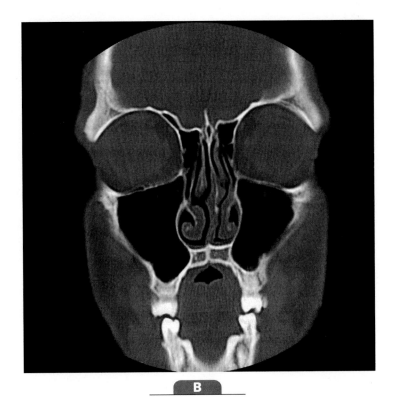

B

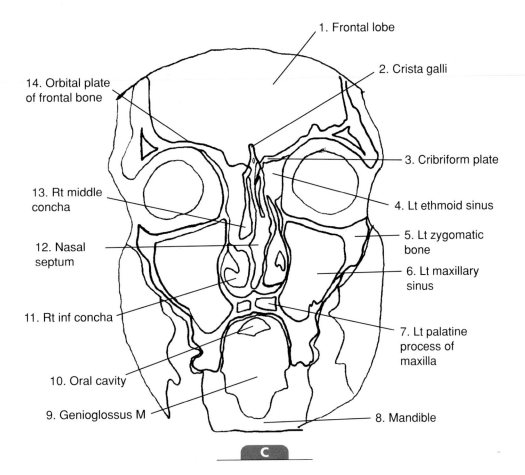

1. Frontal lobe

2. Crista galli

14. Orbital plate of frontal bone

3. Cribriform plate

13. Rt middle concha

4. Lt ethmoid sinus

5. Lt zygomatic bone

12. Nasal septum

6. Lt maxillary sinus

11. Rt inf concha

7. Lt palatine process of maxilla

10. Oral cavity

9. Genioglossus M

8. Mandible

C

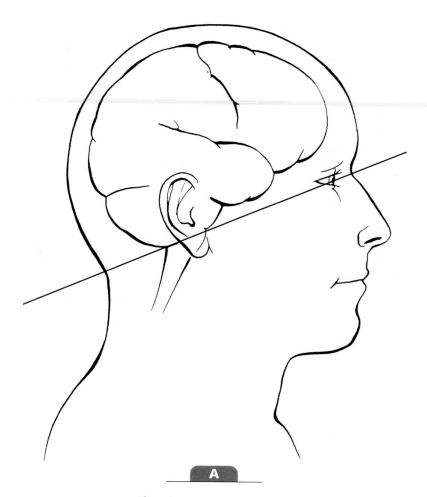

Figure 5-47 Axial CT image 6.

Axial CT Images

The following 16 axial CT images of the head will be described at 8.0 mm intervals from the base to the top of the skull. The sections were taken in a plane 15-20° caudal to the line extending from the infraorbital ridge to the external auditory meatus and the middle of the occipital bone. The images were generated immediately after the administration of venous contrast at the following technical factors: 120 kVp and 250 mA-s. Abbreviations: kVp = kilovolt peak, mA-s = milliampere-second.

Figure 5-47 (A,B,C). Demonstrating the anatomy at the base of the skull, this image would be the first in a series of scans through the region of the head. Most noticeably, the eyes are shown on either side and the lens is apparent on the patient's right side. Between the eyes, the nasal cavity is found, including the medially located vomer bone, which acts to separate much of the right and left nasal cavity. Forming the posterior wall of the bony orbital cavity, the greater wing of the sphenoid is demonstrated. On the left side, the foramen ovale, which transmits the mandibular branch of cranial nerve V, the trigeminal nerve, can be seen. The clivus, formed by the body of the sphenoid bone and the basilar part of the occipital bone, is shown centrally located within the base of the skull. On either side of the clivus, the foramina lacerum are shown at the juncture of the occipital, temporal, and sphenoid bones. Within the petrous portion of the temporal bone, the openings of the internal carotid artery and internal jugular vein can also be seen on the left side of the patient. Lateral to the foramina, the mandibular condyle can be identified within the temporomandibular joint. Within the occipital bone, the hypoglossal canal is demonstrated on either side anterolateral to the foramen magnum. Because this section demonstrates the contents within the base of the skull, the major structure found within the foramen magnum is the medulla oblongata and the vertebral arteries. In this patient, the left vertebral artery is difficult to discern, because it does not appear enhanced by contrast.

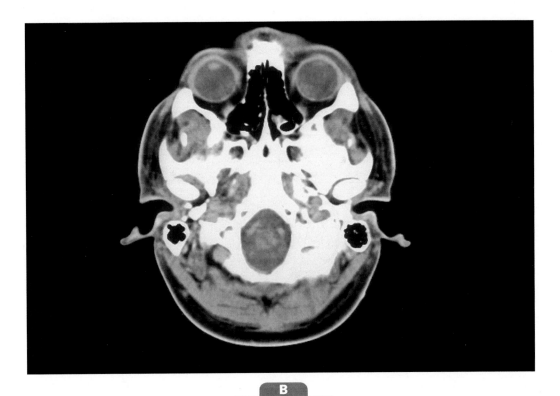

B

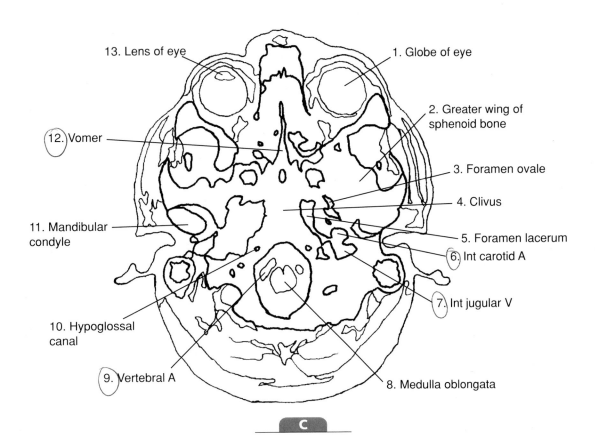

13. Lens of eye

1. Globe of eye

12. Vomer

2. Greater wing of sphenoid bone

3. Foramen ovale

4. Clivus

11. Mandibular condyle

5. Foramen lacerum

6. Int carotid A

7. Int jugular V

10. Hypoglossal canal

9. Vertebral A

8. Medulla oblongata

C

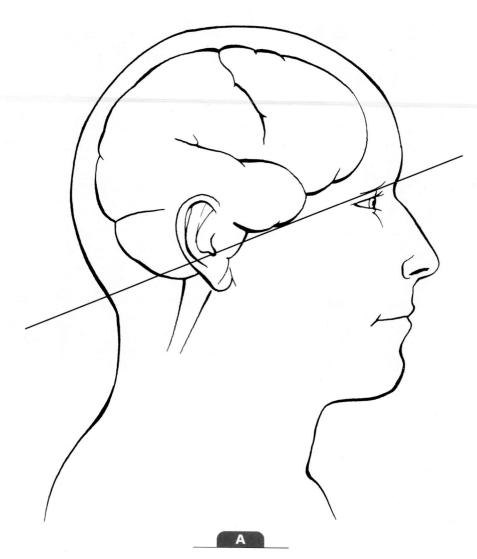

Figure 5-48 Axial CT image 7.

Figure 5-48 (A,B,C). The absence of the foramen magnum and the large petrous part of the temporal bone demonstrated in this image indicate the level of this image is just above the base of the skull. Within the petrous part of the temporal bones, the mastoid air cells are hypodense areas just posterior to the external acoustic meatus and deep to the auricle of the ear. Also within the petrous part of the temporal bone, the opening of the sigmoid sinus can be clearly identified on the left side as it extends from the transverse sinus down to the opening on the inferior surface of the skull where it drains into the internal jugular vein. Anterior to the temporal bones, the sphenoid bone is sectioned at the level of the sphenoid sinus directly behind the ethmoid air cells within nasal cavity. Together, the ethmoid and sphenoid bones make up much of the bony orbital margin, which at this level contains the optic nerve, the medial rectus muscle, and the lateral rectus muscle.

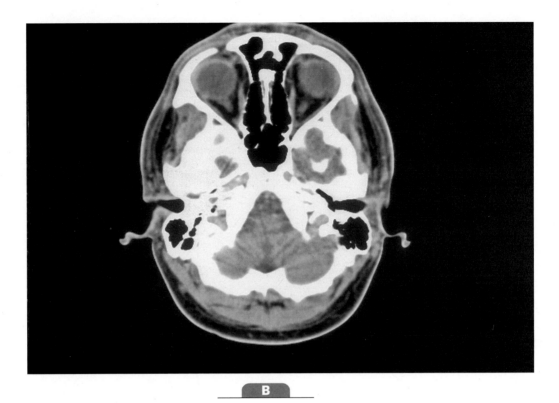

B

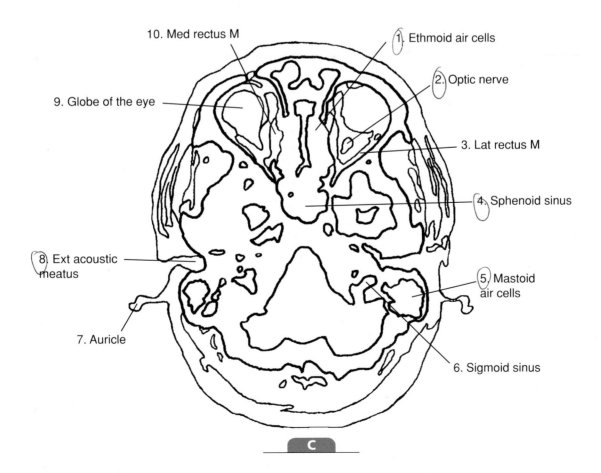

10. Med rectus M

9. Globe of the eye

1. Ethmoid air cells

2. Optic nerve

3. Lat rectus M

4. Sphenoid sinus

8. Ext acoustic meatus

5. Mastoid air cells

7. Auricle

6. Sigmoid sinus

C

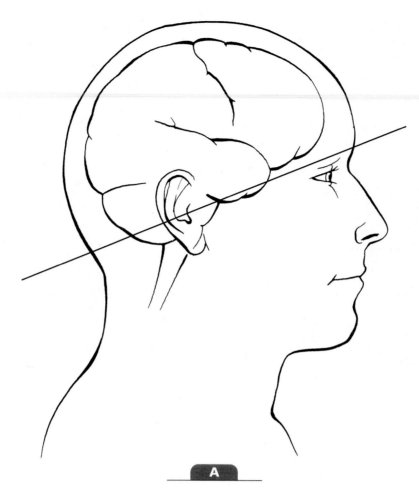

Figure 5-49 Axial CT image 8.

Figure 5-49 (A,B,C). The presence of the frontal and sphenoid sinuses indicate the level of this section to be in a region of the skull near the top of the orbits. Within the nasal cavity, the ethmoid bone is shown on the right side sectioned through the region of the cribriform plate. The foramina within the cribriform plate transmit the olfactory, or the first cranial, nerves from the mucous membranes within the nasal cavity. Within the orbital cavities, the upper part of the globe can be seen on the right side, and the left side is slightly higher, demonstrating the superior rectus muscle. In the posteromedial aspect of the bony orbital margin, the optic foramina are shown on either side between the lesser wings and body of the sphenoid bone. Within the soft tissue structures found within the posterior cranial cavity, a contrast-enhanced vessel, the basilar artery, is found directly posterior to the sphenoid sinus. Although most of the posterior cranial fossa is occupied by the lobes of the cerebellum, much of the region between the petrous parts of the temporal bones is occupied by the pons, which is just anterior to the fourth ventricle. Directly behind the fourth ventricle, the cerebellar vermis is shown to be the constricted region joining the right and left cerebellar hemispheres. On the lateral aspect of the cerebellar hemisphere, the sigmoid sinus is shown sectioned within the petrous part of the temporal bone as it extends downward from the transverse sinus to drain into the internal jugular vein.

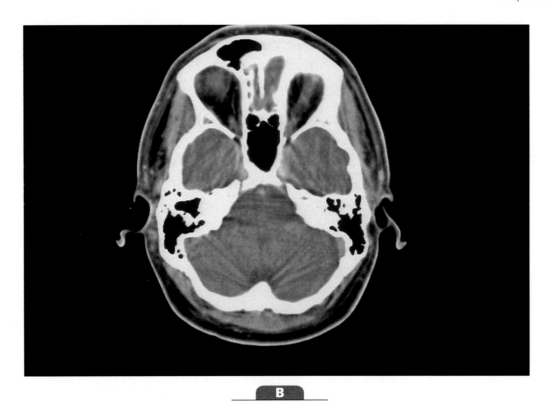

B

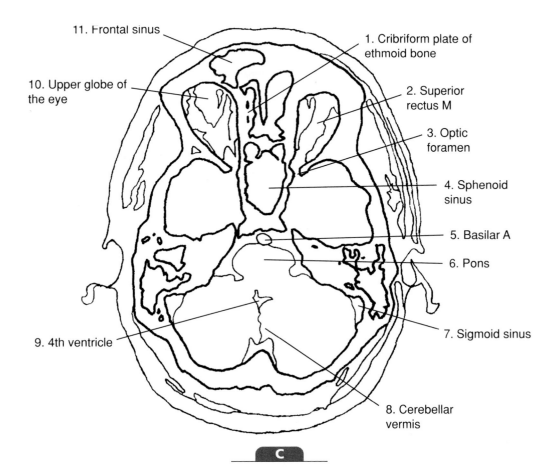

11. Frontal sinus

10. Upper globe of
the eye

1. Cribriform plate of
ethmoid bone

2. Superior
rectus M

3. Optic
foramen

4. Sphenoid
sinus

5. Basilar A

6. Pons

7. Sigmoid sinus

9. 4th ventricle

8. Cerebellar
vermis

C

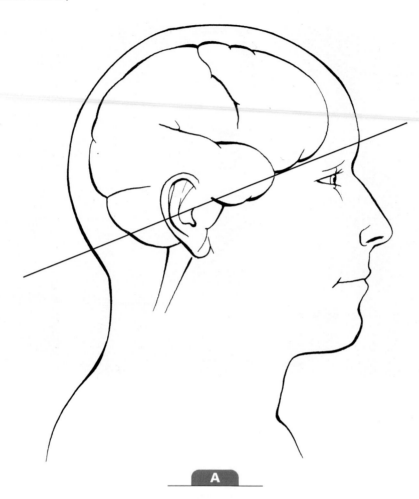

Figure 5-50 Axial CT image 9.

Figure 5-50 (A,B,C). As seen on the right side of this patient, the orbital plate of the frontal bone forms the roof of the bony orbital cavity. Centrally, the anterior clinoid processes are extending toward the dorsum sellae to form the sella turcica. As in the previous images, a small part of the sphenoid sinus can still be seen within the body of the sphenoid bone, and the mastoid air cells can be found within the petrous parts of the temporal bones. Within the sella turcica, the pituitary gland lies behind the internal carotid artery, which is readily identified on the left side owing to contrast enhancement. In this image, the contrast-enhanced vessel is labeled the internal carotid artery, because it has not yet joined the circle of Willis to give rise to the middle cerebral and anterior cerebral arter-ies. On either side of the sella turcica, the neural tissue in the middle cranial fossa represents the lower parts of the temporal lobes of the cerebrum. Similar to the previous image, the contrast-enhanced basilar artery is shown sectioned directly in front of the region of the pons. At this level, the fourth ventricle is again demonstrated between the pons and the cerebellum; however, this image shows the lateral recesses of the fourth ventricle, which extend laterally to join the subarachnoid space on either side through the foramina of Luschka. Between the cerebellum and the petrous part of the temporal bones, the sigmoid sinuses appear as indentations. On the right side of this patient, the dark area within the petrous part of the temporal bone represents the middle ear cavity.

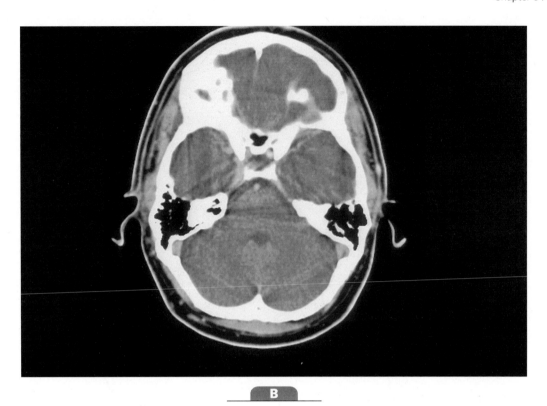

B

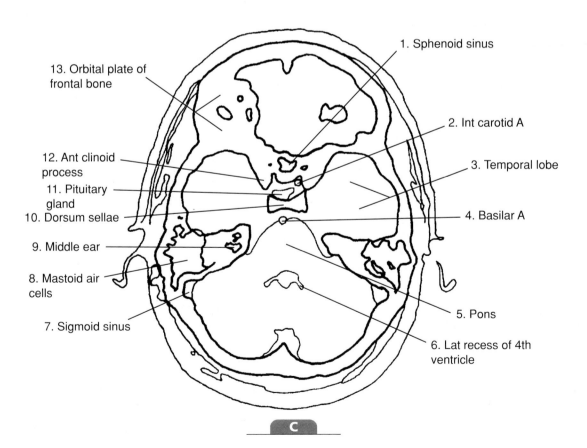

13. Orbital plate of frontal bone

12. Ant clinoid process

11. Pituitary gland

10. Dorsum sellae

9. Middle ear

8. Mastoid air cells

7. Sigmoid sinus

1. Sphenoid sinus

2. Int carotid A

3. Temporal lobe

4. Basilar A

5. Pons

6. Lat recess of 4th ventricle

C

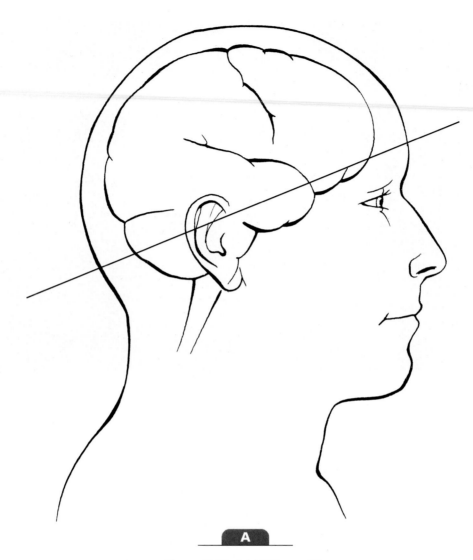

Figure 5-51 Axial CT image 10.

Figure 5-51 (A,B,C). Most of the cranial cavity is occupied by neural tissue, and the only bony parts labeled are the dorsum sellae and the mastoid air cells. Unlike the previous image, in which the pituitary gland was found directly anterior to the dorsum sellae, the stalk or infundibulum of the pituitary gland is now shown in cross-section at a higher level. In the area previously occupied by the internal carotid artery, the middle cerebral artery is now shown obliquely sectioned as it extends laterally through the Sylvian fissure. Directly posterior to the dorsum sellae, the contrast-enhanced basilar artery is shown in cross-section as it lies anterior to the pons. On the right side of the pons, the contrast-enhanced posterior cerebral artery is sectioned as it extends from the circle of Willis located just above the sella turcica to supply blood to the posterior cerebral hemisphere. As in previous images, the fourth ventricle is between the pons and the cerebellum within the posterior cranial fossa.

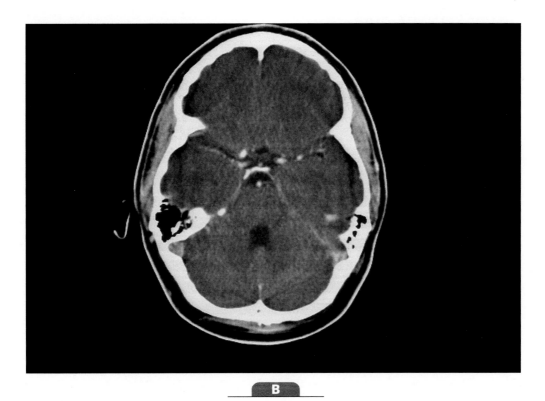

B

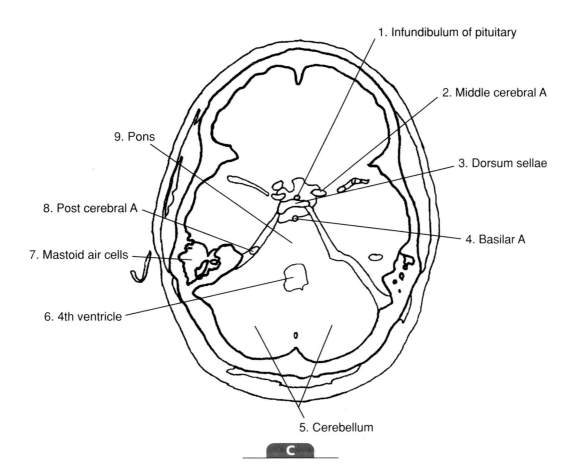

1. Infundibulum of pituitary

2. Middle cerebral A

3. Dorsum sellae

4. Basilar A

5. Cerebellum

6. 4th ventricle

7. Mastoid air cells

8. Post cerebral A

9. Pons

C

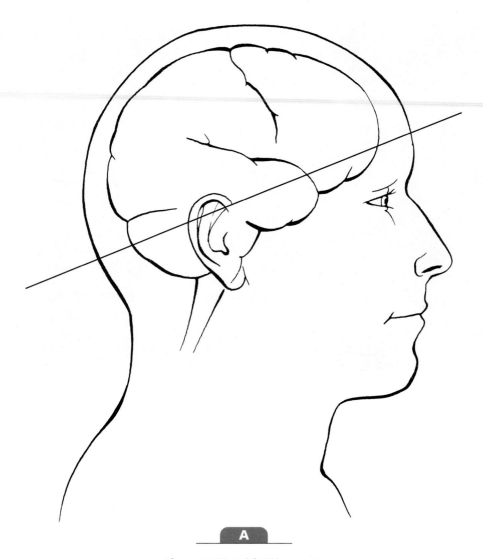

Figure 5-52 Axial CT image 11.

Figure 5-52 (A,B,C). The bony structures making up the base of the skull are no longer seen and the indentations of the inner skull indicate the margins between the neural structures. Anteriorly, the structure found medially extending between the right and left cerebral hemispheres can be identified as the falx cerebri. On the anterolateral aspects of the skull, the Sylvian fissures can be identified near the indentations of the skull as they divide the temporal and frontal lobes of the cerebrum. Posterolaterally, the transverse sinus is demonstrated forming the margin of the tentorium cerebelli that separates the cerebellum from the cerebrum. On the posterior aspect of the skull, the projection between the right and left lobes of the cerebellum can be identified as the falx cerebelli. At this level, the midbrain is found between the cerebrum and cerebellum. In the region of the posterior cerebrum, the contrast-enhanced posterior cerebral arteries are shown sectioned in several places as they extend from the region of the sella turcica to the posterior cerebrum. By comparison, the left middle cerebral artery is longitudinally sectioned, extending from the region previously occupied by the internal carotid artery to the region of the middle cerebrum. Anteriorly, the contrast-enhanced right anterior cerebral artery is also shown projecting from the region of the sella turcica toward the falx cerebri to supply the region of the anterior cerebrum with arterial blood. Although quite small at this level, the midline opening within the cerebrum represents the third ventricle between the right and left hypothalamus.

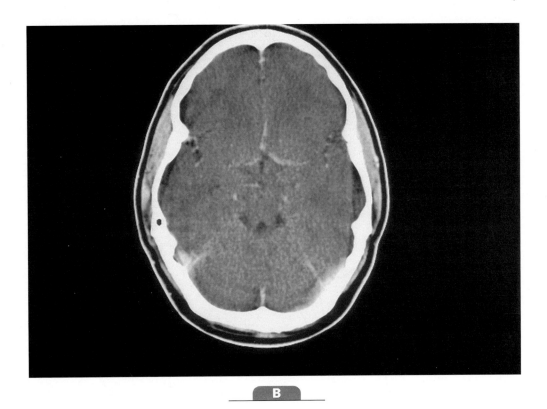

B

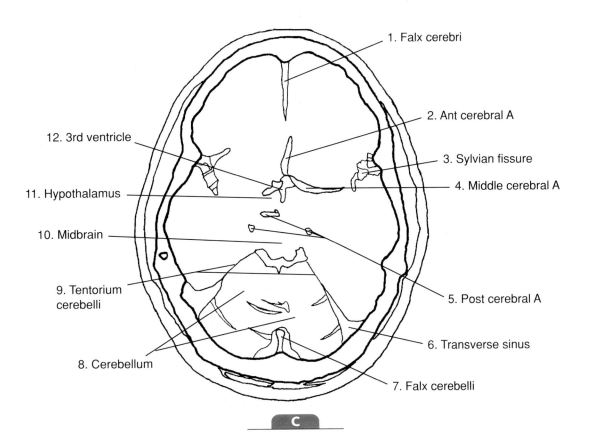

1. Falx cerebri

2. Ant cerebral A

12. 3rd ventricle

3. Sylvian fissure

4. Middle cerebral A

11. Hypothalamus

10. Midbrain

9. Tentorium cerebelli

5. Post cerebral A

8. Cerebellum

6. Transverse sinus

7. Falx cerebelli

C

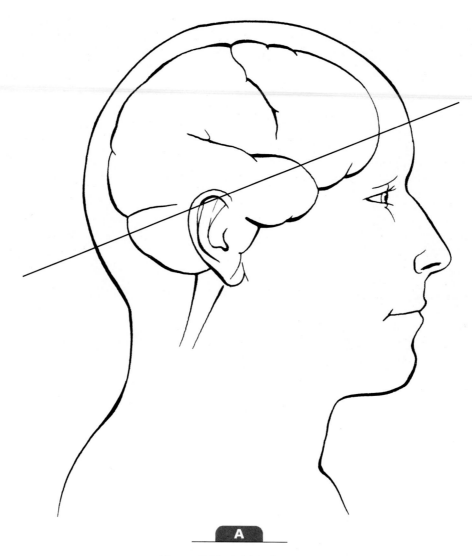

Figure 5-53 Axial CT image 12.

Figure 5-53 (A,B,C). Although a small part of the upper cerebellum can still be seen within the posterior part of this image, the majority of the brain cavity is occupied by the cerebral hemispheres. In the posterior part of the skull cavity, the contrast-enhanced confluence of sinuses marks the boundary between the cerebellar and cerebral hemispheres. Between the hemispheres, the midbrain is sectioned, demonstrating the cerebral peduncles, the cerebral aqueduct, and the posteriorly situated quadrigeminal plate. Within the cerebrum, the most easily identified landmarks are the radiolucent areas of the ventricles. In the midline, the third ventricle is a narrow opening between the thalamic nuclei. Within the cerebral hemispheres, the anterior horns of the lateral ventricles are bounded by the genu of the corpus callosum and the heads of the caudate nuclei. At this level, the inferior horns of the lateral ventricles are not yet sectioned but will appear in the region of the hippocampal formation in the following images. Medial to the hippocampal formation, the contrast-enhanced posterior cerebral artery is obliquely sectioned as it extends from the circle of Willis to the posterior cerebrum.

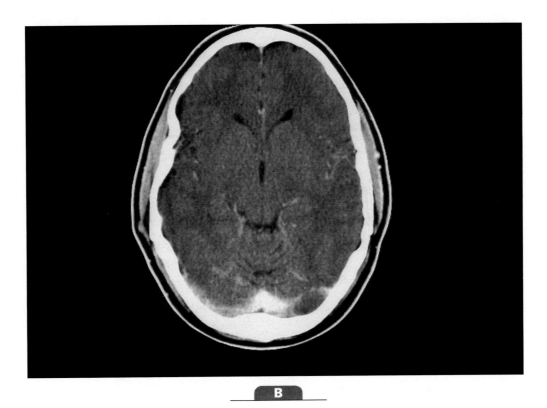

B

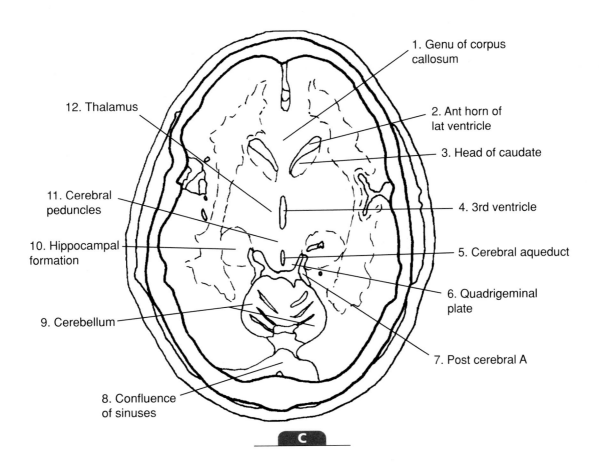

1. Genu of corpus callosum

12. Thalamus

2. Ant horn of lat ventricle

3. Head of caudate

11. Cerebral peduncles

4. 3rd ventricle

10. Hippocampal formation

5. Cerebral aqueduct

6. Quadrigeminal plate

9. Cerebellum

7. Post cerebral A

8. Confluence of sinuses

C

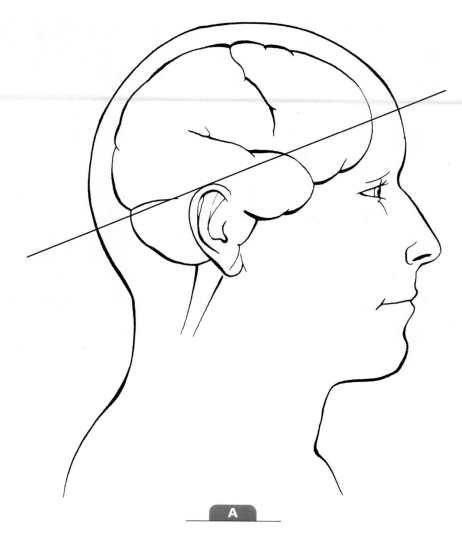

A

Figure 5-54 Axial CT image 13.

Figure 5-54 (A,B,C). At this level, the radiolucent areas of the anterior horns of the lateral ventricles are divided by the fornix, and the inferior horn of the lateral ventricle can now be labeled on the right side of this patient. Between the cerebral hemispheres, the anterior cerebral arteries are cut in cross-section as they ascend from the circle of Willis in the region of the sella turcica to the anterior cerebrum. Near the center of the image, the third ventricle appears as a clearly distinct radiolucent area between the thalamic nuclei, which are surrounded by the internal capsules. Although spots of high density appear to be within the third ventricle, they are calcifications within the pineal gland found outside the third ventricle between the quadrigeminal plate and the splenium of the corpus callosum. Although the radiolucent area between the pineal body and the cerebellar vermis appears the same density as the ventricle previously described, this area is formed by an enlarged part of the subarachnoid space outside of the brain, the superior cistern. Forming the border between the occipital lobes of the cerebrum and the upper part of the cerebellum, the tentorium cerebelli is sectioned, demonstrating the straight sinus and the confluence of sinuses that are formed in part by an extension of dura mater from the tentorium cerebelli.

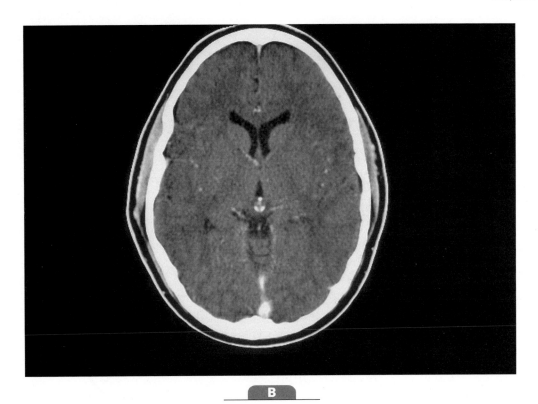

B

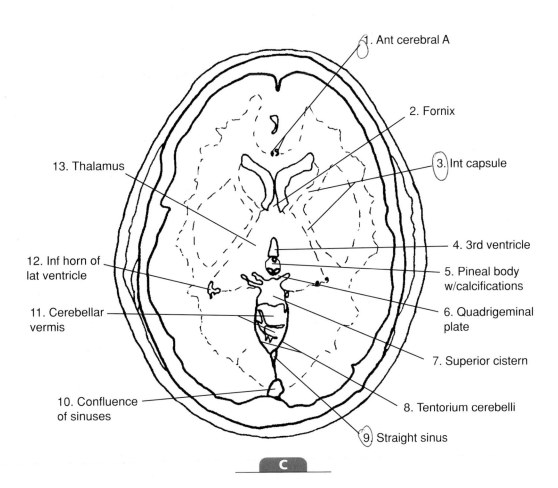

1. Ant cerebral A

2. Fornix

3. Int capsule

13. Thalamus

4. 3rd ventricle

12. Inf horn of
lat ventricle

5. Pineal body
w/calcifications

11. Cerebellar
vermis

6. Quadrigeminal
plate

7. Superior cistern

10. Confluence
of sinuses

8. Tentorium cerebelli

9. Straight sinus

C

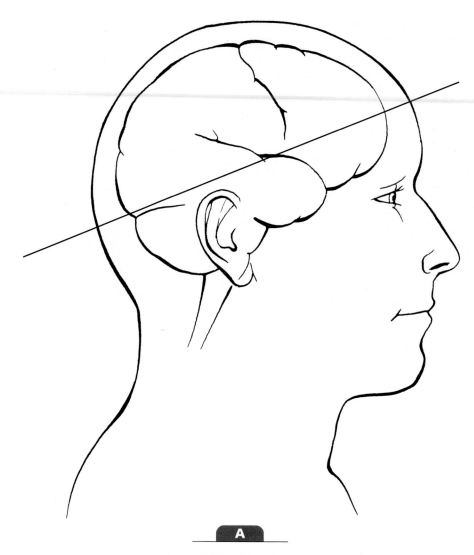

Figure 5-55 Axial CT image 14.

Figure 5-55 (A,B,C). The darkened areas representing parts of the lateral ventricles can be readily identified on either side. Anteriorly, the heads of the caudate nuclei are shown protruding into the anterior horns of the lateral ventricles. Between the cerebral hemispheres, the contrast-enhanced anterior cerebral arteries are shown in cross-section as they extend from the base of the brain where they originate from the circle of Willis to extend upward to supply blood to the anterior cerebral hemispheres. At this level, the midline ventricle previously identified as the third ventricle is sectioned near the top of the opening. Within the ventricles, the choroid plexuses are enhanced by contrast, because they are highly vascular and are responsible for the production of CSF. As described previously, the lateral walls of the third ventricle are formed by the thalamic nuclei. On the opposite side of the thalamic nuclei, the internal capsules act to separate the thalamic nuclei from the basal ganglia: caudate nucleus, globus pallidus, and putamen. Posterior to the thalamic nuclei, the tails of the caudate nuclei are shown in cross-section as they extend toward the inferior horns of the lateral ventricles. In the midline between the cerebral hemispheres, the vein of Galen is shown in cross-section as a large contrast-enhanced vessel directly behind the third ventricle. The vein of Galen drains venous blood into the straight sinus obliquely sectioned between the posterior cerebral hemispheres.

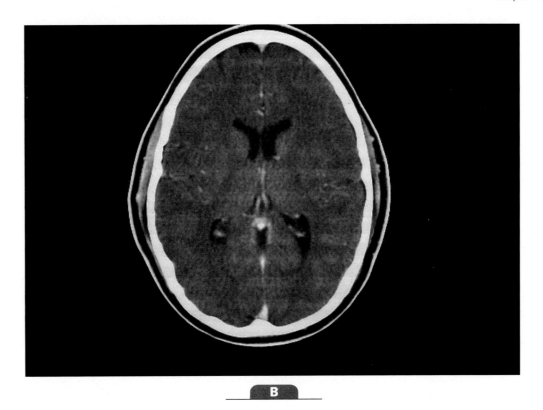

B

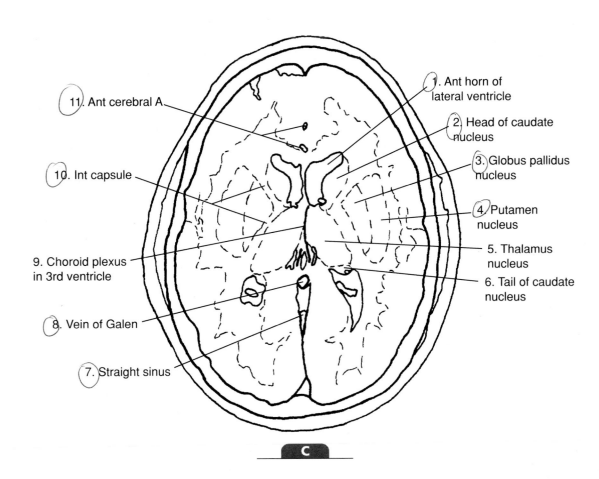

11. Ant cerebral A

10. Int capsule

9. Choroid plexus in 3rd ventricle

8. Vein of Galen

7. Straight sinus

1. Ant horn of lateral ventricle

2. Head of caudate nucleus

3. Globus pallidus nucleus

4. Putamen nucleus

5. Thalamus nucleus

6. Tail of caudate nucleus

C

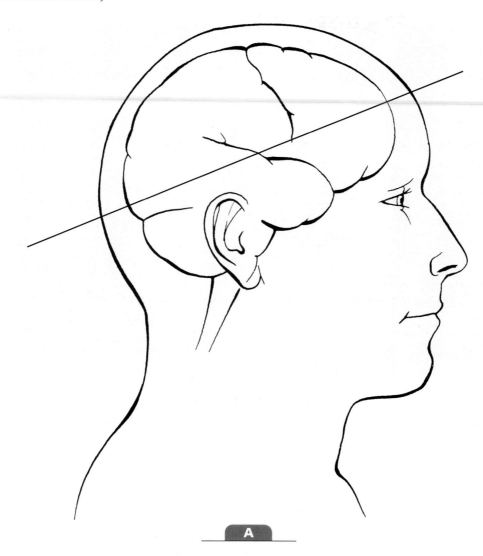

Figure 5-56 Axial CT image 15.

Figure 5-56 (A,B,C). At this level, the third ventricle is no longer seen and has been replaced by the structure forming the roof of the third ventricle, the splenium of the corpus callosum. Similar to previous images, the anterior horns of the lateral ventricles are readily identified as radiolucent areas within the anterior cerebral hemispheres. The anterior horns of the lateral ventricles are separated by the septum pellucidum, which extends between the splenium and genu of the corpus callosum. Between the anterior and posterior horns of the lateral ventricles, the contrast-enhanced choroid plexus lies within the bodies of the lateral ventricles. Similar to the previous image, the contrast-enhanced vein of Galen and straight sinus are sectioned between the posterior cerebral hemispheres.

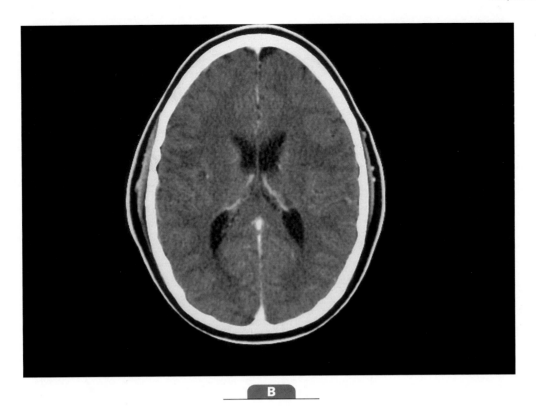

B

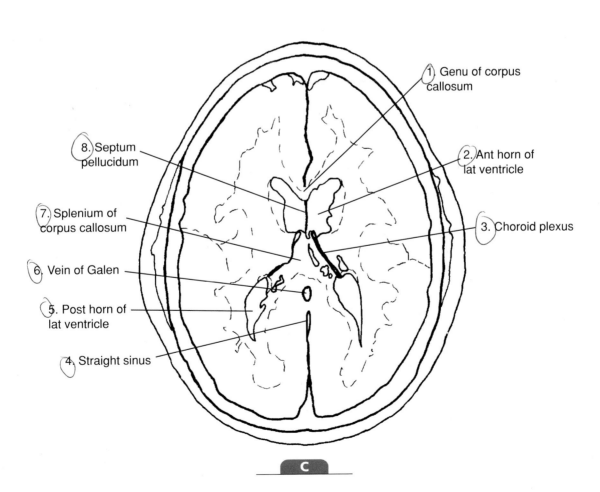

1. Genu of corpus callosum

8. Septum pellucidum

2. Ant horn of lat ventricle

7. Splenium of corpus callosum

3. Choroid plexus

6. Vein of Galen

5. Post horn of lat ventricle

4. Straight sinus

C

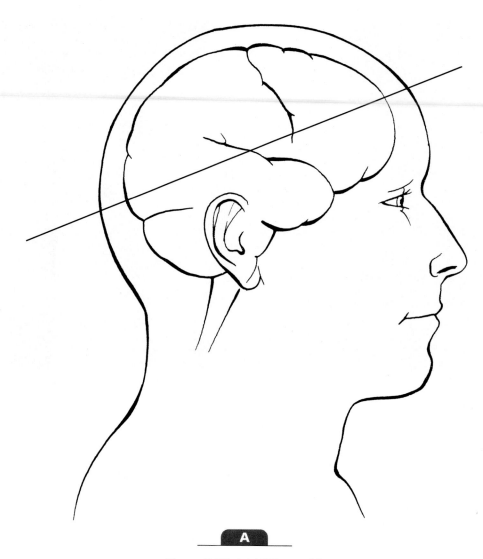

Figure 5-57 Axial CT image 16.

Figure 5-57 (A,B,C). In this image, the bodies of the lateral ventricles are the most readily identifiable landmarks. On the patient's right side, the posterior part of the lateral ventricle is labeled the collateral trigone, which is where the inferior and posterior horns join the body of the lateral ventricle. On either side, the ventricles are surrounded by an area of white matter formed primarily of neural fibers extending to and from the gray matter of the cerebral cortex. Just medial to the lateral ventricles, the region of white matter represents the body of the corpus callosum and consists of a group of nerve fibers extending between the right and left cerebral hemispheres. In the midline, the falx cerebri is formed by a reflection of dura mater separating the right and left cerebral hemispheres.

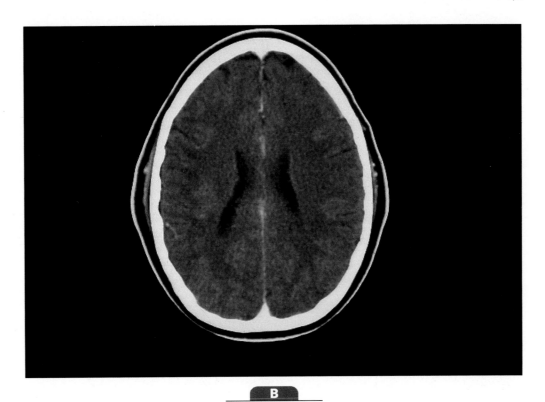

B

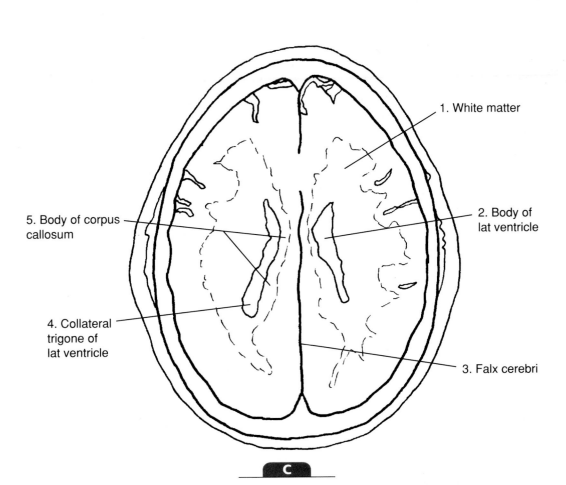

1. White matter

5. Body of corpus callosum

2. Body of lat ventricle

4. Collateral trigone of lat ventricle

3. Falx cerebri

C

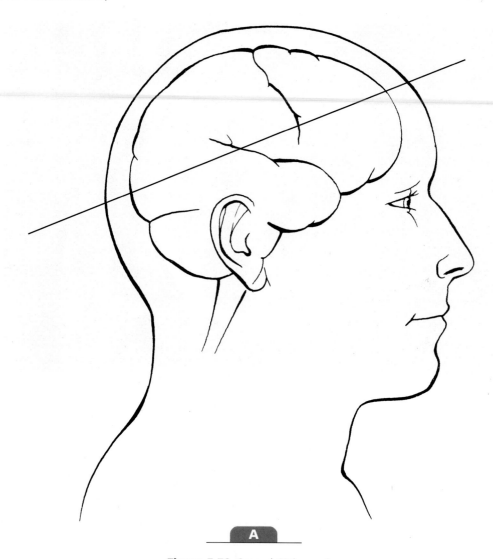

Figure 5-58 Coronal CT image 1.

Figure 5-58 (A,B,C). Owing to the absence of ventricular structures, Figure 5-58 represents the anatomy near the top of the head. Similar to the previous image, the falx cerebri is shown separating the right and left cerebral hemispheres. Along its margin, the falx cerebri forms the superior sagittal sinus and is labeled on the posterior part of the image adjacent to the parietal bone. Within the cerebral hemispheres, the regions of the frontal and parietal lobes are labeled and contain both white and gray matter.

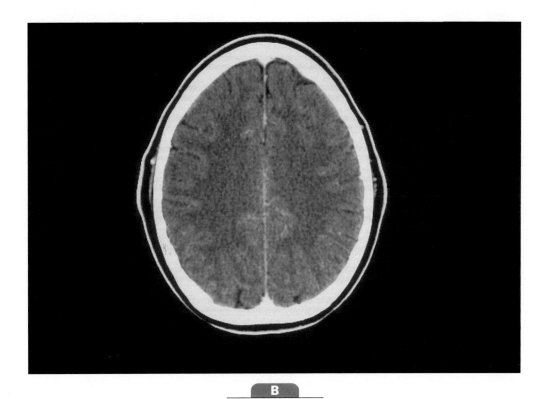

B

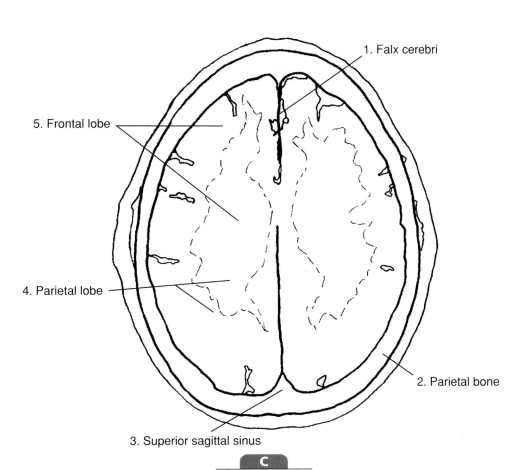

1. Falx cerebri

5. Frontal lobe

4. Parietal lobe

2. Parietal bone

3. Superior sagittal sinus

C

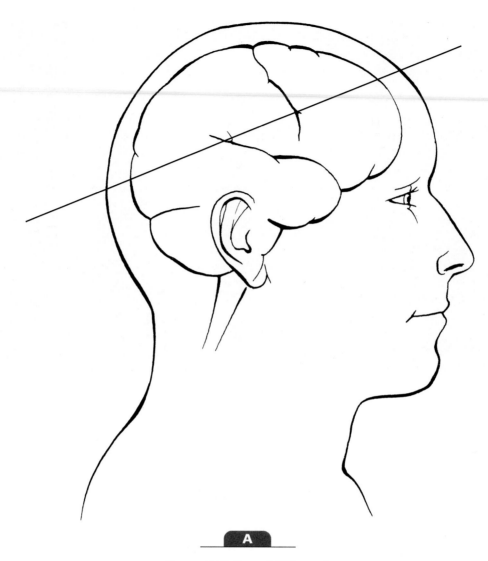

A

Figure 5-59 Coronal CT image 2.

Figure 5-59 (A,B,C). Nearing the top of the head, the falx cerebri is again shown separating the right and left cerebral hemispheres. In this image, the superior sagittal sinus is labeled anteriorly, bounded by the dural reflections from the falx cerebri and the frontal bone. Although it is not labeled, the superior sagittal sinus is also within the posterior margin of the falx cerebri adjacent to the parietal bone. Within the cerebral hemispheres, white matter is shown surrounded by the gray matter following the convoluted appearance of the external cerebral hemispheres. Within this section, the enlarged central sulcus can be identified separating the frontal and parietal lobes of the cerebrum.

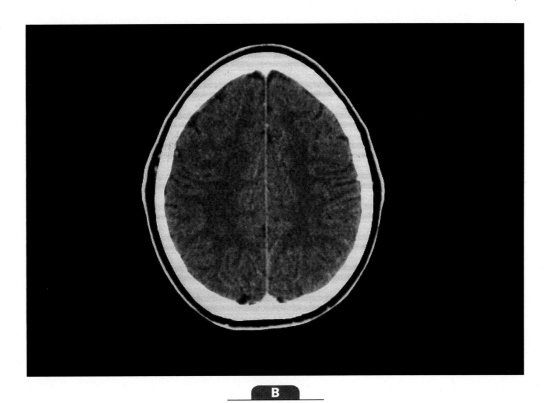

B

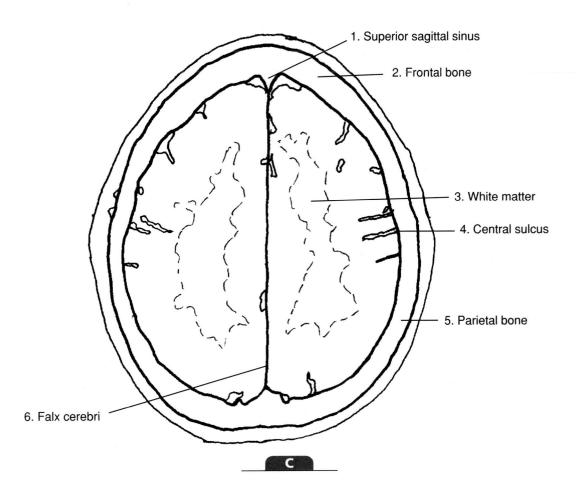

1. Superior sagittal sinus

2. Frontal bone

3. White matter

4. Central sulcus

5. Parietal bone

6. Falx cerebri

C

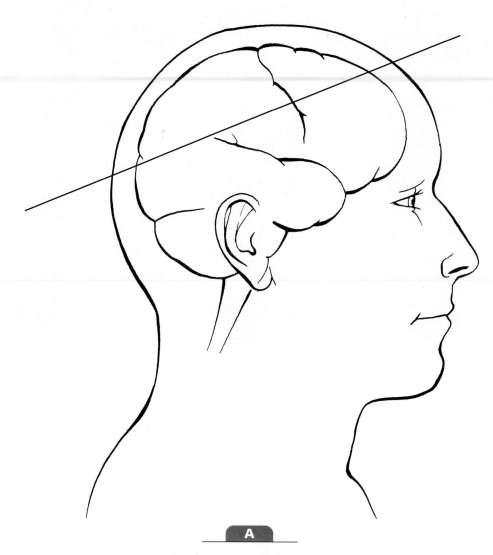

Figure 5-60 Coronal CT image 3.

Figure 5-60 (A,B,C). The convoluted appearance of the neural structures in this image indicates that the section lies near the top of the cerebral hemispheres. Because this section represents the anatomy of the upper head, the frontal bone is labeled anteriorly and the parietal bone is labeled posteriorly, even though the coronal suture cannot be identified. Internally, the central sulcus can be identified and marks the boundary between the frontal and parietal lobes of the cerebrum. In the midline, the superior sagittal sinus is labeled along the margin of the falx cerebri extending between the right and left cerebral hemispheres. Within the cerebral hemispheres, the corona radiata appear as regions of white matter on either side surrounded by the gray matter of the cerebral cortex.

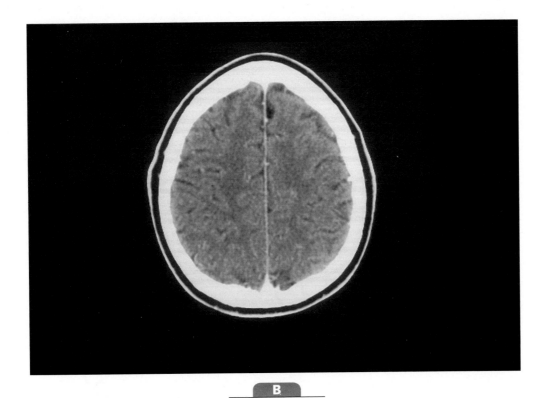

B

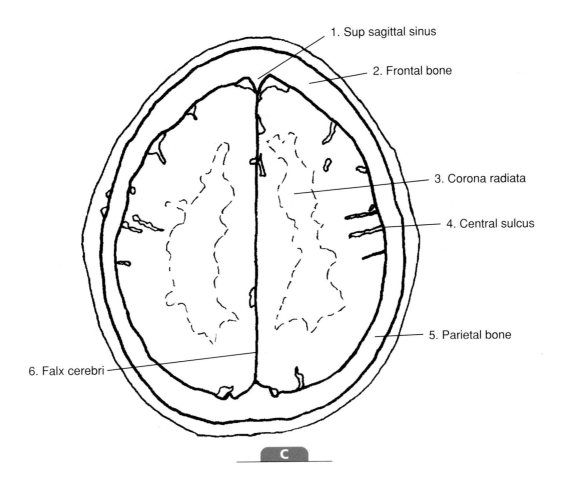

1. Sup sagittal sinus

2. Frontal bone

3. Corona radiata

4. Central sulcus

5. Parietal bone

6. Falx cerebri

C

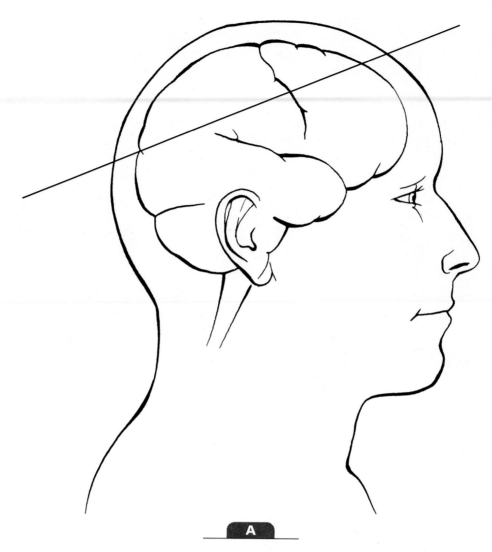

Figure 5-61 Coronal CT image 4.

Figure 5-61 (A,B,C). The appearance of sulci and gyri within the majority of the neural tissue indicates that the image is nearing the top of the brain. Despite the predominance of surface anatomy, a small amount of white matter can be identified on either side within the frontal and parietal lobes of the cerebrum. Similar to previous images, the falx cerebri extends between the parietal and frontal bones and contains the superior sagittal sinus along its bony margin. Surrounding the skull, the scalp appears as two distinct layers: The outer layer of skin is dense and consists primarily of dense connective tissue and skin; and the inner layer consists primarily of loose connective tissue, fat, and blood vessels.

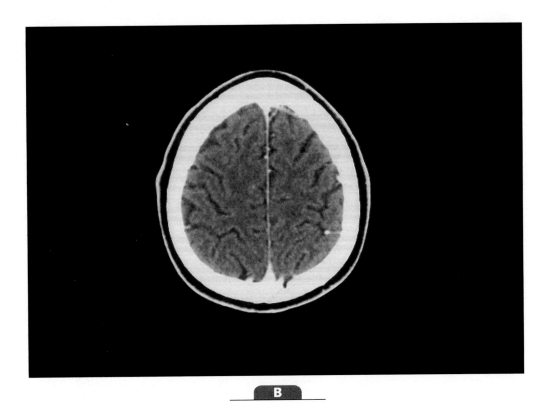

B

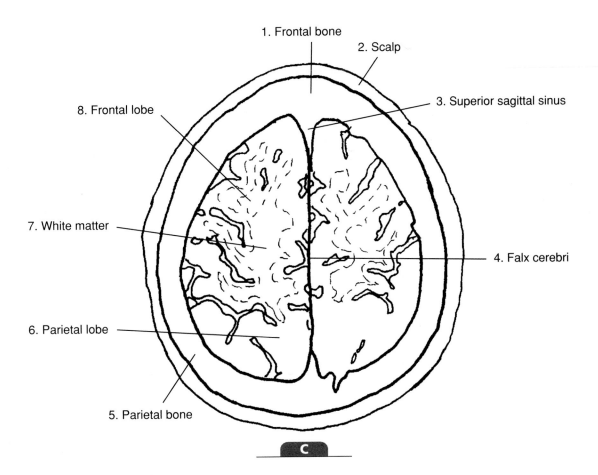

1. Frontal bone

2. Scalp

3. Superior sagittal sinus

8. Frontal lobe

7. White matter

4. Falx cerebri

6. Parietal lobe

5. Parietal bone

C

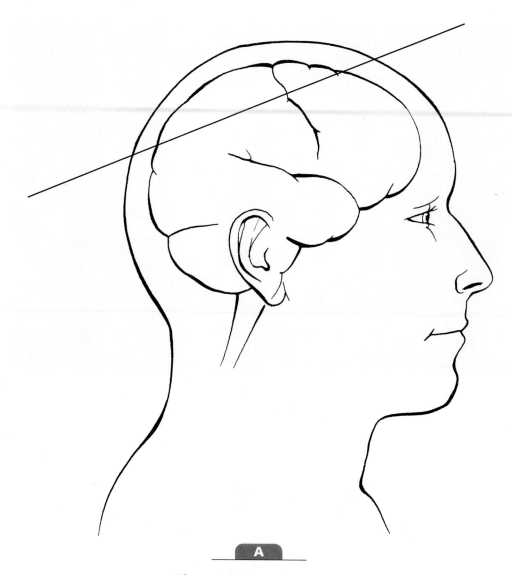

Figure 5-62 Coronal CT image 5.

Figure 5-62 (A,B,C). This section demonstrates the anatomy typically seen in the most superior scan of the head. Within the image, the falx cerebri is again shown containing the superior sagittal sinus within its bony margin, which attaches to the frontal and parietal bones. Outside of the bones of the skull, the scalp appears as two distinct layers; the inner is radiolucent and the outer is radiodense.

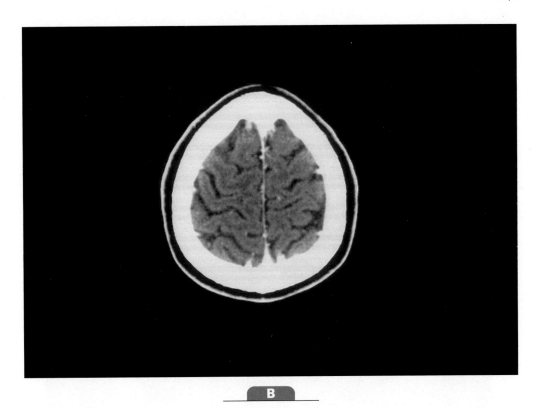

B

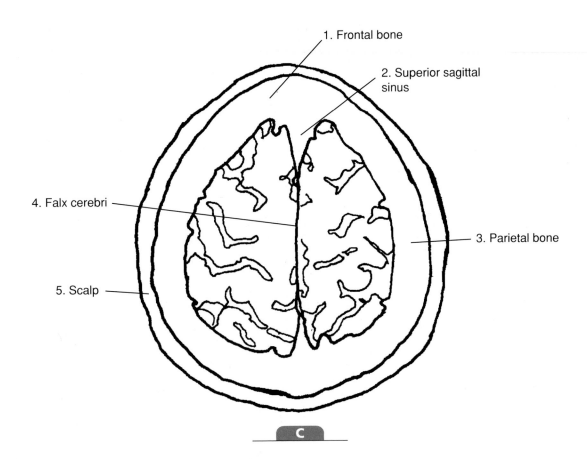

1. Frontal bone

2. Superior sagittal sinus

4. Falx cerebri

3. Parietal bone

5. Scalp

C

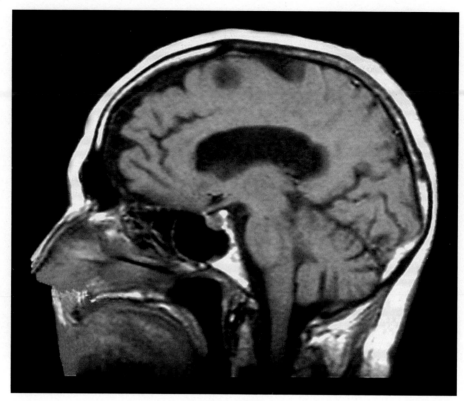

Figure 5-63

Supplement 5-1. *Figure 5-63 is a sagittal T1-weighted MR image of an 82-year-old woman who was suffering from "confusion" and could not remember her name, where she was, or the general time period. In the image, cerebellar atrophy is marked by the enlarged subarachnoid space surrounding the cerebellum. Given the patient's age, the cerebellar atrophy is considered mild. The enlarged subarachnoid spaces surrounding the cerebral cortex and the enlarged ventricles, however, mark severe atrophy of the cerebrum. In this patient, the atrophy or irreversible loss of brain tissue resulted from chronic ischemic changes in the cerebral vascular supply.*

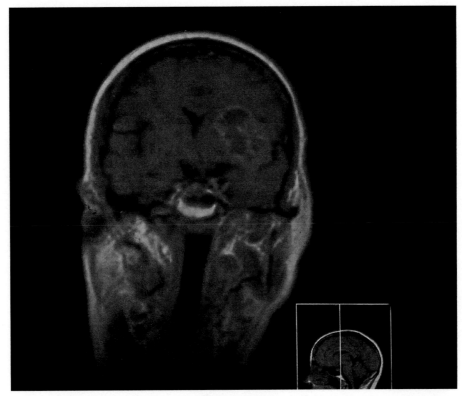

Figure 5-64

Supplement 5-2. *Figure 5-64 shows an MR image of a 73-year-old woman who was suffering from severe headaches and memory loss. T1-weighted coronal MR images were generated after the injection of gadolinium. The sixth slice reveals a large mass that involves most of the left parietal lobe. Located medially within the lobe, the mass is causing a midline shift and compression of the ipsilateral ventricle. Additional tests showed the mass to be metastatic disease from the right breast.*

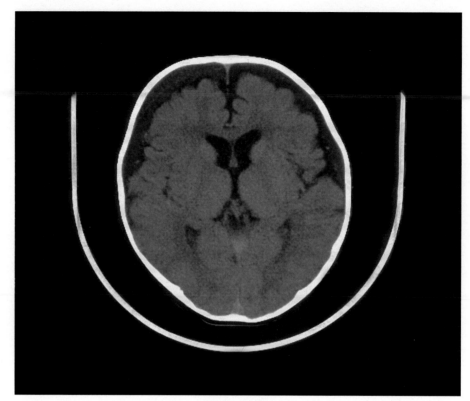

Figure 5-65

Supplement 5-3. *Figure 5-65 shows a CT scan of a 5-month-old boy with an enlarged head owing to suspected child abuse by his mother. In this axial slice, a large hypodense region is seen compressing the brain parenchyma bilaterally, displacing the brain posteriorly. The gyri and sulci do not appear to be compressed by the dura mater, indicating the fluid is within the subdural space. Because the low-density material seen within the subdural space represents a collection of congealed blood, the patient was diagnosed as having a chronic subdural hematoma.*

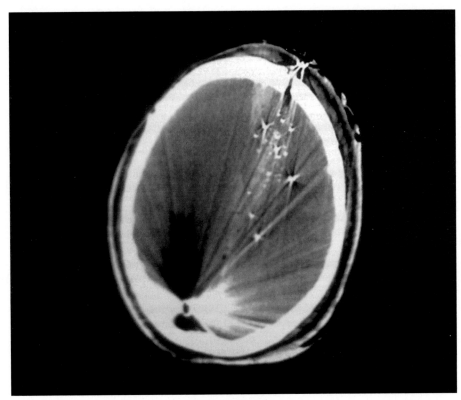

Figure 5-66

Supplement 5-4. *Figure 5-66 shows a CT examination of the head of a 40-year-old man who suffered from a self-inflicted gunshot wound. Within the axial image, numerous metallic fragments and foreign bodies mark the path of the bullet through the frontal and parietal lobes of the cerebrum. The largest fragment is noted in the right occipital region near the calvarium and measures approximately 1 cm in diameter. Originating predominantly from the largest fragment, beam hardening artifacts radiate throughout the image, masking many of the soft tissue structures. Unfortunately, after 2 days of intensive care, the patient succumbed to this critical injury.*

REVIEW QUESTIONS

1. When imaging the head, the_____is considered the inferior boundary of the region.
2. What bones form the bony nasal septum?
3. The_____foramen within the greater wing of the sphenoid bone transmits the mandibular branch of the trigeminal nerve.
4. Describe the palatine bones.
5. Which of the following nuclei appears to be protruding into the lateral ventricles?
   A. Putamen
   B. Caudate
   C. Globus pallidus
   D. Thalamus
6. Describe the location of the insula.
7. The meningeal layers surrounding the central nervous system are the_____, closest to the skull; the_____, the intermediate layer; and the_____, closest to the brain.
8. Which of the following describes the venous sinus between the inferior margin of the falx cerebri and tentorium cerebelli?
   A. Superior sagittal sinus
   B. Sigmoid sinus
   C. Straight sinus
   D. Inferior sagittal sinus
9. Describe the fornix.
10. Which of the following is most laterally situated within the brain?
    A. Putamen
    B. Caudate
    C. Globus pallidus
    D. Thalamus
11. Which of the following is not considered part of the midbrain?
    A. Pineal body
    B. Quadrigeminal plate

C. Red nucleus
D. Substantia nigra
12. Describe the location and function of the hippocampal formation.
13. The_____is an enlarged region of the subarachnoid space between the cerebellum and the tentorium cerebelli.
14. The_____transmits cerebrospinal fluid between the third and fourth ventricles.
    A. Foramen of Magendie
    B. Interventricular foramen
    C. Foramen of Luschka
    D. Cerebral aqueduct
15. The vertebral arteries enter the cranial cavity through the foramen_____.
16. Describe the location of the middle cerebral artery.
17. Which of the following sinuses is located most posteriorly within the skull?
    A. Sphenoid
    B. Maxillary
    C. Ethmoid
    D. Frontal
18. The optic nerve passes through the_____bone to enter the orbital cavity.
19. Which of the following is found closest to the clivus?
    A. Pons
    B. Midbrain
    C. Medulla oblongata
    D. Hypothalamus
20. Which of the following is located most medially within the brain?
    A. Putamen
    B. Caudate
    C. Globus pallidus
    D. Thalamus

Chapter 6

Neck

OBJECTIVES

Upon completion of this chapter, the student should be able to:

1. State the superior and inferior boundaries of the neck.
2. Explain the distinguishing characteristics of the third through sixth cervical vertebrae.
3. Describe the atlas and axis.
4. Describe the glandular structures located within the neck.
5. Identify and describe the cartilaginous structures forming the larynx.
6. Describe the openings within the larynx and pharynx.
7. Identify and describe the folds of skin found within either the larynx or the pharynx.
8. Identify and describe the major vessels within the neck.
9. Describe the position of major vessels within the neck in relation to other structures.
10. Correctly identify anatomical structures on patient CT and MR images of the neck.

ANATOMICAL OVERVIEW

The anatomy within the neck is generally symmetrical and is described as the region between the base of the skull and the bony thoracic cage.

Skeletal

Cervical (*SER-vĭ-kal*) **vertebrae.** The uppermost seven vertebrae located between the base of the skull and the thoracic vertebrae (Fig. 6-1). Easily distinguished from other vertebrae by their small size and the foramina (*fō-RAM-i-nă*) in their transverse processes, the transverse foramina (Figs. 6-2 to 6-4).

Atlas. The first cervical vertebra, which supports the head. Named for Atlas, the mythical Greek Titan who was thought to have supported the world on his shoulders. The most atypical vertebra, because it lacks a body and a true spinous process and is roughly circular in shape (Fig. 6-2). The front and back of the vertebra are formed by the anterior and posterior arches; the lateral masses form the sides.

Anterior arch. Marked feature of the atlas. An arch of bone with a central expanded area, the anterior tubercle (*TŪ-ber-kl*). In the vertebral (*VER-tĕ-brăl*) column, the centrum that would have given rise to the body of the atlas is fused to the second cervical vertebral body and is directly posterior to the anterior arch.

Posterior arch. Does not have a true spinous process, which would be expected; instead, has a much smaller posterior tubercle.

Lateral mass. The bulky bony structures lateral to the vertebral foramen (*fō-RA-men*) with articular facets. The superior articular facets correspond to the occipital condyles (*ok-SIP-i-tăl KON-dilz*) and are large oval-shaped structures facing medially and upward. They are usually constricted in the middle and may be divided in some individuals. The inferior articular facets are also large but are roughly round in shape.

Axis. The second cervical vertebra, or epistropheus (*ep-i-STRŌ-fē-ŭs*), forms the pivot for rotation of the atlas and head. It is easily distinguished by the body, which is long and extends cranially, forming the dens, or odontoid process (Fig. 6-3).

Dens. A bony structure, roughly 1.5 cm long, that projects from the vertebral body of the axis and acts as the body for the atlas. Highly involved in the rotational and nodding movements of the head and is often the sight of trauma. When the head is forced into hyperflexion or hyperextension, as in whiplash injuries, it may become fractured. Because it forms the anterior wall of the spinal foramen, a fracture may be life-threatening if the spinal cord is involved. Hence, immobilization is critical when neck injury is suspected.

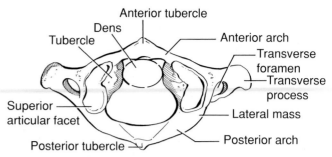

Figure 6-2 Superior view of the atlas.

C3 through C6. The typical cervical vertebrae can be divided into two main parts: a body and a vertebral arch, which surround and house the spinal cord (Fig. 6-4).

Vertebral foramina. Large and triangular openings within the cervical vertebrae between the body and the vertebral arch. Although thoracic and lumbar vertebrae are larger than cervical vertebrae, their vertebral foramina are smaller and rounder.

Spinous processes. The terminal processes of cervical vertebrae are usually bifid, resulting in tubercles of unequal size. Except for C6 and C7, cervical vertebrae have shorter spinous processes than other vertebrae. The spinous processes of C6 and C7 are longer than those of other vertebrae and extend caudally in the median plane.

Transverse processes. The most distinctive feature of cervical vertebrae are the transverse foramina, which are located centrally in the processes and encase the vertebral arteries and veins.

Articular (ar-TIK-yū-lăr) processes. The bony structures directly lateral to the vertebral foramen. They extend upward and downward from the points where the pedicles (*PED-ĭ-klz*) and laminae (*LAM-i-nē*) join. The upward projection, the superior articular process, has the articular surface facing posteriorly. The adjacent surface, the inferior articular process, is the downward projection of bone that faces anteriorly. Together, the processes form the zygapophysial (*ZĪ-gă-pō-FIZ-ē-ăl*) joints between adjacent vertebrae.

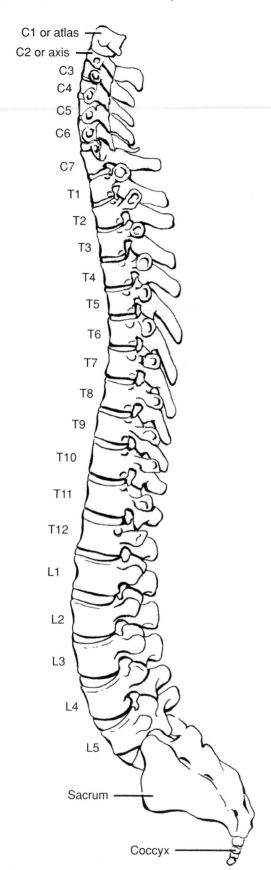

Figure 6-1 Lateral view of entire vertebral column.

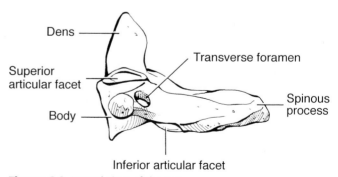

Figure 6-3 Lateral view of the axis.

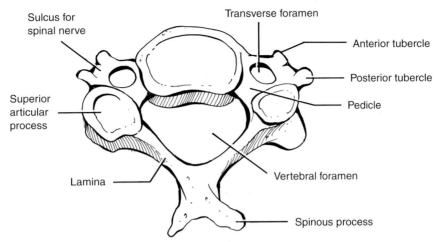

Figure 6-4 Superior view of a cervical vertebra.

Vertebra prominens (*PROM-i-nens*). C7 is the most distinctive of the lower cervical vertebrae, owing primarily to its large spinous process. The process is a thick bony projection that extends in a horizontal fashion posteriorly and can be easily palpated on the posterior base of the neck. In contrast to the typical vertebrae, the spinous process is not bifid, but ends in a single tubercle. Because this structure is easily distinguished on a lateral radiograph and can be easily palpated, it is often used as a landmark for the separation between the cervical and thoracic vertebrae.

Hyoid. (*HĪ-oyd*). A U-shaped bone located just below the mandible at the level of C3 (Fig. 6-5). It can be located by placing the thumb under the chin and moving it backward until it stops at the angle of the neck. This angle is formed by a series of flat muscles that originate at the mandible and thoracic cage and insert on the hyoid bone. The bone also has ligamentous attachments with the larynx, or the voice box (Fig. 6-6).

Cartilage and Other Structures

Larynx (*LAR-ingks*). Commonly called the voice box. Part of the air passageway in the anterior neck. Averages approximately 4.5 cm in length, but is typically shorter in women and children, and extends from the level of C3 to C6 (Figure 6-5). Although its framework is composed of cartilages similar to other parts of the airway, the laryngeal (*lă-RIN-jē-ăl*) cartilages are uniquely arranged and are interconnected by a series of ligaments and muscles capable of voice production (Fig. 6-6).

Thyroid (*THĪ-royd*) **cartilage.** Found just below the hyoid bone. The largest of the cartilaginous structures within the larynx. Similar to the hyoid, it is roughly U shaped, is open posteriorly, and has an irregular surface. Anteriorly, its superior margin forms the laryngeal prominence (commonly called the Adam's apple) at the approximate level of C4 (Fig. 6-5).

Epiglottis (*ep-i-GLOT-is*). Single spoon-shaped cartilage that closes the opening of the larynx when food or drink is moved down the pharynx (Fig. 6-6). As seen posteriorly, its inferior part is narrow and anchors to the thyroid cartilage. Superiorly, it is larger, extending upward adjacent to the hyoid bone to a position posterior to the tongue. As food or drink is swallowed, the tongue moves posteriorly, bending the epiglottis over the opening of the larynx.

Cricoid (*KRĪ-royd*) **cartilage.** Single cartilage found in the larynx just below the thyroid cartilage. It encircles the airway. Seen from above, it is circular; when viewed from the lateral aspect, the ring is much wider posteriorly. Consequently, the posterior cricoid cartilage may be visualized without the anterior portion in axial sections.

Arytenoid (*ar-i-TĒ-noyd*) **cartilages.** From a posterior view of the larynx, the two pyramidal-shaped cartilages are found resting on the posterior cricoid cartilage. Owing to the wide posterior arch of the cricoid cartilage, these cartilages are just below the laryngeal prominence of the thyroid cartilage.

Aryepiglottic (*AR-ē-ep-i-GLOT-ik*) **folds.** As seen in median section, a fold of skin on each side extends between the arytenoid cartilage and the margin of the epiglottis. Besides covering the ligaments connecting the cartilaginous structures, they mark the lateral boundaries between the larynx and the pharynx.

Vocal cords (or folds). The ligaments extending between the arytenoid cartilages and the thyroid cartilage covered with a mucous membrane. Muscles acting on the cartilages move them with respect to one another, changing the tension of the ligaments and modulating the sound emitted when air moves through the larynx.

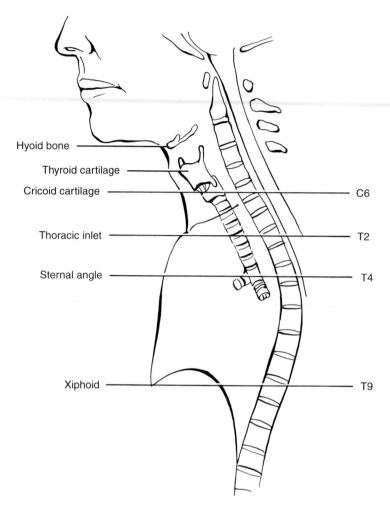

Figure 6-5 Relationships of cervical and thoracic vertebrae to the major airway structures.

Vestibular (*ves-TIB-yū-lăr*) **folds.** Often called the false vocal cords. The mucous membrane structures situated just above the glottic space. Unlike the vocal folds, they do not have an underlying ligament and have little to no role in voice production.

Laryngeal vestibule. A space within the upper larynx bounded by the aryepiglottic folds, epiglottis, arytenoid cartilages, and vestibular folds. In sectional images, it is seen immediately behind the epiglottis.

Glottic (*GLOT-ik*) **space.** Also called the ventricle (*VEN-tri-kl*). The space within the larynx bounded by the vestibular folds and the vocal folds.

Infraglottic space. The opening within the larynx below the vocal folds that is continuous inferiorly with the opening of the trachea.

Trachea (*TRă-kē-ă*). The major airway, extending from the larynx and terminating in the main bronchi (*BRONG-ki*),

from approximately the level of C6 to T4. Centrally located in the neck and immediately anterior to the esophagus and the vertebral bodies.

Pharynx (*FAR-ingks*). A muscular tube extending from the base of the skull to the level of approximately C6, where it is continuous with the esophagus (Fig. 6-7). Lies adjacent to the vertebral bodies and is divided into several parts: nasopharynx, oropharynx, and laryngeal pharynx.

Nasopharynx (*NĀ-zō-FAR-ingks*). The first division of the pharynx. Located posterior to the nasal cavity and extending from the base of the skull to the soft palate.

Oropharynx (*ŌR-ō-FAR-ingks*). The second division of the pharynx. Located posterior to the oral cavity and extending from the soft palate to the tip of the epiglottis.

Median glossoepiglottic (*GLOS-ō-ep-i-GLOT-ik*) *fold.* The fold of skin that extends between the posterior tongue and the tip of the epiglottis (Fig. 6-8).

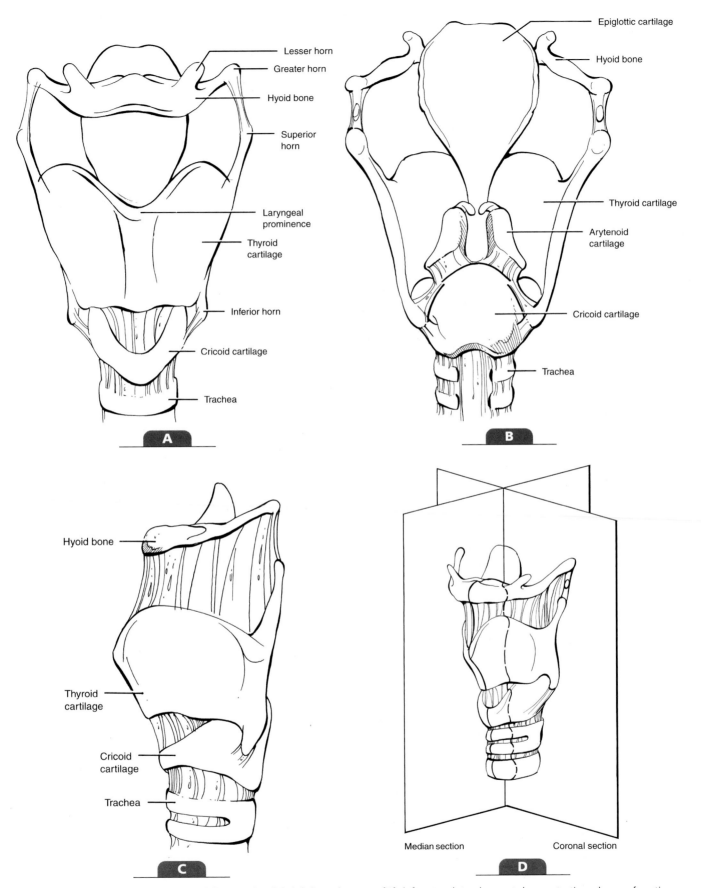

Figure 6-6 The larynx: **(A)** anterior, **(B)** posterior, **(C)** left lateral aspect, **(D)** left anterolateral aspect demonstrating planes of section, **(E)** coronal section, and **(F)** median section.

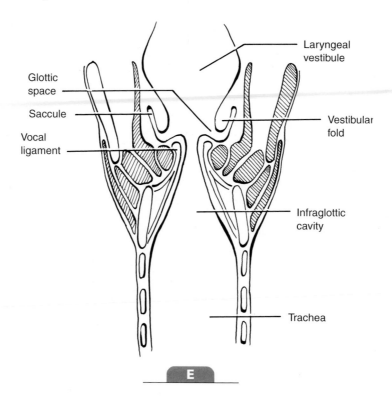

Laryngeal
vestibule

Glottic
space

Saccule

Vocal
ligament

Vestibular
fold

Infraglottic
cavity

Trachea

E

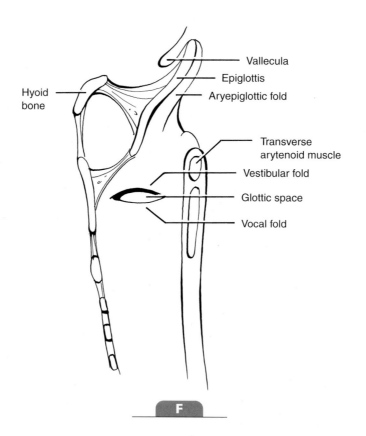

Vallecula

Epiglottis

Aryepiglottic fold

Hyoid
bone

Transverse
arytenoid muscle

Vestibular fold

Glottic space

Vocal fold

F

Valleculae (vă-LEK-yū-lē). Spaces on either side of the median glossoepiglottic fold, between the posterior tongue and the epiglottis. During swallowing, the tongue moves backward folding the valleculae and bending the epiglottis to close the opening to the larynx.

Laryngeal pharynx. The third division of the pharynx. Located posterior to the larynx (Fig. 6-7). In a coronal section through the posterior pharynx, the aryepiglottic folds are bilaterally situated around the inlet of the larynx, marking the boundary between the pharynx and larynx.

Piriform (PIR-i-fōrm) sinuses. Within the laryngeal pharynx, a sinus can be found on either side of the larynx.

Esophagus (ē-SOF-ă-gŭs). Originates at the level of C6, at the end of the pharynx. Situated medially, just anterior to the vertebral bodies, and descends inferiorly to terminate at the stomach. In sectional images, it is between the trachea and the vertebral bodies near the median plane of the body.

Other Viscera *(VIS-er-ă)*

Submandibular *(sŭb-man-DIB-yū-lăr)* **glands.** A pair of glands just below the mandible *(MAN-di-bl)*, on either side,

that are easily palpable as a spongy area just below the posterior half of the mandible (Fig. 6-9). They are the second largest salivary glands, about the size of a walnut. Secretions from the glands are drained by the submandibular duct (Wharton's duct) to an opening in the anterior floor of the mouth.

Thyroid gland. U-shaped single gland, just inferior to the larynx in the anterior neck, that surrounds the upper region of the trachea. Its two lobes are situated on either side of the trachea, connected by a narrowed region, called the isthmus, on the anterior trachea.

Arteries

Common carotids *(ka-ROT-idz).* On the right side, originates from the brachiocephalic artery; on the left side, is the second major branch off the aortic arch. On both sides, they ascend through the neck, with the internal jugular veins, beside the trachea. Above the thyroid cartilage, or at approximately the level of the intervertebral disk between C3 and C4, they bifurcate into the internal and external carotid arteries.

Internal carotids. Originating from the common carotid arteries, they ascend through the neck next to the internal

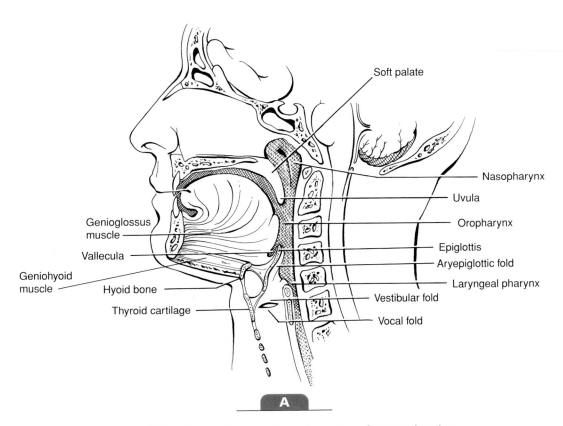

Figure 6-7 The pharynx: **(A)** median section and **(B)** posterior view of a coronal section.

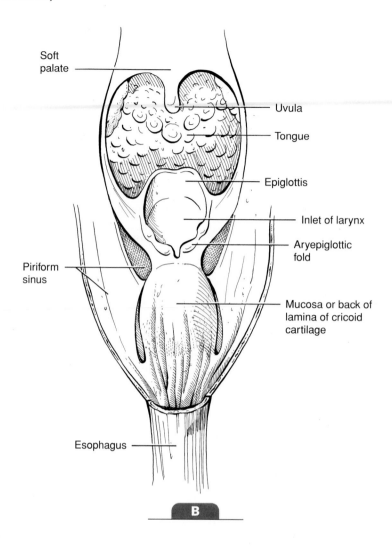

Soft palate

Uvula

Tongue

Epiglottis

Inlet of larynx

Aryepiglottic fold

Piriform sinus

Mucosa or back of lamina of cricoid cartilage

Esophagus

B

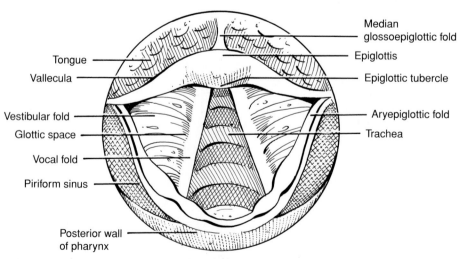

Tongue

Vallecula

Vestibular fold

Glottic space

Vocal fold

Piriform sinus

Posterior wall of pharynx

Median glossoepiglottic fold

Epiglottis

Epiglottic tubercle

Aryepiglottic fold

Trachea

Figure 6-8 Superior aspect of the larynx during inspiration.

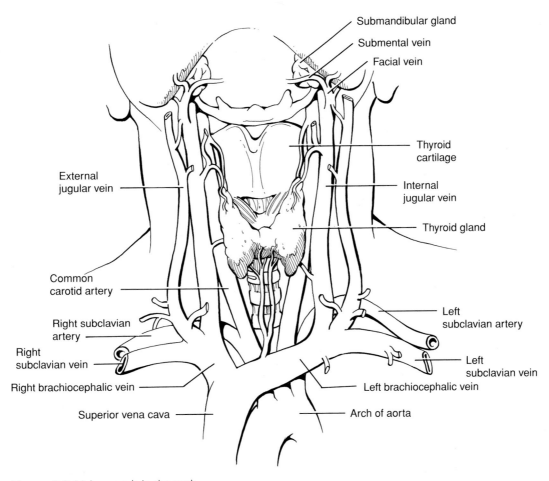

Figure 6-9 Major vessels in the neck.

jugular veins. At the base of the skull, they exit the upper neck through the carotid foramen to supply blood to the middle and anterior cerebrum (*SER-ĕ-brŭm*) (Fig. 6-10).

External carotids. Arising from the common carotid arteries, they ascend through the upper neck to supply blood to the external head. They are more superficially located in the anterior neck than the internal carotids.

Vertebrals. As the name implies, they are closely associated with the vertebral column and ascend through the transverse foramina of the cervical vertebrae. On both sides, they originate from the subclavian (*sŭb-KLA-vē-an*) arteries and enter the skull through the foramen magnum (*MAG-nŭm*) to supply blood to the posterior brain.

Veins

Internal jugulars (*JŬG-yū-larz*). Two major veins located on either side of the neck next to the common carotid

arteries. They are more superficial and usually larger than the adjacent arteries (Figs. 6-9 and 6-11).

External jugulars. Originating from the superficial head, they descend superficially through the neck and terminate in the subclavian vein. Their slow gentle pulse can usually be felt near the middle of the sternocleidomastoid muscle. Besides providing a reference for palpating the vein, the sternocleidomastoid muscle is also a useful landmark for identifying the external jugular vein in sectional images.

Retromandibular (*RE-trō-man-DIB-yū-lăr*). Two smaller veins on either side of the head just posterior to the mandible. Originate from smaller veins in the temporal (*TEM-pō-răl*) and maxillary (*MAK-si-lār-ē*) regions; descend to terminate in the external jugular veins. During their course, they pass within the parotid (*pă-ROT-id*) glands and are superficial to the external carotid arteries.

Vertebrals. The venous plexuses (*PLEK-sŭs-ez*) within the transverse foramina surrounding the vertebral arteries on either side of the neck. Drain blood from the spine and

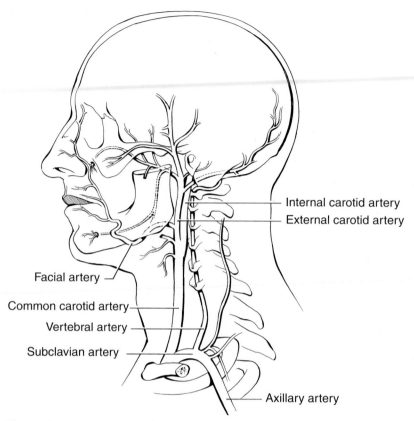

Figure 6-10 Major arteries of the head and neck from the left lateral aspect.

Internal carotid artery
External carotid artery
Facial artery
Common carotid artery
Vertebral artery
Subclavian artery
Axillary artery

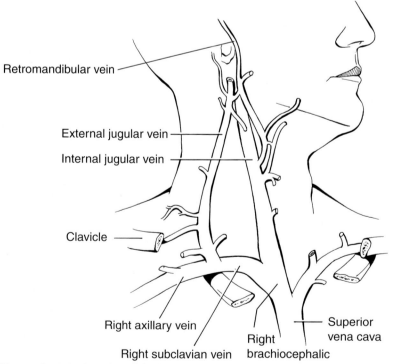

Figure 6-11 Major veins of the head and neck from the right anterolateral aspect.

Retromandibular vein
External jugular vein
Internal jugular vein
Clavicle
Right axillary vein
Right subclavian vein
Right brachiocephalic
Superior vena cava

descend into the chest, emptying into the subclavian veins.

Muscles

All are bilateral.

Genioglossus (*JĔ-ni-ō-GLOS-ŭs*). Originate from the superior mental spine on the posterior aspect of the mandible and insert on the hyoid bone. Large, thick muscles that form the majority of the musculature of the tongue.

Geniohyoid (*jĕ-NĪ-ō-HĪ-oyd*). Originate from the inferior mental spine and insert on the hyoid bone just below the genioglossus muscle. Thin strap muscles that act to raise the hyoid and depress the mandible.

Sternocleidomastoid (*STER-nō-KLĪ-dō-MAST-toyd*). Originate from the sternum and clavicle and insert on the mastoid process of the temporal bone. Their action is generally described as bending and rotating the head. Owing to their superficial location, they provide landmarks for identifying superficial structures within the neck.

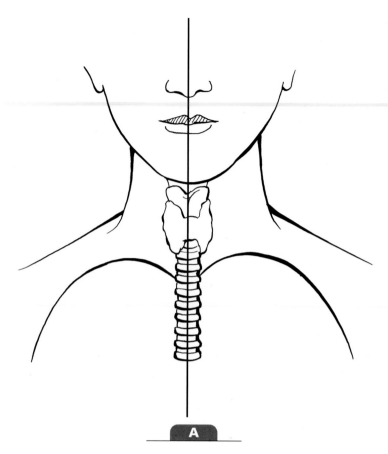

Figure 6-12 Sagittal MR image 1.

Sagittal MR Images

The following two sagittal MR images of the neck are described at 5.0 mm intervals from the midsagittal plane to the left side. The right side is not described, because the structures are similar to those described on the left side. The images were generated at the following technical factors: TR = 500, TE = 20, RF = 90°, FOV = 30 cm. Abbreviations: TR = repetition time, TE = echo-time, RF = radiofrequency, FOV = field of view.

Figure 6-12 (A,B,C). Near the center of the image, the bodies of the cervical and thoracic vertebrae are shown in cross-section to form a highly organized pattern. Just behind the vertebral bodies, the subarachnoid space is shown on either side of the spinal cord. Based on the thickness of the spinal cord and its presence through most of the image, this anatomy lies near the midsagittal plane. Posterior to the spinal canal, the spinous processes of the cervical and thoracic vertebrae are seen projecting posteriorly and are covered by a layer of superficial fat. Anterior to the vertebral column, the openings of the pharynx, larynx, and surrounding soft tissue structures are cross-sectioned. In the region of the nasopharynx, the soft palate projects posteriorly from the hard, or bony, palate to separate the nasopharynx from the oropharynx. Directly below the soft palate, the genioglossus muscle is shown to be the largest muscle found within the tongue. On the lower aspect of the genioglossus muscle, the cartilage of the epiglottis can be identified, forming part of the anterior wall of the oropharynx. As described earlier, the epiglottis attaches inferiorly to the thyroid cartilage, which is located just below the hyoid bone. Although both these structures are U shaped, the thickness of the image demonstrates only their most anterior parts, causing them to appear irregular, or oval. The thyroid cartilage forms part of the upper larynx and contains the laryngeal vestibule. Because this section is taken through the midsagittal plane, the vestibular and vocal folds are not seen. The arytenoid and the cricoid cartilages, however, are cross-sectioned adjacent to the lower laryngeal space. Below the larynx, the isthmus of the thyroid gland is cross-sectioned as it extends between the lobes located on either side of the trachea. Between the trachea and the vertebral column, the esophagus is labeled as it extends from the region of the laryngeal pharynx down to the stomach.

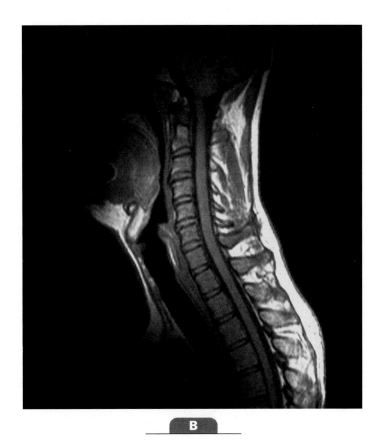

B

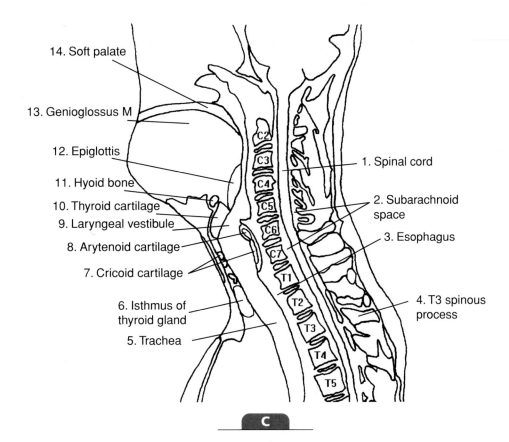

14. Soft palate

13. Genioglossus M

12. Epiglottis

11. Hyoid bone

10. Thyroid cartilage

9. Laryngeal vestibule

8. Arytenoid cartilage

7. Cricoid cartilage

6. Isthmus of
thyroid gland

5. Trachea

1. Spinal cord

2. Subarachnoid
space

3. Esophagus

4. T3 spinous
process

C

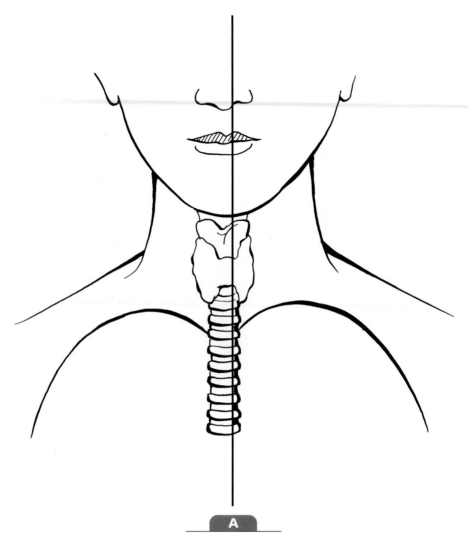

Figure 6-13 Sagittal MR image 2.

Figure 6-13 (A,B,C). As in the previous image, this image shows the regular pattern of the cervical and thoracic vertebrae; however, here the spinal cord is slightly thicker superiorly where it joins the brainstem, located within the skull cavity. In this image, the medulla oblongata and the pons are shown just anterior to the cerebellum. Lying just below the skull, a projection of bone (the dens) is sectioned, extending upward from the body of C2 to form the body of C1, the atlas. The dark area behind the nasal cavity, representing the nasopharynx, lies above the soft palate and is shown with its most caudal extension, the uvula (YŪ-vyū-lǎ). Below the nasopharynx, the oropharynx is the space posterior to the tongue between the uvula and the epiglottis. Below the level of C4, the spinal cord begins to narrow and is absent through much of the thoracic region, indicating that the lower half of the image demonstrates structures on the patient's left side. Because this image is slightly to the left of the midsagittal plane, we can now identify the vestibular fold above the vocal fold, or true vocal cord. Both these folds extend between the thyroid and the arytenoid cartilages. As described earlier, the arytenoid cartilage is found resting on the posterior part of the ring-shaped cricoid cartilage. Between the folds of skin, the middle laryngeal space can now be labeled the glottic space. As in the previous image, the trachea can be seen as it extends downward from the larynx between the isthmus of the thyroid gland and the esophagus.

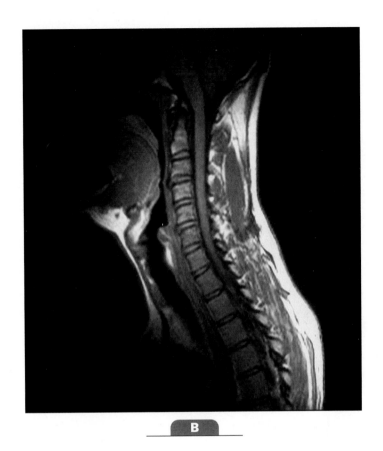

B

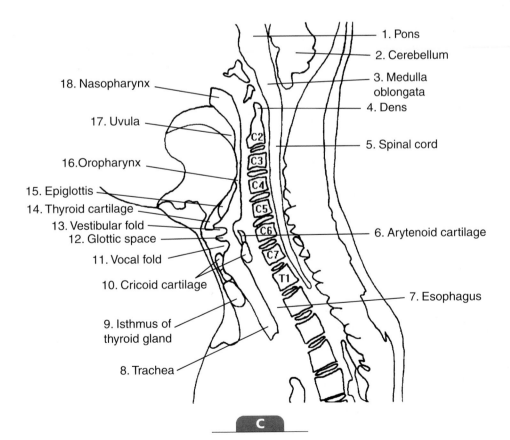

1. Pons
2. Cerebellum
3. Medulla oblongata
4. Dens
5. Spinal cord
6. Arytenoid cartilage
7. Esophagus

18. Nasopharynx
17. Uvula
16. Oropharynx
15. Epiglottis
14. Thyroid cartilage
13. Vestibular fold
12. Glottic space
11. Vocal fold
10. Cricoid cartilage
9. Isthmus of thyroid gland
8. Trachea

C

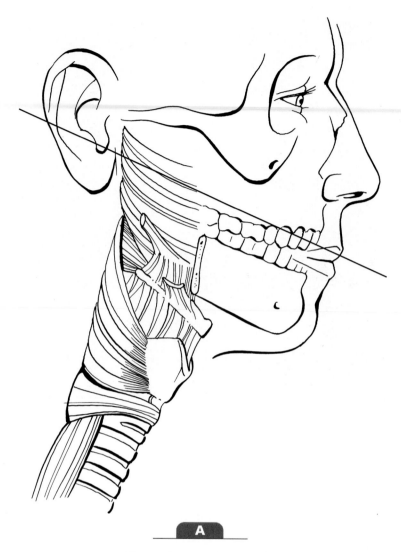

Figure 6-14 Axial CT image 1.

Axial CT Images

The following 18 axial CT images of the neck are described at 5.0 mm intervals from superior to inferior. The images were generated immediately after the administration of 100 mL venous contrast at the following scanning factors: 120 kVp and 150 mA-s. Abbreviations: kVp = kilovolt peak, mA-s = milliampere-second.

Figure 6-14 (A,B,C). When looking at the bony anatomy in this image, one can readily identify the lower teeth in front of the rami of the mandible. Within the temporal bone, the mastoid air cells can be easily identified on either side. Medially, projections from the occipital bone appear continuous with the anterior arch of the atlas, which surrounds the dens that projects upward from the vertebral body of C2. Surrounded by the occipital bone, the contents of the lower posterior cranial fossa are labeled the cerebellum and the medulla oblongata. On either side of the medulla oblongata, the vertebral arteries should be found; however, only the contrast-enhanced right vertebral artery can be identified in this patient. The sigmoid sinus is found on either side in what appears as a notch in the lower petrous part of the temporal bone; it will be shown at lower levels to drain into the internal jugular vein. Anteriorly, the internal carotid arteries are the contrast-enhanced structures near the atlas, or C1. Superficial to these vessels, the parotid gland can be identified by its characteristic consistency on either side postero-lateral to the rami of the mandible. Similar to the sagittal sections, the soft tissue structure within the mouth is labeled the genioglossus muscle.

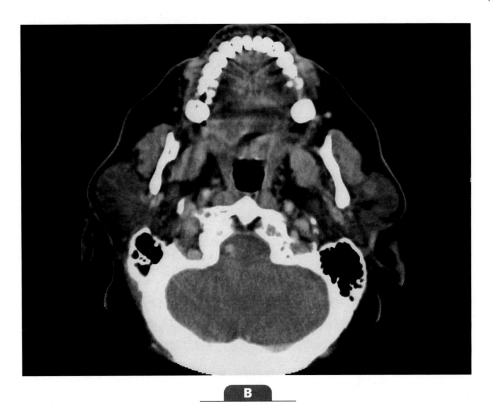

B

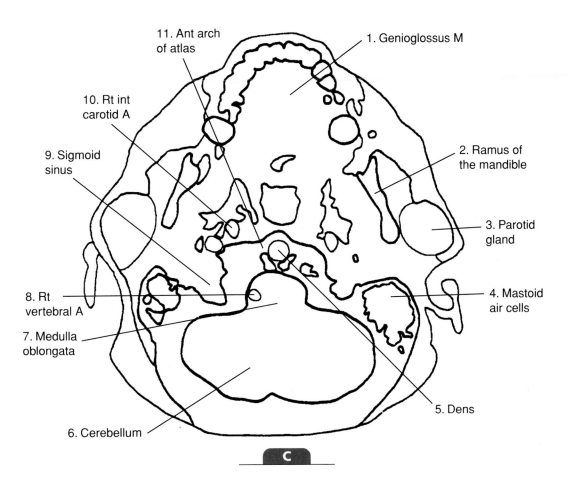

11. Ant arch of atlas

1. Genioglossus M

10. Rt int carotid A

9. Sigmoid sinus

2. Ramus of the mandible

3. Parotid gland

8. Rt vertebral A

4. Mastoid air cells

7. Medulla oblongata

5. Dens

6. Cerebellum

C

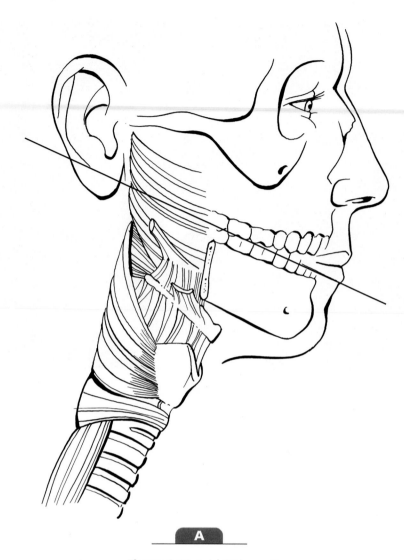

A

Figure 6-15 Axial CT image 2.

Figure 6-15 (A,B,C). The lower teeth and the mandibular rami can be readily identified on the anterior part of this image. Posteriorly, the lower parts of the occipital and temporal bones are shown with the anterior part of C1, the atlas; and the dens is seen projecting from the body of C2, the axis. The vertebral artery can be seen on the right side of the patient; the left does not appear enhanced by contrast. Within what appears as a notch in the lower petrous part of the temporal bone, the sigmoid sinus is now labeled the internal jugular vein, because it is exiting the skull. On the left side of the patient, a small section of the styloid process of the temporal bone is sectioned between the atlas and the superficially situated parotid gland. Medially, the oropharynx appears as a radiolucent area directly behind the soft palate.

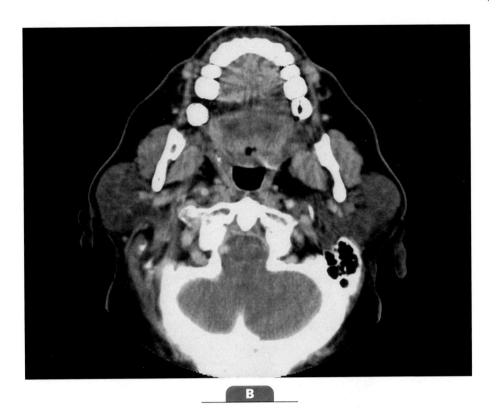

B

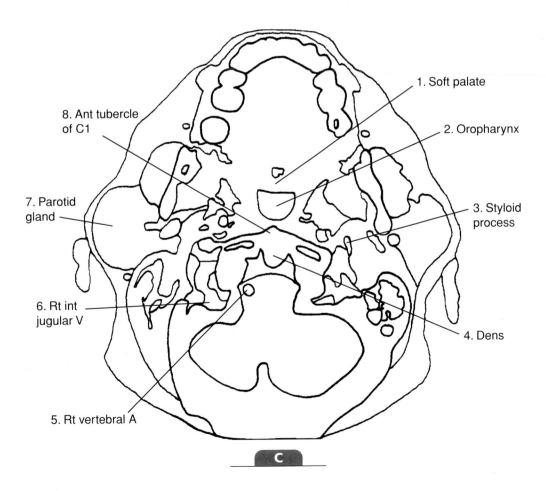

1. Soft palate

8. Ant tubercle
of C1

2. Oropharynx

7. Parotid
gland

3. Styloid
process

6. Rt int
jugular V

4. Dens

5. Rt vertebral A

C

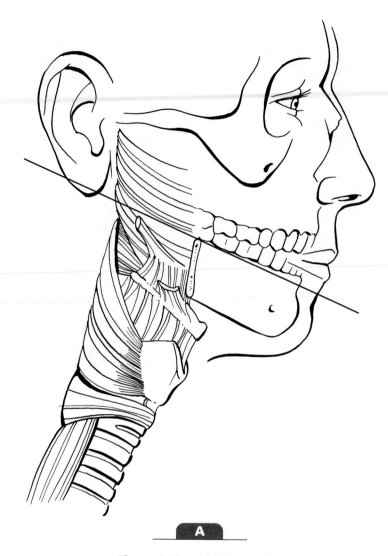

Figure 6-16 Axial CT image 3.

Figure 6-16 (A,B,C). Similar to previous images, the dens can readily be identified centrally along with the adjacent atlas, C1. At this level, the spinal cord is found between the cervical spine structures and the lower part of the occipital bone, because it lies below the level of the foramen magnum. Anterior to the cervical spine, the contrast-enhanced internal carotid artery and internal jugular vein can be identified on the right. In general, the carotid artery will lie deep to the internal jugular vein as the vessels extend through the region of the neck. Within the parotid gland, the retromandibular vein is shown in cross-section below its origin from the smaller veins in the temporal and maxillary regions. In lower images, the retromandibular vein will be shown to drain into the external jugular vein. Between the cervical spine structures and the genioglossus muscle, the extension of the soft palate known as the uvula is labeled within the opening of the oropharynx.

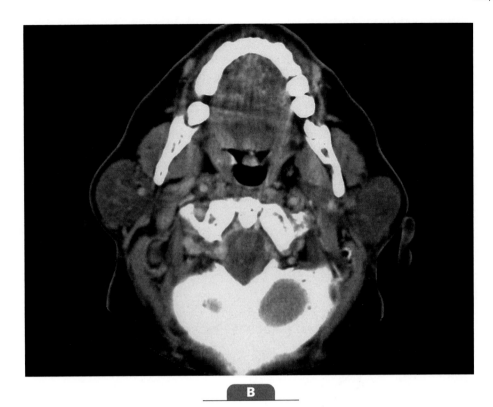

B

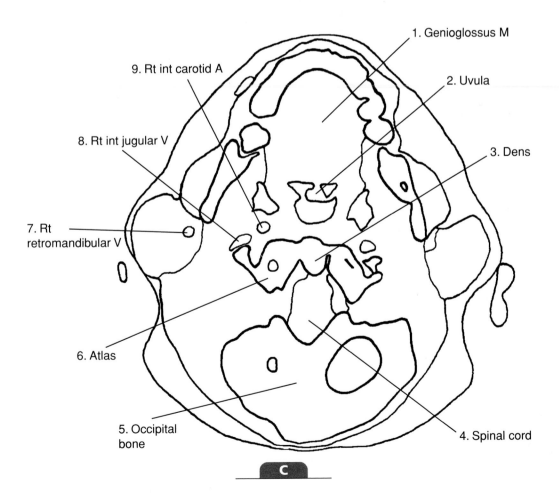

1. Genioglossus M

9. Rt int carotid A

2. Uvula

8. Rt int jugular V

3. Dens

7. Rt retromandibular V

6. Atlas

5. Occipital bone

4. Spinal cord

C

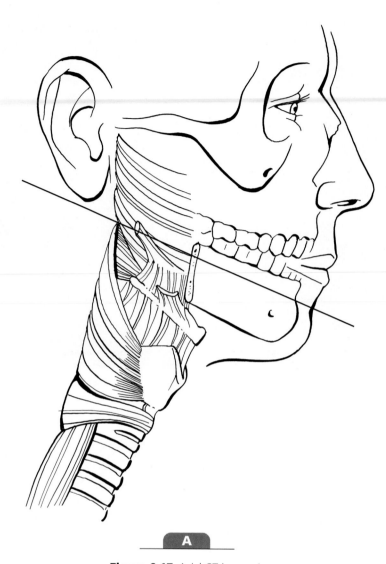

Figure 6-17 Axial CT image 4.

Figure 6-17 (A,B,C). At this level, the lower teeth are joining the body of the mandible and the rami can no longer be clearly identified as separate structures. Between the mandible and the cervical spine, the genioglossus and oropharynx can again be seen. On either side of C2, the contrast-enhanced internal carotid arteries are found deep to the internal jugular veins. Superficially, the characteristic consistency of the parotid gland is again shown to include the contrast-enhanced retromandibular veins. Posterior to the left parotid gland, a small part of the auricle of the ear is shown, sectioned separate from the other structures within this image. The occipital bone is again found posterior to the cervical spine but here has an irregular appearance, because the image demonstrates the lower-most part of the bone.

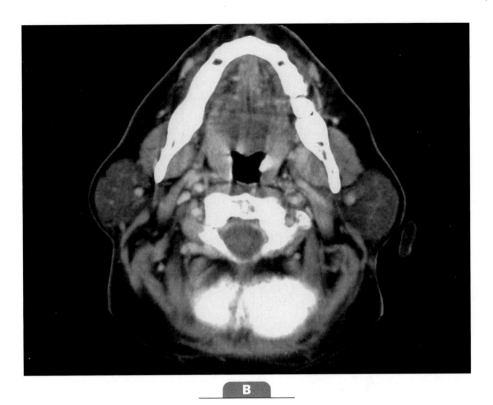

B

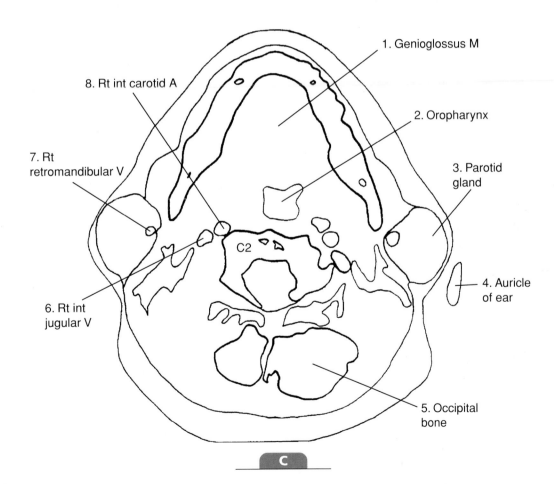

1. Genioglossus M

8. Rt int carotid A

2. Oropharynx

7. Rt
retromandibular V

3. Parotid
gland

C2

4. Auricle
of ear

6. Rt int
jugular V

5. Occipital
bone

C

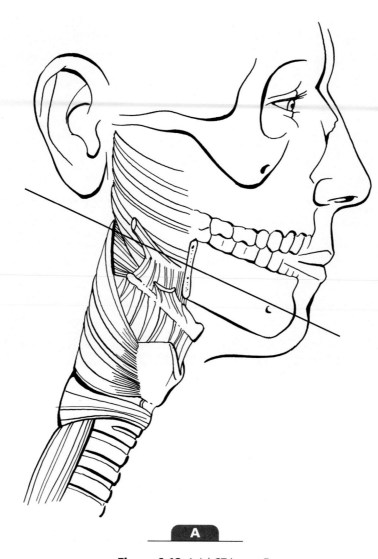

A

Figure 6-18 Axial CT image 5.

Figure 6-18 (A,B,C). The occipital bone is no longer seen, and the teeth have been replaced by the body of the mandible. Centrally, the spinal cord is separating the body and laminae of C2. Similar to previous images, the oropharynx is located anterior to the cervical spine. Anterolateral to the body of C2, the internal carotid arteries and internal jugular veins are readily distinguished from surrounding structures by contrast enhancement. Superficially, the characteristic consistency of the parotid gland can be found on either side encompassing the retromandibular veins.

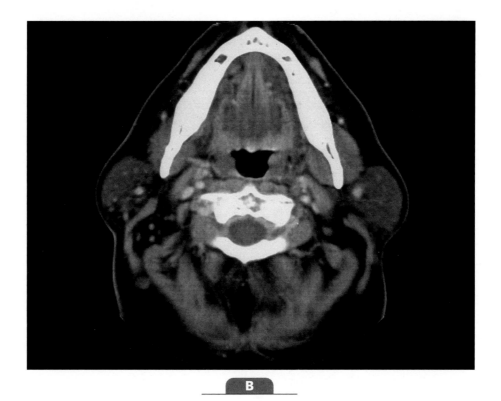

B

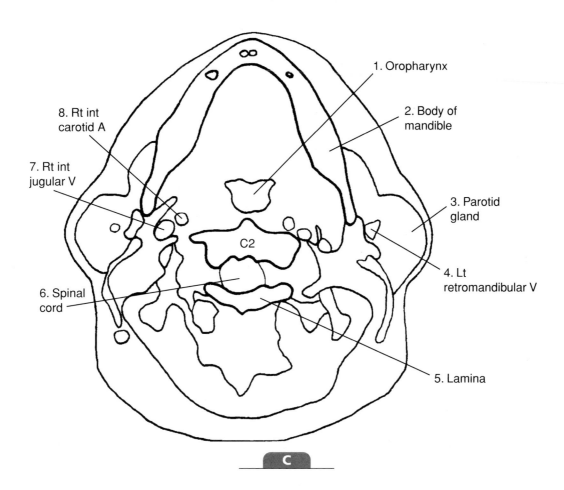

1. Oropharynx

2. Body of mandible

8. Rt int carotid A

7. Rt int jugular V

3. Parotid gland

C2

4. Lt retromandibular V

6. Spinal cord

5. Lamina

C

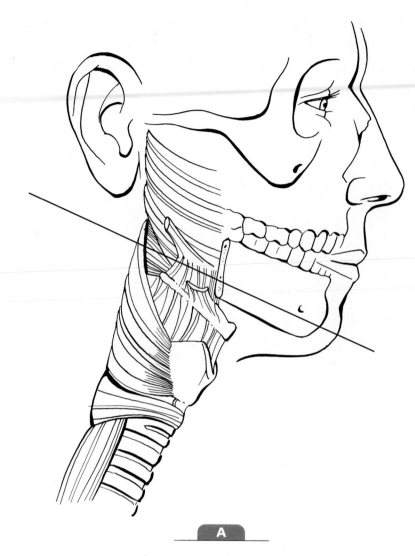

Figure 6-19 Axial CT image 6.

Figure 6-19 (A,B,C). The bony structures in this image can be labeled the body of the mandible and the third cervical vertebra. Although the oropharynx is again found just anterior to the body of C3, the genioglossus muscle seen in higher images has been replaced by the thinner geniohyoid muscles that extend between the inferior mental spine on the mandible to the hyoid bone, forming the floor of the mouth. On the right side of C3, the internal carotid artery is labeled deep to the internal jugular vein, and the right retromandibular vein is labeled within the parotid gland.

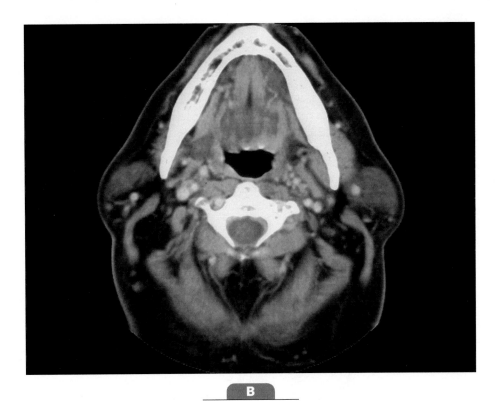

B

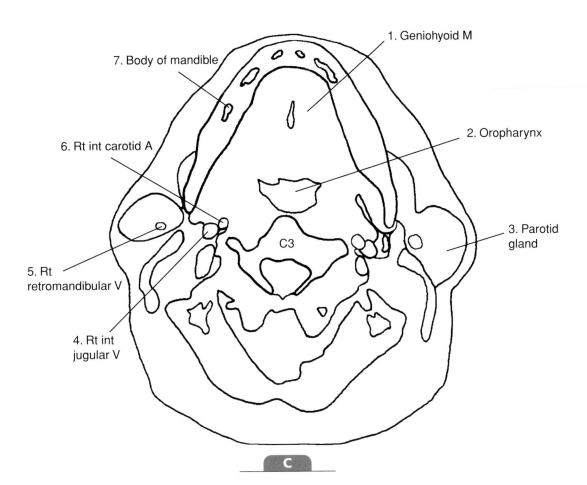

1. Geniohyoid M

7. Body of mandible

2. Oropharynx

6. Rt int carotid A

3. Parotid gland

5. Rt retromandibular V

C3

4. Rt int jugular V

C

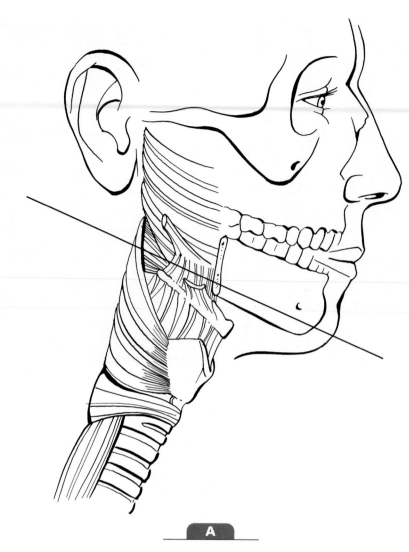

Figure 6-20 Axial CT image 7.

Figure 6-20 (A,B,C). In regard to bony anatomy structures, the body of the mandible is shown in its entirety anterior to C3. In this image, the body of C3 is found directly behind the oropharynx and is separated from the vertebral arch by the intervertebral foramina. On the right side of the patient, the right vertebral artery can be seen as a contrast-enhanced vessel sectioned near the transverse foramen. Lateral to the vertebral body, the internal carotid artery is again demonstrated deep to the internal jugular vein. However, the external carotid artery can now be seen as a contrast-enhanced vessel anterior to the internal carotid artery. Superficially, the retromandibular vein is now found outside of the parotid gland and will be seen in subsequent sections to drain into the external jugular vein.

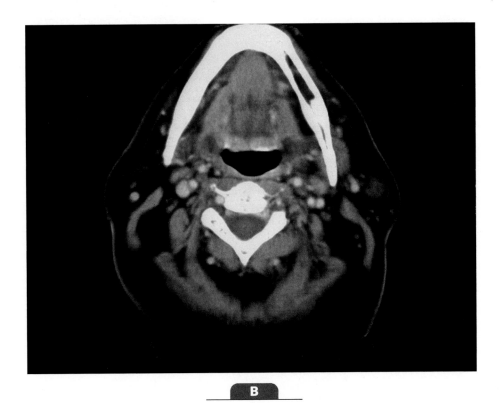

B

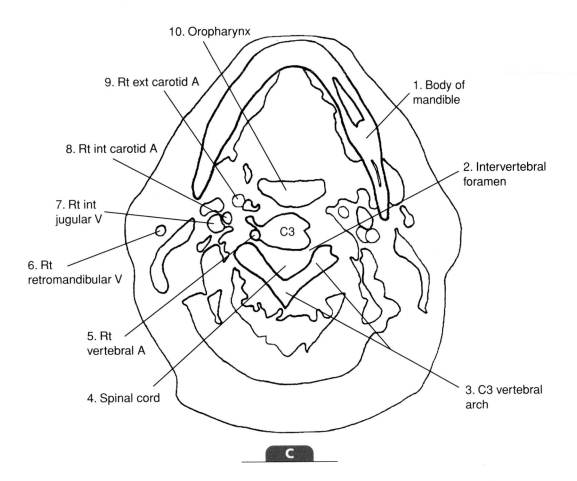

10. Oropharynx

9. Rt ext carotid A

8. Rt int carotid A

7. Rt int jugular V

6. Rt retromandibular V

5. Rt vertebral A

4. Spinal cord

1. Body of mandible

2. Intervertebral foramen

C3

3. C3 vertebral arch

C

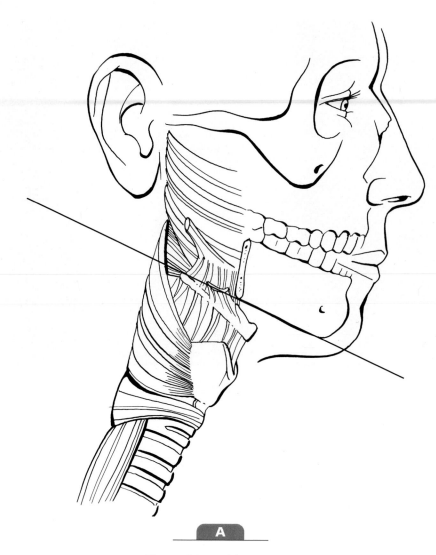

Figure 6-21 Axial CT image 8.

Figure 6-21 (A,B,C). The muscles of the tongue and the oropharynx are found between the body of the mandible and C3. On the right side of the patient, the right vertebral artery is the contrast-enhanced vessel within the transverse foramen. Lateral to the cervical vertebra, the internal carotid artery can be distinguished from the adjacent internal jugular vein, because the vein is larger and more superficially located. Compared with the previous image, the external carotid artery and the internal carotid artery are somewhat closer together, but the external carotid artery still occupies a more anterior position. Separated from these vessels by the sternocleidomastoid muscle, the retromandibular vein is found on the side of the neck in a superficial position below the level of the parotid gland.

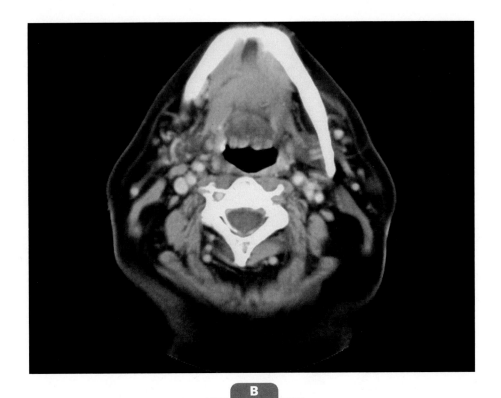

B

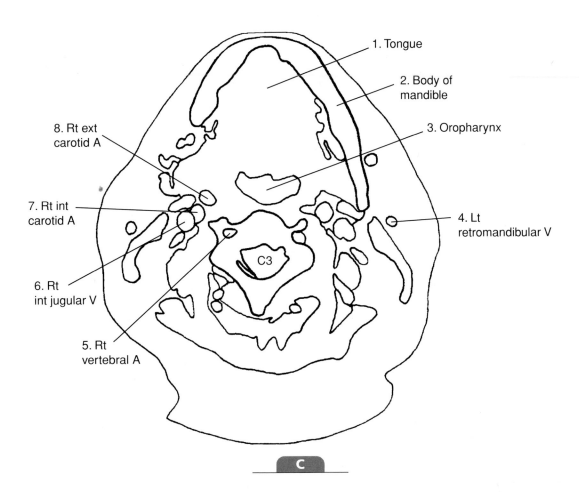

1. Tongue

2. Body of mandible

3. Oropharynx

4. Lt retromandibular V

8. Rt ext carotid A

7. Rt int carotid A

6. Rt int jugular V

5. Rt vertebral A

C3

C

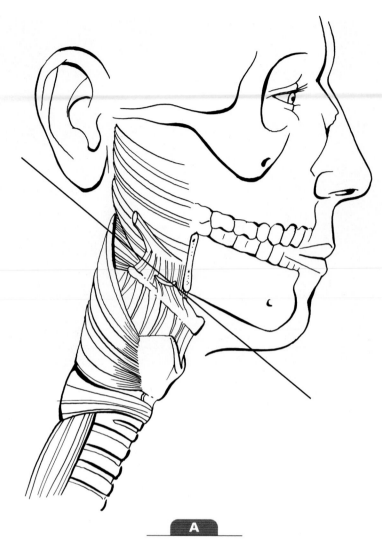

Figure 6-22 Axial CT image 9.

Figure 6-22 (A,B,C). At this level in the neck, the body of the mandible is no longer seen. Owing to the downward projection of the spinous processes of the cervical vertebrae, the bifid spinous process is demonstrated posterior to C4 extending from C3. On either side of the vertebral body, the vertebral arteries are contrast enhanced and are demonstrated emerging from the transverse foramina. Anterior to the vertebral body, the upper tip of the epiglottis is within the pharynx, indicating the radiolucent area is the laryngeal pharynx. Between the epiglottis and the muscles of the tongue, the valleculae are spaces on either side and are continuous with the more posteriorly located laryngeal pharynx. The characteristic consistency of the submandibular gland can be identified on either side of the pharynx, just anterior to the major vessels of the neck. At this level, the external and internal carotid arteries have joined to form the contrast-enhanced common carotid artery deep to the internal jugular veins. Because we are now below the level of the mandible, the retromandibular vein has given rise to the external jugular vein, which continues in a superficial location in the anterolateral neck.

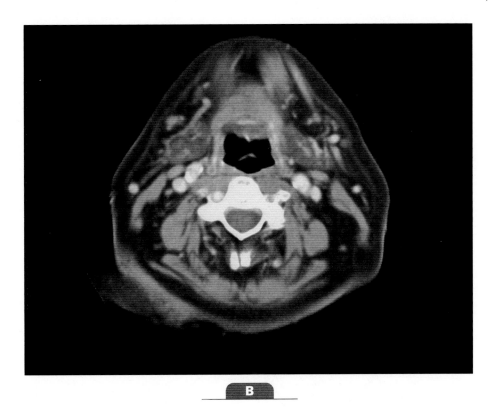

B

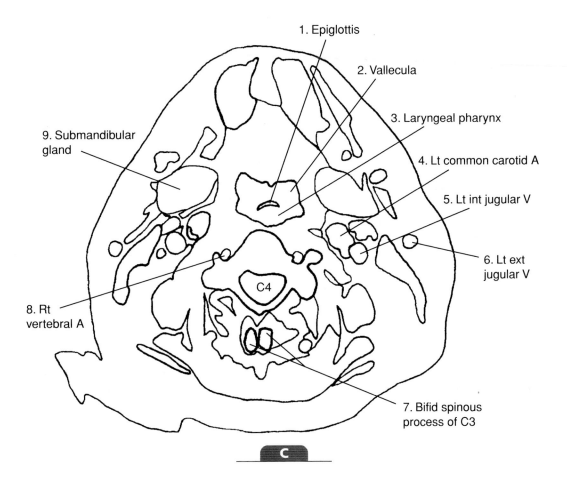

1. Epiglottis

2. Vallecula

3. Laryngeal pharynx

4. Lt common carotid A

5. Lt int jugular V

6. Lt ext jugular V

9. Submandibular gland

8. Rt vertebral A

C4

7. Bifid spinous process of C3

C

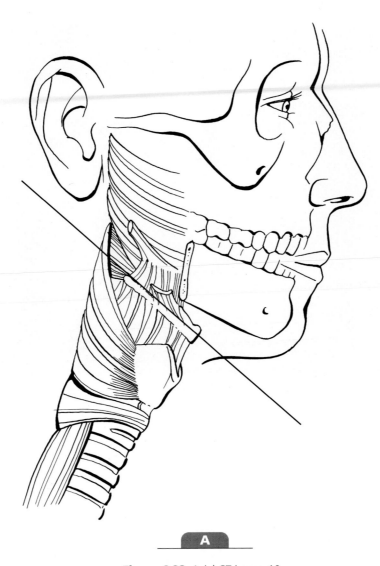

A

Figure 6-23 Axial CT image 10.

Figure 6-23 (A,B,C). Centrally, C4 is shown anterior to the spinous process of C3, which projects inferiorly into this section. On the right side of the body of C4, the contrast-enhanced vertebral artery is labeled in the location previously described as the transverse foramen. Anterior to the cervical vertebra, the small U-shaped hyoid bone is seen surrounding the pharynx and, because of its smaller size and deeper location within the neck, should not be confused with the mandible. Similar to the previous image, the upper epiglottis is sectioned and divides the laryngeal pharynx from the valleculae. At this lower level, the valleculae are on either side of the median glossoepiglottic fold and extend from the posterior tongue to the epiglottis. Outside of the hyoid bone, the characteristic consistency of the submandibular gland is seen anterior to the contrast-enhanced external jugular veins. Deep to the external jugular veins, the internal jugular veins are cross-sectioned posterolateral to the common carotid arteries.

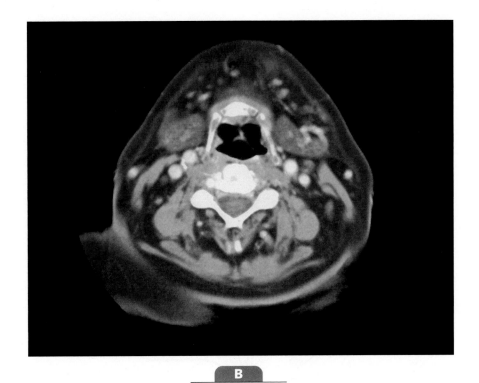

B

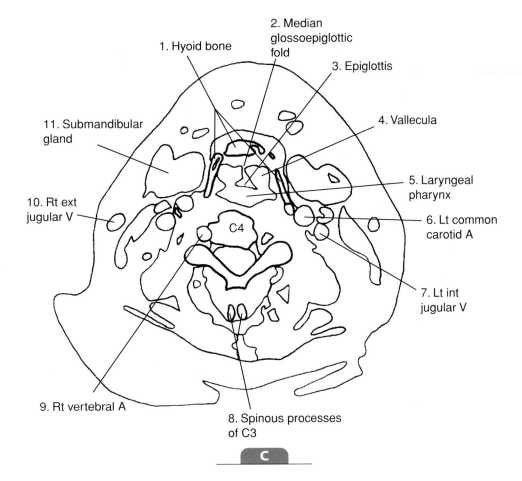

C

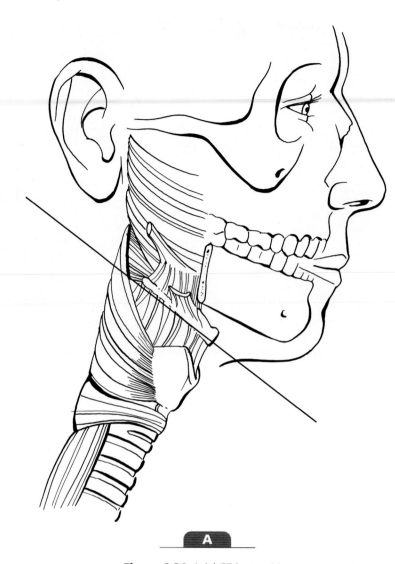

Figure 6-24 Axial CT image 11.

Figure 6-24 (A,B,C). This image clearly demonstrates the bony anatomy of C5, which contains a fracture in the posterior lamina on the right side. On either side of the vertebral body, the vertebral arteries are contrast-enhanced structures within the transverse foramina. As indicated in previous images, the size and contrast enhancement of the right vertebral artery is normal. On the left side, the vertebral artery is smaller than normal, indicating reduced blood flow. Anteriorly, the U-shaped hyoid bone arches around the epiglottis and laryngeal vestibule. On the lateral side of the neck, the deep contrast-enhanced vessels can be labeled the common carotid artery and the more superficially located internal jugular vein. On the other side of the sternocleidomastoid muscle, the vessel just below the skin is the external jugular vein.

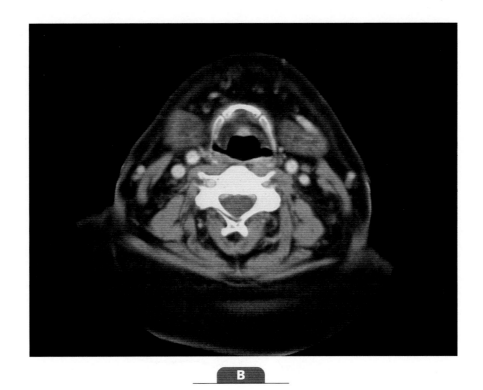

B

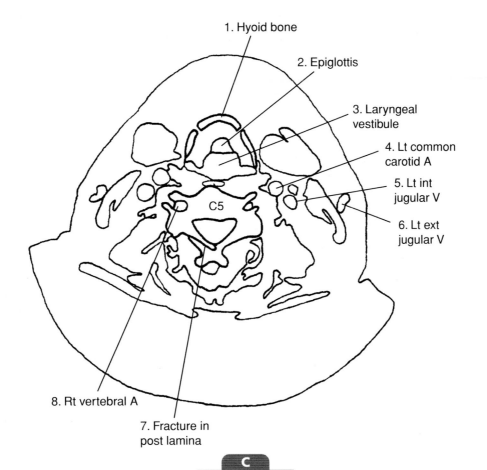

1. Hyoid bone

2. Epiglottis

3. Laryngeal vestibule

4. Lt common carotid A

5. Lt int jugular V

6. Lt ext jugular V

C5

8. Rt vertebral A

7. Fracture in post lamina

C

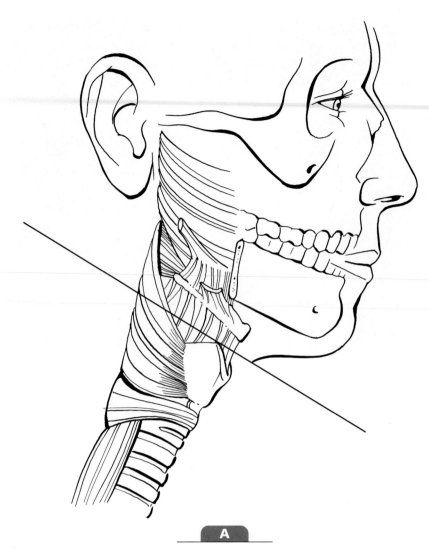

A

Figure 6-25 Axial CT image 12.

Figure 6-25 (A,B,C). The fifth cervical vertebra occupies a central position in this image. As for other cervical vertebrae, the vertebral arteries are located within the transverse foramina on either side of the vertebral body. Owing to the downward projection of the spinous processes in the cervical vertebrae, the spinous process of C4 is labeled posterior to C5. Anteriorly, the laryngeal openings are now divided into three separate spaces by the aryepiglottic folds. As described earlier, the aryepiglottic folds of skin extend from the margins of the epiglottis to the posteriorly located arytenoid cartilages. Within the aryepiglottic folds, the laryngeal vestibule is the larger opening, which will be seen in subsequent sections to lead to the vocal cords. Lateral to the aryepiglottic folds, the piriform sinuses are formed on either side outside of the larynx. When food is swallowed, the tongue moves posteriorly pushing the epiglottis down over the laryngeal vestibule so that the food continues down outside the larynx into the esophageal opening. On the lateral part of the neck, the external jugular vein is again seen more superficially located than the common carotid arteries and internal jugular veins.

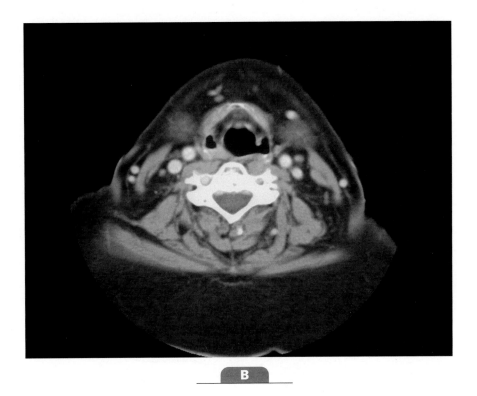

B

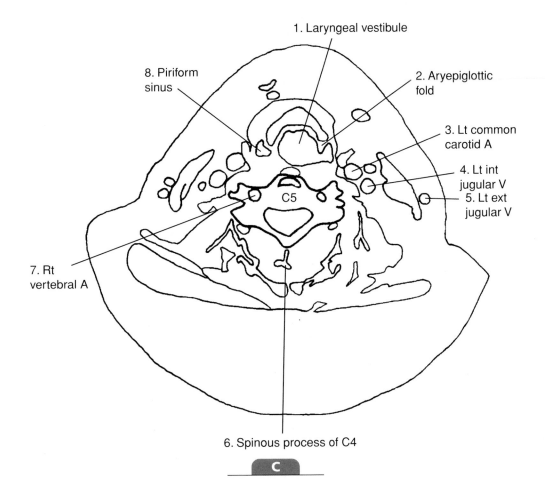

1. Laryngeal vestibule

8. Piriform sinus

2. Aryepiglottic fold

3. Lt common carotid A

4. Lt int jugular V

5. Lt ext jugular V

C5

7. Rt vertebral A

6. Spinous process of C4

C

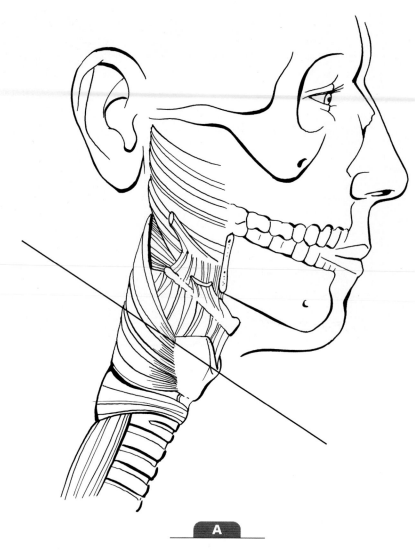

Figure 6-26 Axial CT image 13.

Figure 6-26 (A,B,C). The lower part of C5 is centrally located in this image, and the contrast-enhanced vertebral arteries are on either side of the vertebral body. The right vertebral artery, which is normal in size, appears considerably larger than the diminished left vertebral artery in this patient. Anterior to the cervical vertebra, the U-shaped thyroid cartilage surrounds the contents of the larynx. The main opening leading into the larynx, the laryngeal vestibule, is centrally located between the piriform sinuses on either side. On the right side of the patient, the arytenoid cartilage is found on the posterolateral aspect of the laryngeal vestibule and will be shown in subsequent sections as the posterior attachment for the vocal cords. On the lateral side of the neck, the common carotid artery is found anteromedial to the internal jugular vein, both of which are deeper than the superficially located external jugular vein.

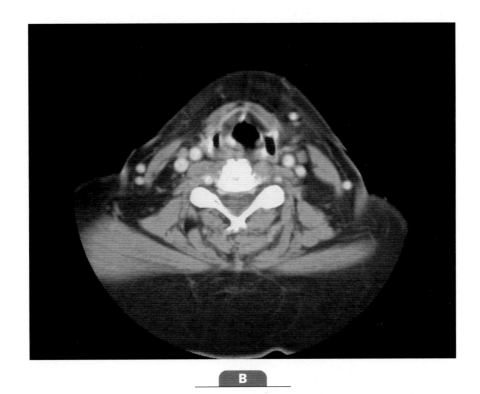

B

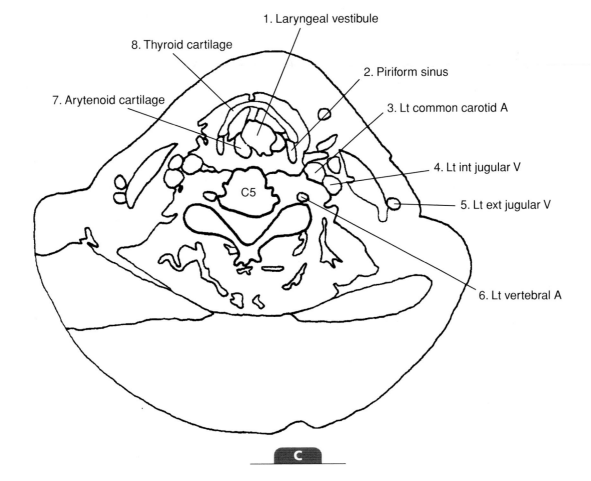

8. Thyroid cartilage

1. Laryngeal vestibule

2. Piriform sinus

7. Arytenoid cartilage

3. Lt common carotid A

4. Lt int jugular V

C5

5. Lt ext jugular V

6. Lt vertebral A

C

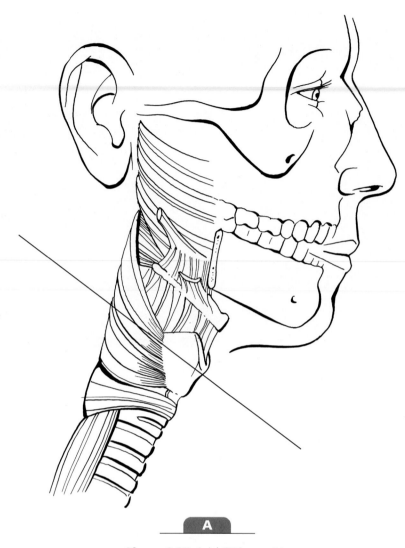

A

Figure 6-27 Axial CT image 14.

Figure 6-27 (A,B,C). C6 is in the center of this image and is demonstrated forming a complete enclosure around the vertebral foramen. Owing to the cervical curvature, the lower cervical vertebrae occupy a more horizontal position, as demonstrated in this image, because the spinous process of C6 is demonstrated along with the vertebral body. Similar to other cervical vertebrae, the vertebral arteries are found on either side within the transverse processes. In this patient, the left vertebral artery is significantly smaller than the normal right vertebral artery. In the anterior neck, the thyroid cartilage arches over the contents of the larynx. The main opening extending into the larynx, the laryngeal vestibule, is found between the thyroid and arytenoid cartilages. Located between the vestibular and vocal folds, the glottic space is shown on the left side continuous with the laryngeal vestibule. The spaces on either side of the laryngeal vestibule outside of the larynx represent the piriform sinuses. Located outside the larynx, the piriform sinuses are continuous with the esophageal opening posterior to the arytenoid cartilages. On the lateral aspect of the neck, the external jugular vein again occupies a superficial location and the internal jugular vein and common carotid artery are more deeply situated under the superficial musculature of the neck.

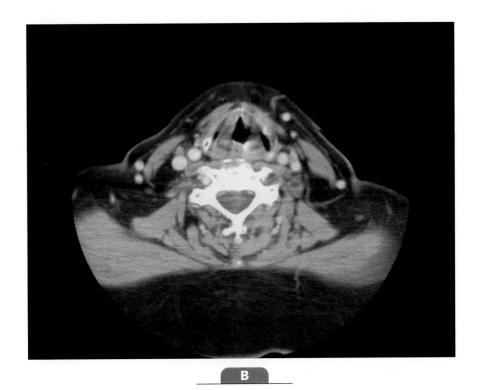

B

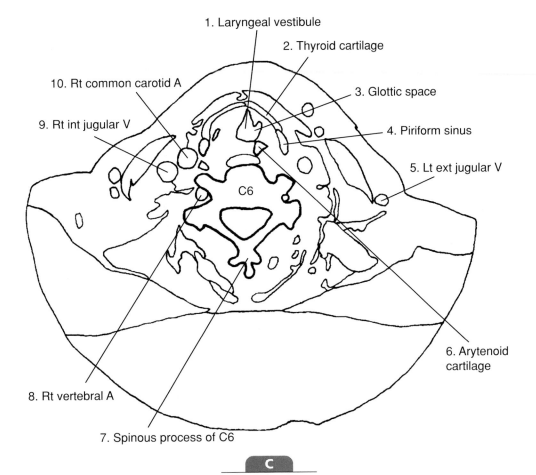

1. Laryngeal vestibule

2. Thyroid cartilage

10. Rt common carotid A

3. Glottic space

9. Rt int jugular V

4. Piriform sinus

5. Lt ext jugular V

C6

6. Arytenoid cartilage

8. Rt vertebral A

7. Spinous process of C6

C

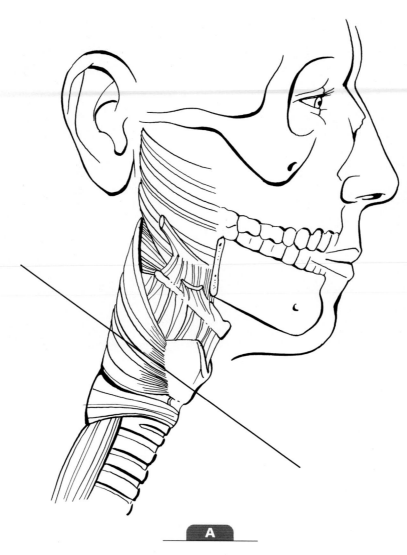

Figure 6-28 Axial CT image 15.

Figure 6-28 (A,B,C). Owing to the larger size of the lower cervical vertebrae, C6 is again seen centrally located in this image, and the vertebral arteries are located in the transverse processes on either side. At this level, the thyroid cartilage is found anterior to the radiolucent area representing the openings within the larynx. Within the larynx, the space is now labeled the infraglottic space, because we are at a level below the vocal cords, which are labeled on the right side. Between the body of the cervical vertebra and the infraglottic space, the oval-shaped region of musculature is formed by the walls of the esophagus, which are collapsed (thus the esophageal opening is not shown in this image). On the lateral aspect of the neck, the common carotid artery is found deep to the adjacent internal jugular vein, and both vessels lie deeper within the neck than the superficially located external jugular vein.

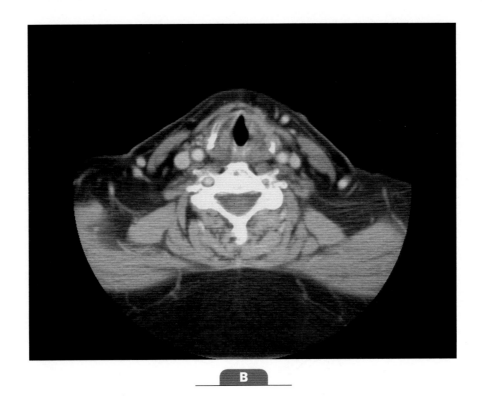

B

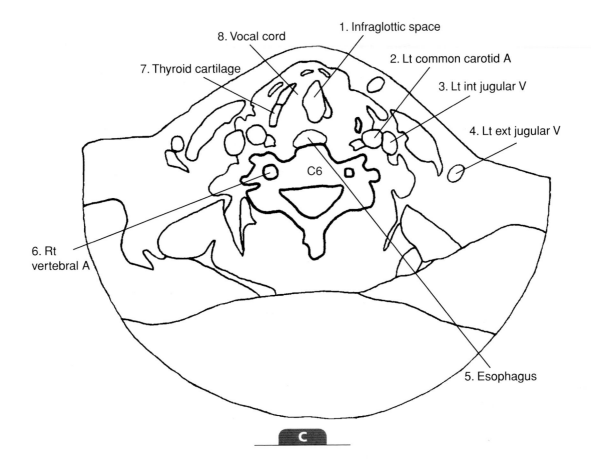

8. Vocal cord

1. Infraglottic space

7. Thyroid cartilage

2. Lt common carotid A

3. Lt int jugular V

4. Lt ext jugular V

C6

6. Rt
vertebral A

5. Esophagus

C

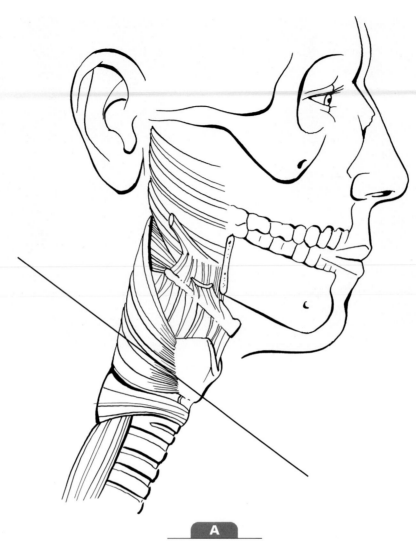

A

Figure 6-29 Axial CT image 16.

Figure 6-29 (A,B,C). The bony anatomy in this image again demonstrates the lower part of C6. Similar to the previous images, the right vertebral artery appears as a normal-sized contrast-enhanced vessel, whereas the left vertebral artery is difficult to distinguish because it is so small. Directly in front of the vertebral body, the esophagus and trachea are cross-sectioned within the deep neck. In the anterior neck, the thyroid cartilage is sectioned on either side of the opening of the trachea. On the lateral aspect of the neck, the common carotid artery is again found deep to the internal jugular vein, and together they are covered by the musculature of the superficial neck. Compared to previous images, the superficially located external jugular vein now occupies a more lateral location as it extends downward to the subclavian vein of the chest.

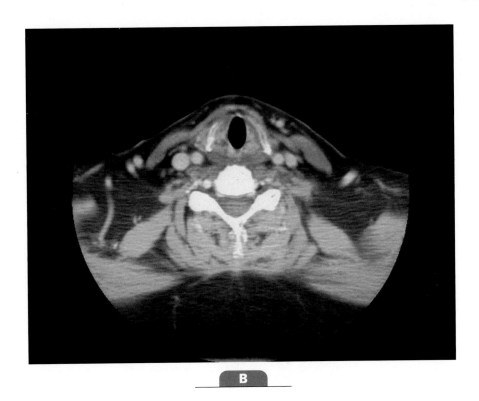

B

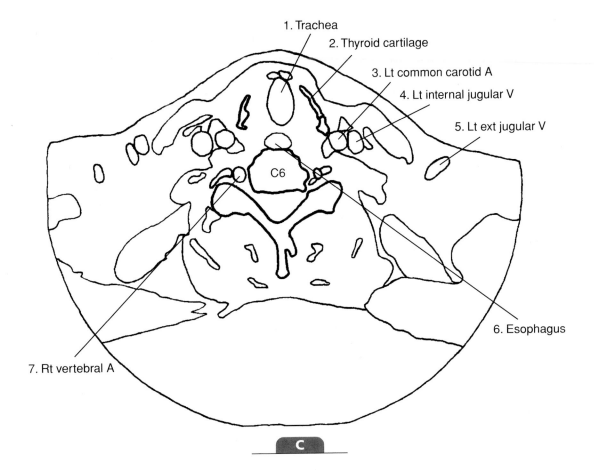

1. Trachea
2. Thyroid cartilage
3. Lt common carotid A
4. Lt internal jugular V
5. Lt ext jugular V

C6

6. Esophagus

7. Rt vertebral A

C

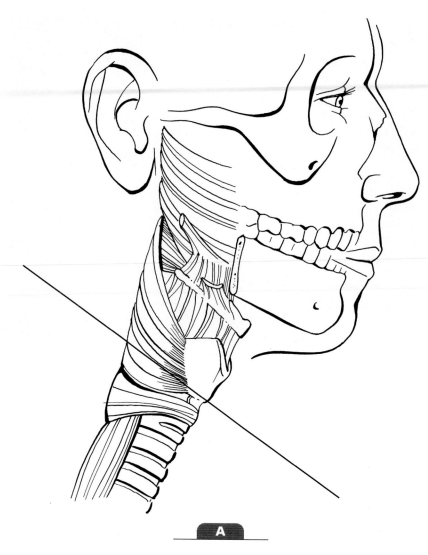

Figure 6-30 Axial CT image 17.

Figure 6-30 (A,B,C). The upper part of C7 can be seen centrally in this image. Although this section shows only the upper part of C7, the spinous process appears quite large compared to the other cervical vertebrae. Similar to previous images, the vertebral arteries are located in the transverse processes on either side, and the left vertebral artery is significantly diminished in size. Anterior to the vertebral body, the oval-shaped musculature of the esophagus lies directly behind the opening of the trachea. On either side of the trachea, the lower parts of the thyroid cartilage are sectioned anterior to the common carotid arteries and internal jugular veins. Similar to the previous image, the external jugular veins are found laterally as they extend toward the subclavian veins in the chest.

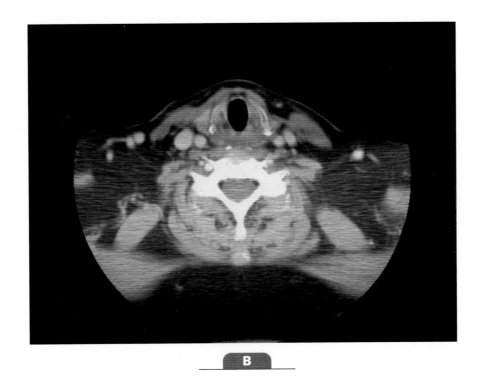

B

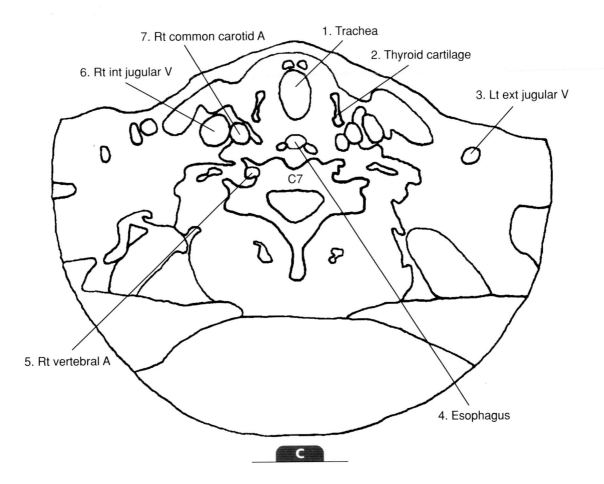

7. Rt common carotid A

1. Trachea

6. Rt int jugular V

2. Thyroid cartilage

3. Lt ext jugular V

C7

5. Rt vertebral A

4. Esophagus

C

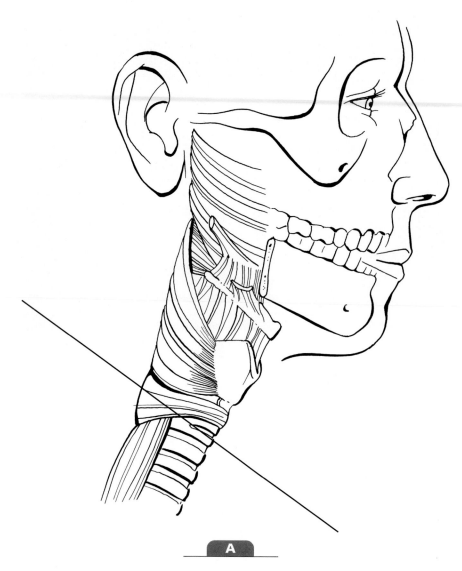

Figure 6-31 Axial CT image 18.

Figure 6-31 (A,B,C). This image clearly demonstrates the enlarged spinous process of C7, known as the vertebra prominens. The inferior location of C7 makes it difficult to image, because it is at the juncture of the neck with the torso. Aliasing or beam-hardening artifacts are frequently seen in CT images as a result of the thickness of the shoulders compared to the neck. Like all cervical vertebrae, the transverse processes of C7 contain transverse foramina. However, the vertebral arteries are not found within the foramina, because they pass in front of the transverse processes of C7. Between the opening of the trachea and the vertebral body, the esophagus appears as an oval-shaped muscular tube and is difficult to discern from the surrounding soft tissue structures. Lateral to the esophagus, the common carotid artery is found deep to the internal jugular vein below the superficial musculature of the neck. In the superficial neck, the external jugular veins occupy a lateral position at this level, because they are nearing the subclavian veins in the chest.

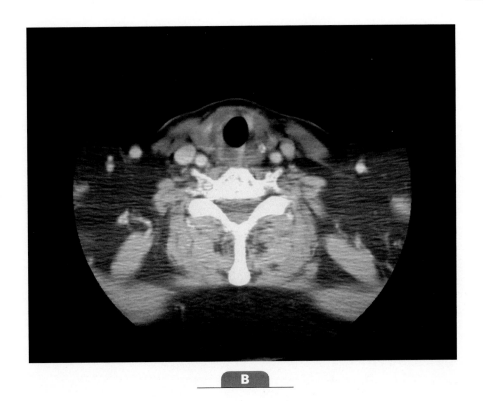

B

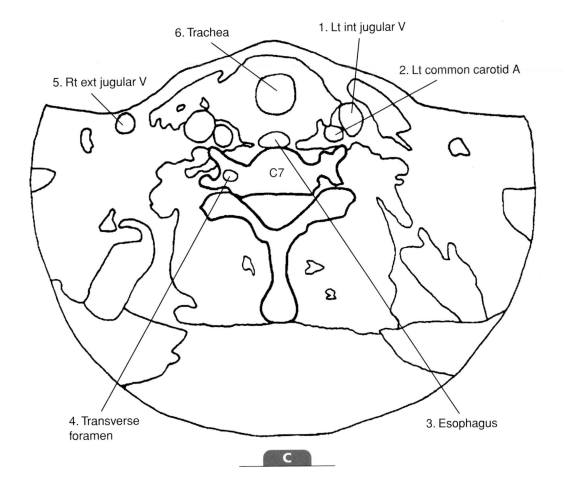

6. Trachea

1. Lt int jugular V

5. Rt ext jugular V

2. Lt common carotid A

C7

4. Transverse
foramen

3. Esophagus

C

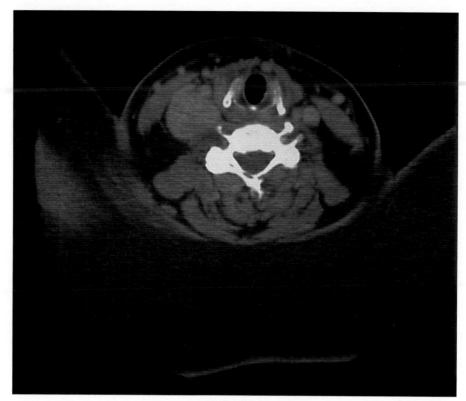

Figure 6-32

Supplement 6-1. *Figure 6-32 shows a CT scan of the neck of a 48-year-old woman. The image reveals a carotid body tumor that involves the right deep cervical region. The mass is located within the region of the vascular sheath and is roughly spherical in shape, measuring 3 cm in diameter. The abnormal tissue is well defined, demonstrates moderate contrast enhancement, and is mildly heterogeneous. The tumor is compressing the internal jugular vein, which appears flattened on its anterior surface. There is also a mass effect on the common carotid artery, seen on the anteromedial aspect of the mass.*

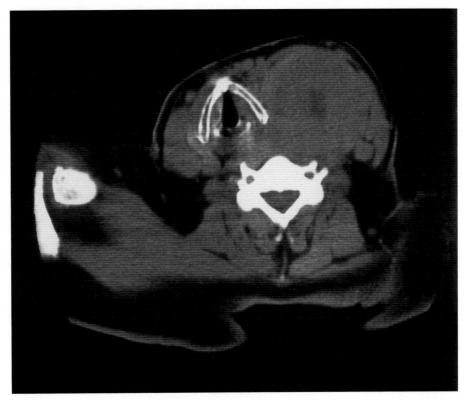

Figure 6-33

Supplement 6-2. *Figure 6-33 is a CT scan of a 67-year-old man. The examination was performed to evaluate a large tumor, 7 cm in diameter, on the left side of his neck. The large mass is well defined and shows a central low-density region consistent with necrosis. In this image, the mass is shown to have a considerable mass effect on the larynx, which remains patent. On the left side, the common carotid artery and the internal jugular vein are displaced laterally but are not encased by the mass. A CT scan of the abdomen and a biopsy result determined the cervical mass to be metastatic disease from a renal cell carcinoma.*

REVIEW QUESTIONS

1. The neck is the region of the body between the_____and the_____.
2. C2 is also called the_____.
3. Which of the following vertebrae is described as not having a vertebral body?
   A. Thoracic
   B. Axis
   C. C3 through C6
   D. Atlas
4. The hyoid bone is found at a level corresponding to the_____cervical vertebra.
5. Which of the following is described as a ring-shaped cartilage forming part of the larynx?
   A. Arytenoid
   B. Thyroid
   C. Cricoid
   D. Epiglottis
6. List the three spaces within the larynx:_____is superior,_____is in the middle, and_____is inferior.
7. Briefly describe the location of the valleculae.
8. The vestibular folds are located superior to the vocal folds. True or false
9. The common carotid arteries bifurcate into the internal and external branches at the level of the intervertebral disk between_____and_____.
10. The left vertebral artery originates from which of the following?
    A. Aortic arch
    B. Axillary
    C. Subclavian
    D. Common carotid
11. Describe the glottic space.
12. Which of the following best describes the piriform sinuses?
    A. Between the epiglottis and tongue
    B. Below the vocal fold
    C. On either side of the larynx
    D. Between the vestibular and vocal folds
13. The aryepiglottic folds are also known as the false vocal cords. True or false
14. The epiglottis attaches inferiorly to the_____ and forms part of the [anterior / posterior] wall of the opening within the larynx.
15. The_____are the spaces on either side of the median glossoepiglottic fold.
16. The_____cartilages are pyramidal shaped and rest on the posterior arch of the_____cartilage.
17. Which of the following vessels is located most anteriorly in the upper neck?
    A. External carotid artery
    B. Internal carotid artery
    C. Internal jugular vein
    D. Vertebral artery
18. List the three parts of the pharynx:_____is superior,_____is in the middle, and_____is inferior.
19. The U-shaped_____gland is located just below the larynx and has two large lobes on either side of the upper trachea.
20. The external jugular veins drain into the_____ veins on either side of the neck.

Chapter 7

Spine

OBJECTIVES

Upon completion of this chapter, the student should be able to:

1. State the number of vertebrae in each region of the spine.

2. Explain the distinguishing characteristics of the vertebrae in each region.

3. Identify and describe the relationships between vertebrae.

4. Describe the components of the intervertebral disk.

5. Describe the ligaments of the spine.

6. Identify and describe the openings within the spine.

7. Describe the parts of the spinal cord.

8. Identify and describe the meningeal coverings of the spinal cord and nerve roots.

9. Describe the position of nerve roots within the spine in relation to other structures.

10. Correctly identify anatomical structures on patient CT and MR images of the spine.

ANATOMICAL OVERVIEW

The anatomy of the spine is symmetrical and is described as the assemblage of vertebrae below the cranium and including the coccyx.

Skeletal

Cervical vertebrae (*SER-vĭ-kal VER-tĕ-brē*). The uppermost seven vertebrae, located between the cranium and the thoracic vertebrae (Fig. 7-1). They are easily distinguished from other vertebrae by their small size and the foramina in the transverse processes. See chapter 6 for more details.

Thoracic (*thō-RAS-ik*) **vertebrae.** The 12 vertebrae of the chest, found in the spine forming the posterior border of the thoracic cage. They are of average size and are distinguishable by the presence of costal facets for articulation with the ribs. See Chapter 2 for more details.

Lumbar (*LŬM-bar*) **vertebrae.** The vertebrae that form the posterior border of the abdominal cavity. Five are usually found; however, four and six are common anomalies, which may confuse the viewer when determining image location. They can be distinguished by their large size and the absence of costal facets and transverse foramina.

Vertebral (*VER-tĕ-brăl*) **structures.** With the exception of the atlas (C1), all vertebrae contain a body, two pedicles, two laminae, and seven processes (two transverse, four articular, and one spinous).

Vertebral body. The largest and heaviest portion of the vertebra. Located anterior to the vertebral arch, forming the anterior margin of the vertebral foramen (*fō-RA-men*). Their size increases as one moves down the vertebral column (Fig. 7-1). The bodies of thoracic vertebrae have superior and inferior costal facets for articulating with the ribs.

Pedicles (*PED-ĭ-klz*). Bony projections that form the lateral walls of the vertebral foramen and connect the vertebral body to the transverse processes.

Laminae (*LAM-i-nē*). The remainder of the vertebral arch. They form the posterolateral walls of vertebral foramen, connecting the transverse processes with the spinous process.

Transverse processes. Bony structures originating from the juncture of the laminae and pedicles that project laterally and provide a site of attachment for the deep muscles of the back. Cervical vertebrae have transverse foramina and thoracic vertebrae have articular facets for the tubercles of the ribs.

Articular processes. Bony structures that are directly lateral to the vertebral foramen and extend upward and downward from the points at which the pedicles and laminae join. On the superior articular process, the upward projection, the articular surface faces posteriorly. The inferior articular

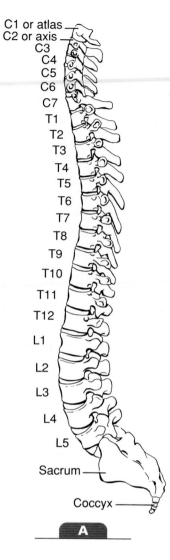

Figure 7-1 A. Lateral view of entire vertebral column with assorted views of individual vertebrae. **B.** Superior view of a cervical vertebra. **C.** Lateral view of a thoracic vertebra. **D.** Lateral view of a lumbar vertebra. **E.** Posterior view of the sacrum.

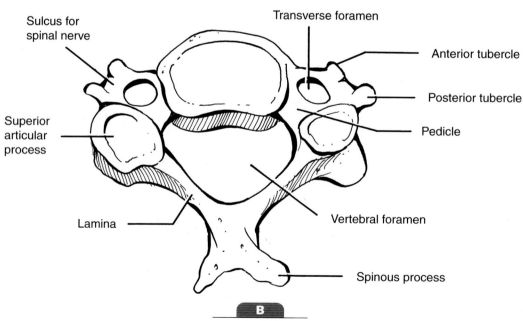

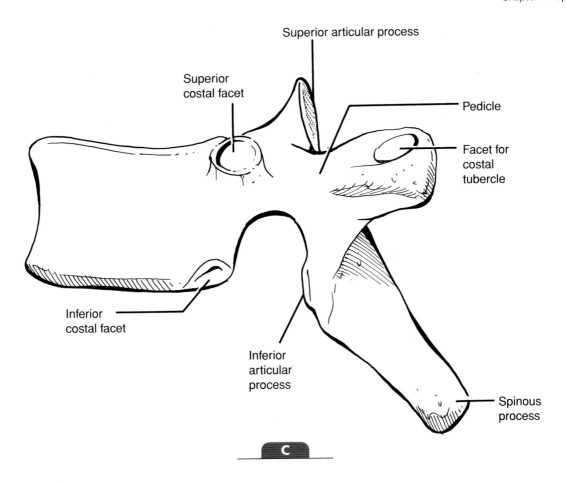

Superior articular process

Superior costal facet

Pedicle

Facet for costal tubercle

Inferior costal facet

Inferior articular process

Spinous process

C

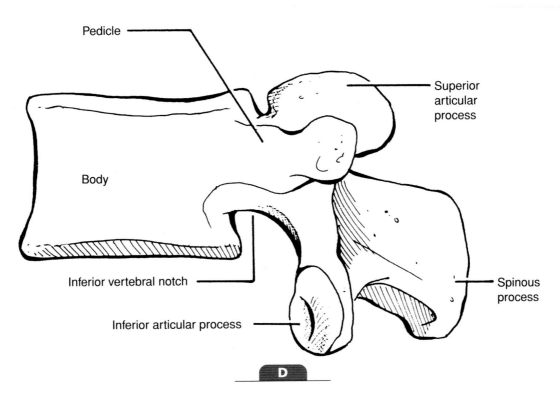

Pedicle

Superior articular process

Body

Inferior vertebral notch

Inferior articular process

Spinous process

D

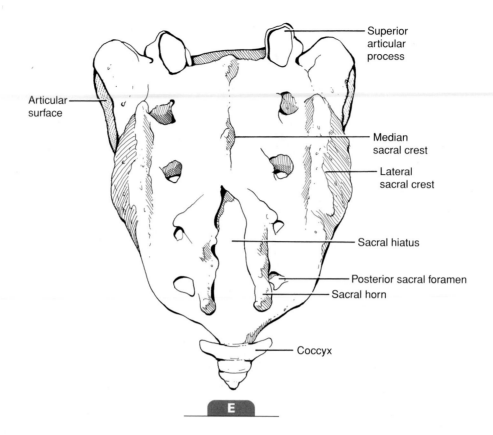

process, the downward projection of bone, faces anteriorly. Together, they form the zygapophyseal (*ZĪ-gă-pō-FIZ-ē-ăl*) joints between adjacent vertebrae.

Spinous processes. Originate from the posterior union of the laminae. Bony processes that extend posteriorly and provide a site of attachment for the muscles of the back. Those on cervical vertebrae are shorter than those on thoracic and lumbar vertebrae, with the exception of the vertebra prominens on C7. The terminal processes of cervical vertebrae are usually bifid, unlike the single processes of other vertebrae.

Sacrum (*SĀ-krŭm*). Composed of five fused vertebral segments. The triangular bone that forms the posterior portion of the pelvis. Because the sacrum articulates with the fused ilia on either side, the foramina for the sacral spinal nerves open both anteriorly and posteriorly.

Coccyx (*KOK-siks*). Usually composed of four small rudimentary vertebral segments that form the caudal end of the spinal column. Common anomalies include three and five vertebral segments.

Foramina (*fō-RAM-i-nă*) of the Spine

Vertebral foramina. The large triangular openings within the vertebrae between the body and the vertebral arch. Together, they create the opening for the spinal cord. Because the opening narrows as it extends downward, the foramina in the thoracic and lumbar vertebrae are smaller and rounder than those in the cervical vertebrae.

Intervertebral foramina. Between the vertebrae, the opening formed on either side of the vertebral foramen that allows nerve roots to enter and exit the spinal column. Their size and shape depend on the alignment of the two adjoining vertebrae (Fig. 7-2).

Intervertebral Joints

Zygapophysis (*ZĪ-gă-POF-i-sis*). The joint between the superior and inferior articular processes of adjacent vertebrae. In axial or sagittal section, the superior articular process is found anterior and lateral to the inferior articular process.

Anterior longitudinal ligament. The layer of dense connective tissue tightly attached to the anterior surfaces of vertebrae and intervertebral disks extending from C2 to the sacrum.

Posterior longitudinal ligament. The layer of dense connective tissue tightly attached to the posterior surfaces of vertebrae and intervertebral disks extending from C2 to the sacrum.

Intervertebral disks. Connective tissue found between the vertebral bodies from C2 to the sacrum. They are of different sizes and help form the curvatures of the spine. They make up approximately one-quarter of the length of the vertebral column. Although their primary function is to form

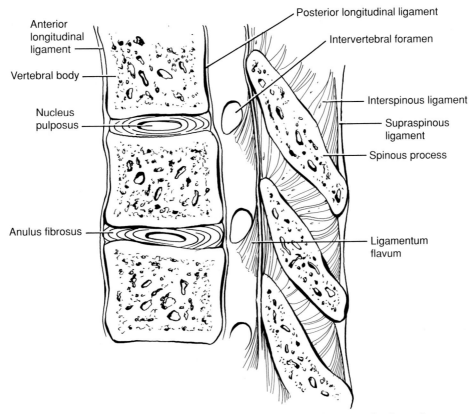

Anterior longitudinal ligament

Vertebral body

Nucleus pulposus

Anulus fibrosus

Posterior longitudinal ligament

Intervertebral foramen

Interspinous ligament

Supraspinous ligament

Spinous process

Ligamentum flavum

Figure 7-2 Mid-sagittal section thorough the vertebral column demonstrating bone, ligaments, and foramina.

part of the amphiarthrodial (*AM-fi-ar-THRO-de-ăl*) joints within the spine, they are also important in absorbing shock to the spine.

Anulus fibrosus (*AN-yū-lŭs fi-brō-sŭs*). A concentric ring of fibrous tissue and fibrocartilage that forms the periphery of the disk.

Nucleus pulposus (*NŪ-klē-ŭs pŭl-PŌ-sŭs*). The soft, pulpy, elastic material found within the center of the disk.

Spinal Cord and Coverings

Conus medullaris (*KŌ-nŭs MED-ŭ-LĂ-ris*). The caudal tip of the spinal cord found between L1 and L3 (Fig. 7-3).
Cauda equina (*KAW-dă E-kwin*). Within the dural sheath, the bundle of lumbar and sacral nerves descending below the termination of the spinal cord. Resembles the caudal end of a horse (a horse's tail).
Nerve roots. At each vertebral level, a pair of nerve roots exit the spine through the intervertebral foramina on either side to form the right and left spinal nerves (Fig. 7-4). They originate from the spinal cord and are separated into anterior and posterior roots. Surrounded by a sleeve of meninges, they join together outside the intervertebral

foramen to form a spinal nerve. With the exception of the cervical vertebrae, the spinal nerves exit below the corresponding vertebrae (Fig. 7-3). In the cervical region, there are eight spinal nerves, because the C1 spinal nerves are found between the skull and C1. Consequently, cervical spinal nerves are above the corresponding vertebrae and spinal nerve 8 is found between C7 and T1.

Posterior (dorsal) nerve root. Nerve fibers originating from the posterior spinal cord. Responsible for carrying motor stimuli to muscles within the body (Fig. 7-4).
Posterior (dorsal) root ganglion (*GANG-glē-on*). Formed by the collection of motor nerve cell bodies as the nerves pass through the intervertebral foramen.
Anterior (ventral) nerve root. Nerve fibers carrying sensory signals and terminating in the anterior spinal cord.

Spinal meninges (*mě-NIN-jēz*). A continuation of the meningeal layers described within the head that surround and protect the spinal cord. As nerve roots exit through the intervertebral foramina, they are protected by a sleeve of meningeal layers that terminates as the spinal nerves are formed outside the spine.

Pia mater (*PĪ-ă MA-ter*). The innermost layer. Continuous with the surface of the spinal cord and nerve roots.

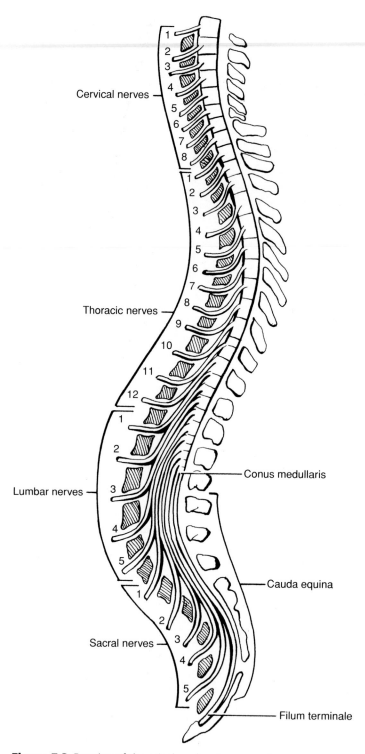

Figure 7-3 Drawing of the spinal cord and nerve roots.

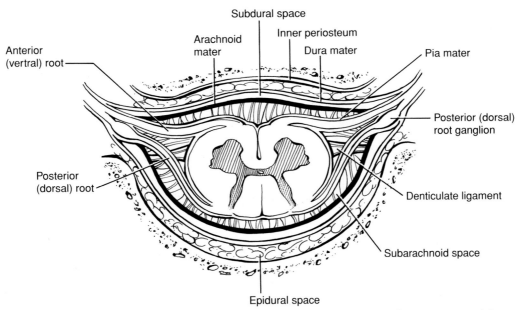

Figure 7-4 Axial drawing of the vertebral foramen demonstrating the spinal cord, nerve roots, and the surrounding meninges.

Arachnoid (ă-RAK-noyd) mater. The middle covering. Composed of thin, delicate fibers known as arachnoid trabeculae *(tră-BEK-yū-lē)*.

Subarachnoid space. Between the arachnoid mater and the pia layer. Continuous with the space of the cranium and filled with cerebrospinal fluid (CSF).

Dura (Dū-ră) mater. The tough outer layer; surrounded by fat in the epidural space within the vertebral foramen. Like the other meningeal layers, it forms a sheath around the nerve roots within the intervertebral foramen.

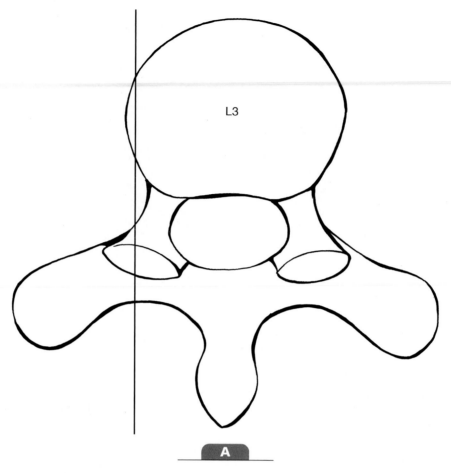

L3

A

Figure 7-5 Sagittal MR image 1.

SAGITTAL MR IMAGES

Although a typical scan of the spine would generate a series of images throughout the entire region, the following are eight selected sagittal MR images of the lumbar spine. The images are generated at 5.0 mm intervals from right to left at the following technical factors: TR = 500, TE = 20, RF = 90°, FOV = 30 cm, Abbreviations: TR = repetition time, TE = echo-time, RF = radiofrequency, FOV = field of view.

Figure 7-5 (A,B,C). Because of the absence of the spinal cord within the vertebral foramina, this image demonstrates structures found on the right side of the vertebral column. The noticeable angle between the lower vertebral bodies demarcates the L5-S1 intervertebral joint. Below this joint, the tilted orientation of the vertebral body of S1 is characteristic of the upper sacral segments within the pelvis. Above the level of the sacrum, the vertebral bodies of L1 through L5 are separated by the intervertebral disks. At the level of L5, a bony process can be seen projecting posteriorly from the vertebral body as the pedicle of L5. As described earlier, the intervertebral foramina are located between the pedicles of adjacent vertebra. Several areas of intense signal found within the intervertebral foramina are labeled the nerve roots of L3 through L5. As described earlier, the nerve roots are found just below the corresponding pedicle. For example, the L5 nerve roots are found just below the pedicle of L5.

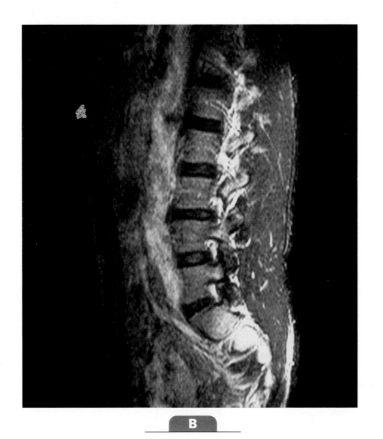

B

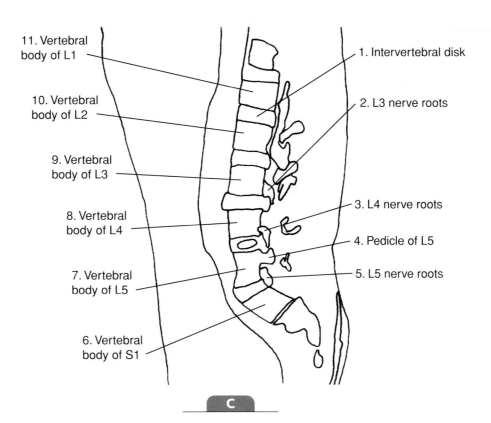

11. Vertebral body of L1

10. Vertebral body of L2

9. Vertebral body of L3

8. Vertebral body of L4

7. Vertebral body of L5

6. Vertebral body of S1

1. Intervertebral disk

2. L3 nerve roots

3. L4 nerve roots

4. Pedicle of L5

5. L5 nerve roots

C

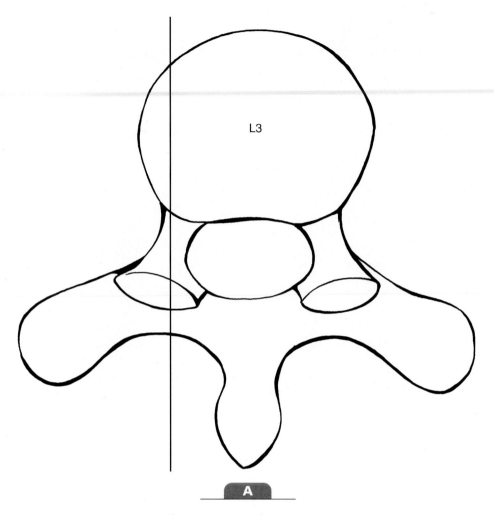

L3

A

Figure 7-6 Sagittal MR image 2.

Figure 7-6 (A,B,C). Compared to the previous image, the visualization of the lumbar pedicles along with the intervertebral foramina indicate that this image is nearing the contents of the spinal canal. Similar to the previous image, nerve roots are labeled as the intense signal areas within the intervertebral foramina corresponding to the vertebral body located just above. Because this image is closer to the midline, the margins of the vertebral bodies are more clearly demonstrated adjacent to the intervertebral disks. As demonstrated in L1, each of the vertebral bodies have a region of cortical bone surrounding the periphery of the body. The superior and inferior regions of cortical bone form the vertebral end plates that are located adjacent to the intervertebral disks.

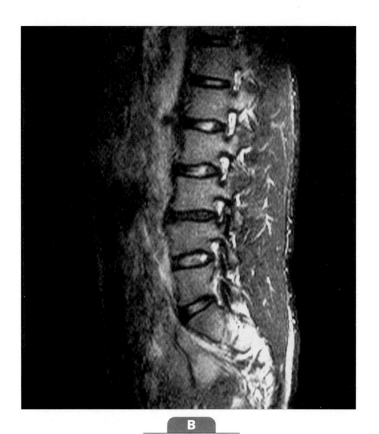

B

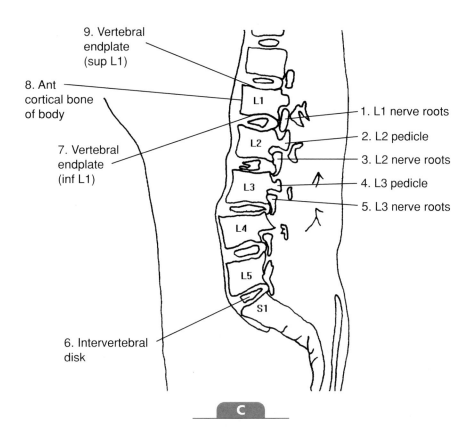

9. Vertebral
endplate
(sup L1)

8. Ant
cortical bone
of body

7. Vertebral
endplate
(inf L1)

1. L1 nerve roots

2. L2 pedicle

3. L2 nerve roots

4. L3 pedicle

5. L3 nerve roots

6. Intervertebral
disk

C

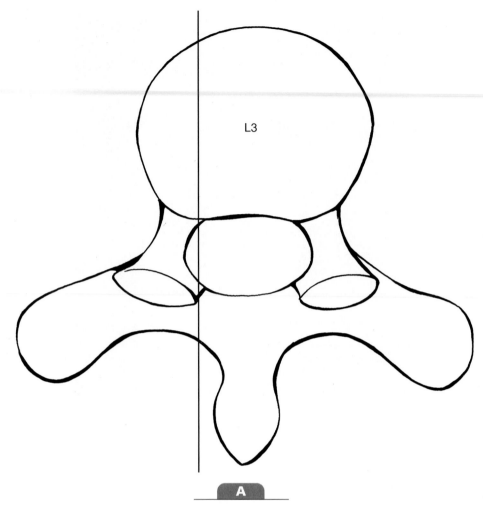

Figure 7-7 Sagittal MR image 3.

Figure 7-7 (A,B,C). Although the vertebral bodies of L1 through S1 are again shown separated by the intervertebral disks, the pedicles are no longer seen indicating that the plane of section is through the spinal canal. In the area previously occupied by the pedicles, a low signal area can be identified directly posterior to the vertebral bodies, representing the edge of the dural sac. Within the vertebral column, the superior end plate of L4 has an irregular appearance owing to the adjoining herniated disk. Within a normal intervertebral disk, demonstrated in this image between L1 and L2, the boundary between the nucleus pulposus and the anulus fibrosus is not clearly discernible. However, the nucleus pulposus has slightly less signal intensity than the surrounding anulus fibrosus.

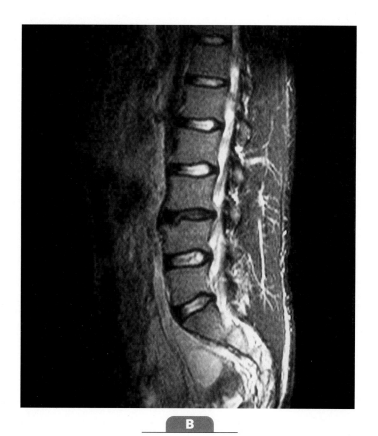

B

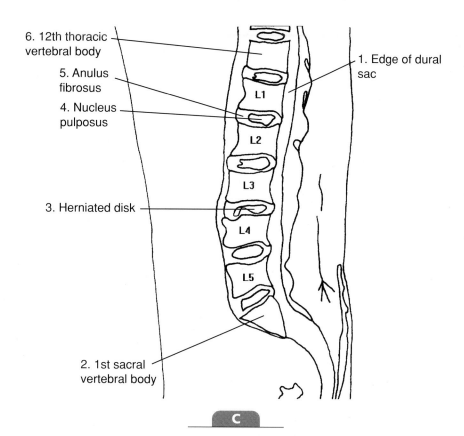

6. 12th thoracic
vertebral body

5. Anulus
fibrosus

4. Nucleus
pulposus

3. Herniated disk

2. 1st sacral
vertebral body

1. Edge of dural
sac

L1

L2

L3

L4

L5

C

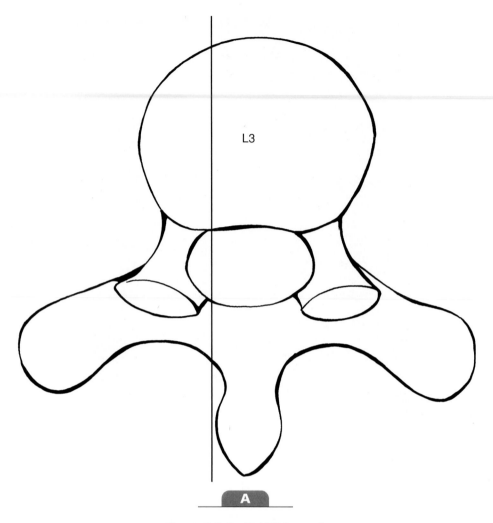

L3

A

Figure 7-8 Sagittal MR image 4.

Figure 7-8 (A,B,C). Within the spinal canal, the spinal cord can be seen within the dural sac on the superior part of this image. As the spinal cord descends below the upper lumbar vertebrae, the spinal cord terminates and gives rise to bundles of nerve roots extending to the lower lumbar and sacral regions, collectively known as the cauda equina. Surrounding the cauda equina, the CSF-filled subarachnoid space has a low signal activity. Between the dural sac and the vertebral column, the posterior longitudinal ligament is labeled as it covers the posterior surface of the vertebral column. Anterior to the vertebral column, the anterior longitudinal ligament is not clearly separable from the intervertebral disks and the anterior cortical margins of the vertebral bodies.

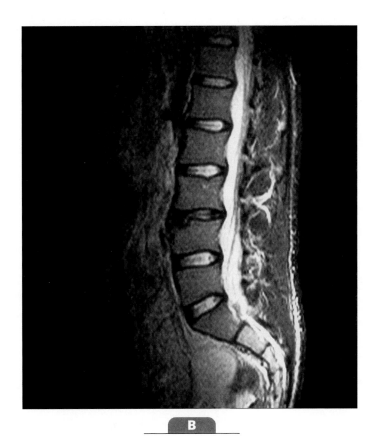

B

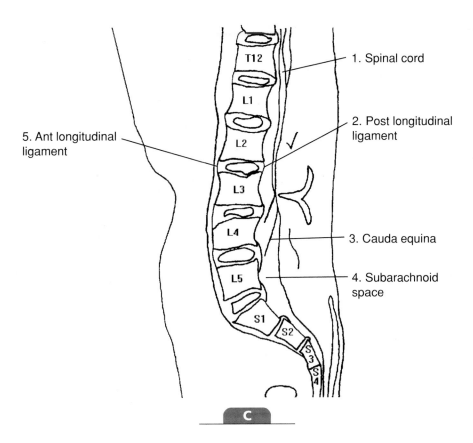

5. Ant longitudinal
ligament

1. Spinal cord

2. Post longitudinal
ligament

3. Cauda equina

4. Subarachnoid
space

T12

L1

L2

L3

L4

L5

S1

S2

S3

S4

C

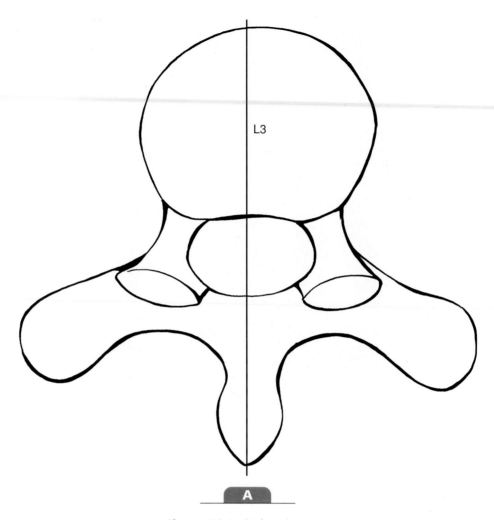

Figure 7-9 Sagittal MR image 5.

Figure 7-9 (A,B,C). In this image, most of the lower spinal cord is demonstrated in cross-section, including its termination at the conus medullaris at the L1-L2 vertebral level. Below the termination of the spinal cord, the lower lumbar and sacral spinal nerve roots continue as the cauda equina. All of the spinal nerve structures just described are surrounded by the low-signal subarachnoid space that lies within the dural sac between the pia mater and arachnoid mater, which is closely associated with the dura mater. In this near mid-sagittal image, the small basivertebral veins can be seen extending into the posterior cortical margin of the vertebral bodies of L2 and L3. Although this appearance could be misinterpreted as a fracture within the vertebral body, the presence of the basivertebral veins is a normal finding and should not be confused with any sort of patho-logic condition. The characteristic angulation in the intervertebral joint between L5 and S1 demonstrates a normal intervertebral disk. Owing to the angulation of this joint, the L5-S1 intervertebral disk is often wedge-shaped and thicker adjacent to the anterior longitudi-nal ligament. Similar to other intervertebral disks, the less-intense nucleus pulposus is surrounded by the anulus fibrosus.

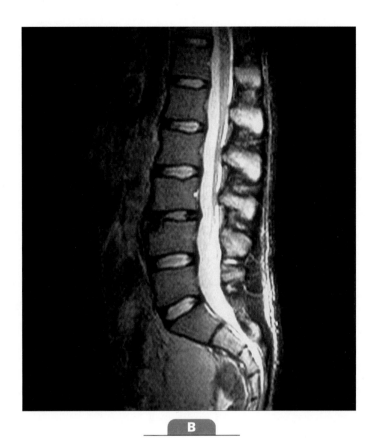

B

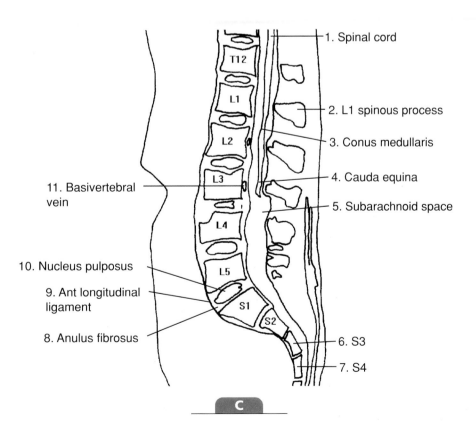

1. Spinal cord

2. L1 spinous process

3. Conus medullaris

4. Cauda equina

5. Subarachnoid space

11. Basivertebral vein

10. Nucleus pulposus

9. Ant longitudinal ligament

8. Anulus fibrosus

6. S3

7. S4

C

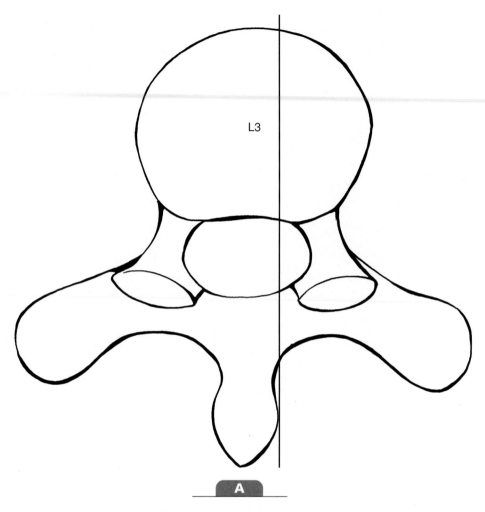

L3

A

Figure 7-10 Sagittal MR image 6.

Figure 7-10 (A,B,C). This image shows the spinal cord in cross-section terminating at the conus medullaris posterior to L1-L2. The nerve roots exiting the spine at the lower lumbar and sacral levels originate above the conus medullaris (L1-L2), forming the cauda equina. Considered part of the CNS, all of the structures just described are surrounded by CSF within the subarachnoid space. The vertebral column appears much like it did in previous images, bounded by the anterior and posterior longitudinal ligaments. A ruptured disk is again demonstrated between L3 and L4. The normal, wedge-shaped intervertebral disk found between L5 and S1 consists of a nucleus pulposus surrounded by an anulus fibrosus.

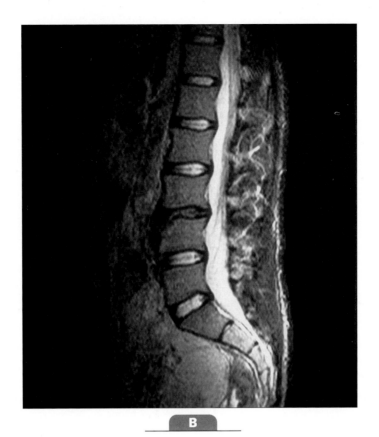

B

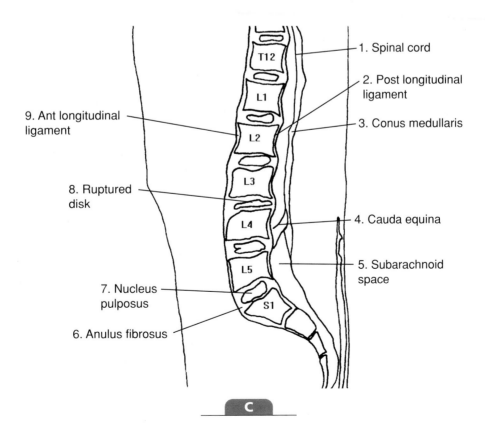

9. Ant longitudinal
ligament

8. Ruptured
disk

7. Nucleus
pulposus

6. Anulus fibrosus

1. Spinal cord

2. Post longitudinal
ligament

3. Conus medullaris

4. Cauda equina

5. Subarachnoid
space

C

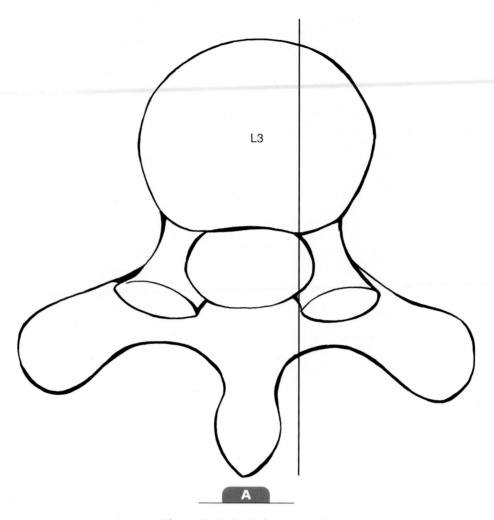

L3

A

Figure 7-11 Sagittal MR image 7.

Figure 7-11 (A,B,C). Because only the edge of the dural sac is seen in this image, the anatomy demonstrated is found along the left side of the spinal canal. Similar to previous images, the vertebral column is bounded on either side by the anterior and posterior longitudinal ligaments. The intervertebral disks, consisting of the nucleus pulposus and the anulus fibrosus, are normal at all levels except L3-L4, where a herniated disk can be identified.

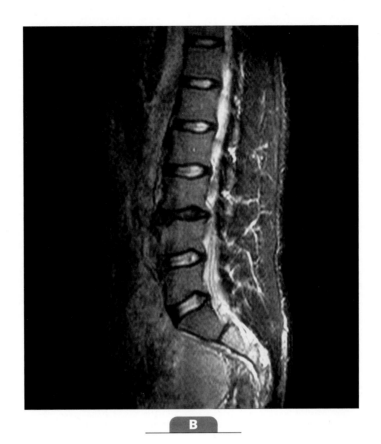

B

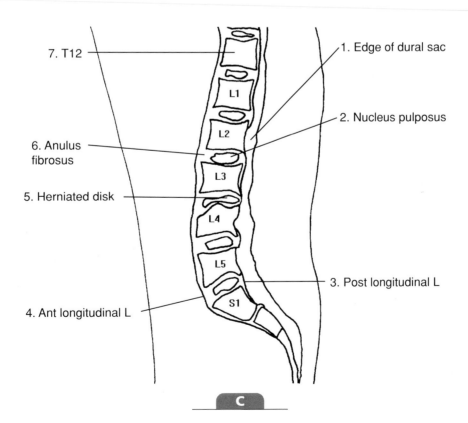

7. T12

1. Edge of dural sac

L1

2. Nucleus pulposus

L2

6. Anulus fibrosus

L3

5. Herniated disk

L4

L5

3. Post longitudinal L

4. Ant longitudinal L

S1

C

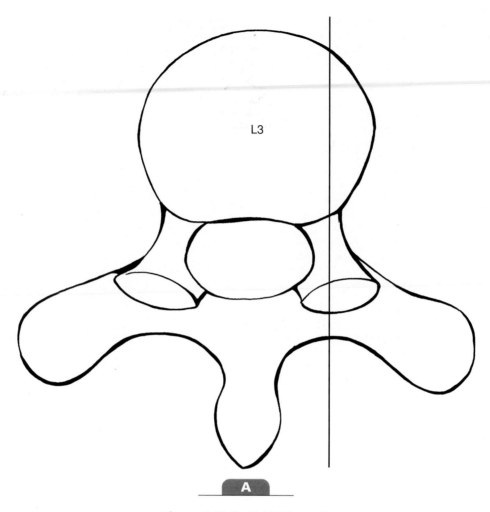

L3

A

Figure 7-12 Sagittal MR image 8.

Figure 7-12 (A,B,C). Owing to the presence of pedicles extending posteriorly from the vertebral bodies in this image, the anatomy demonstrated lies outside of the spinal canal. Between the pedicles, high-intensity signal areas represent the nerve roots within the intervertebral foramina. At the termination of the pedicle, the superior articular process articulates with the inferior articular process of the adjoining vertebra. Each nerve root lies just below the corresponding vertebra and consists of an anterior and posterior root as described earlier. Surrounded by a sheath of dura mater, the nerve roots terminate outside the intervertebral foramina at the origin of the spinal nerve.

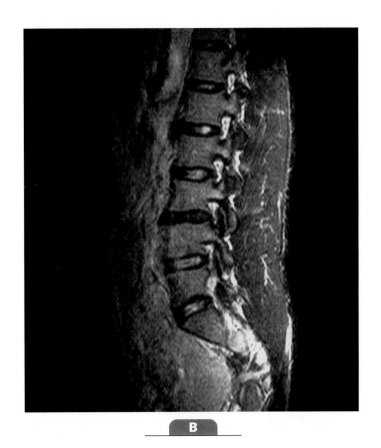

B

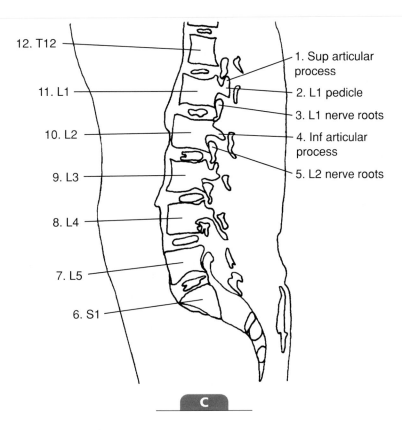

12. T12

11. L1

10. L2

9. L3

8. L4

7. L5

6. S1

1. Sup articular process

2. L1 pedicle

3. L1 nerve roots

4. Inf articular process

5. L2 nerve roots

C

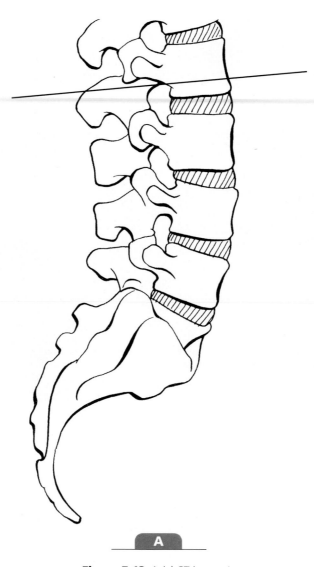

Figure 7-13 Axial CT image 1.

AXIAL CT IMAGES

The following nine selected CT images of the lumbar and sacral regions of the spine will be described at 8 mm intervals from superior to inferior. In a typical scan of the spine using a disk protocol, the images are generated at 4 mm intervals through the intervertebral disk and the cortical margins of the adjacent vertebrae. To reduce density-averaging artifacts caused by slice thickness, the plane of section is set parallel to the cortical margin of the vertebrae for each intervertebral disk. To enhance visualization of the dural sac, the following images were generated immediately after the administration of 5 mL 180 Iohexol into the subarachnoid space. The patient was rolled and then taken to CT where the scans were obtained via a disk protocol at the following technical factors: 130 kVp, 300 mA-s, and TH = 4.0 mm. Abbreviations: kVp = kilovolt peak, mA-s = milliampere-second, TH = slice thickness.

Figure 7-13 (A,B,C). Between the vertebral body and the laminae, the pedicle is seen on only the left side of the vertebral foramen, indicating the level of section is through the middle of L2. Within the vertebral foramen, the epidural space is visualized just outside of the dural sac. Extending posteriorly from the vertebral foramen, the large singular spinous process of L2 is demonstrated between the muscles of the back.

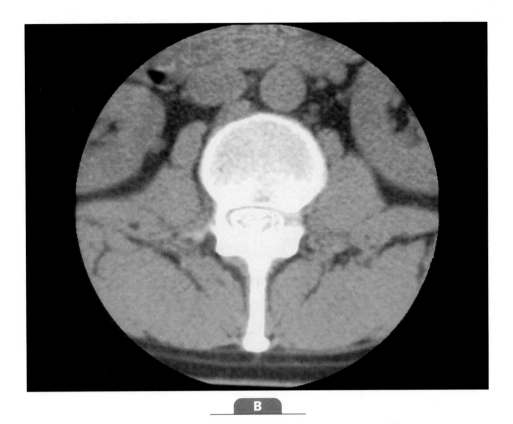

B

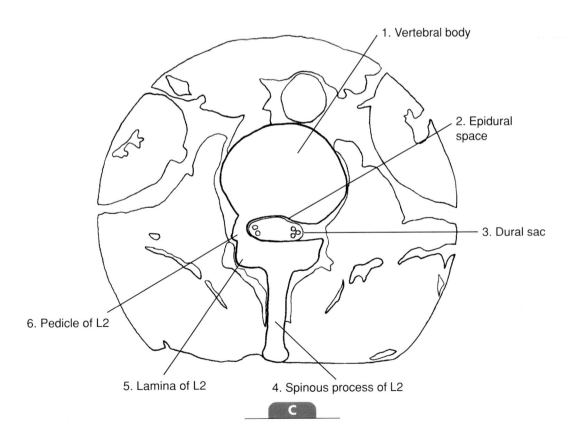

1. Vertebral body

2. Epidural space

3. Dural sac

6. Pedicle of L2

5. Lamina of L2

4. Spinous process of L2

C

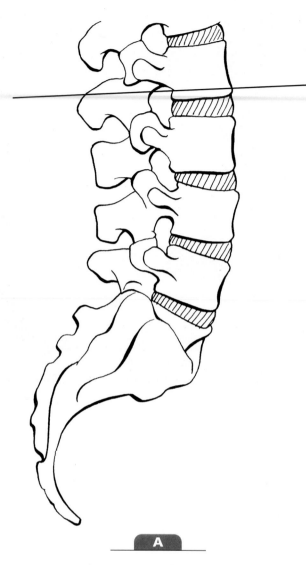

Figure 7-14 Axial CT image 2.

Figure 7-14 (A,B,C). At this level, no pedicles are seen connecting the laminae with the vertebral body, indicating that the level of this section is in the lower part of the L2 vertebral body. In the areas previously occupied by the pedicles, the intervertebral foramina now form openings through which spinal nerves can enter or exit the vertebral foramen. Similar to the previous image, the dural sac is within the vertebral foramen and is clearly demonstrated, because contrast has been injected into the subarachnoid space. Although it is difficult to clearly discern each nerve bundle, nerve roots can be seen within the dural sac and are collectively referred to as the cauda equina. On the right side, an oval-shaped region is enhanced by contrast and represents the area of the posterior (dorsal) root ganglia, which is a collection of motor nerve cell bodies.

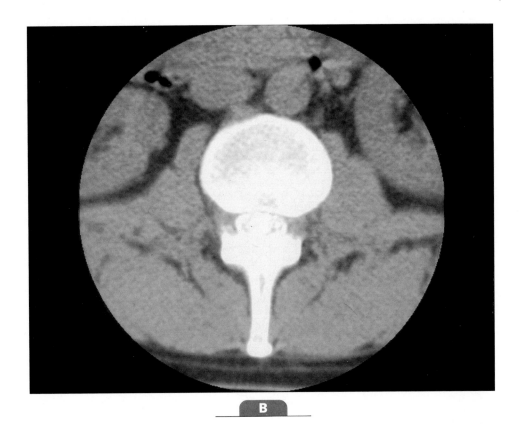

B

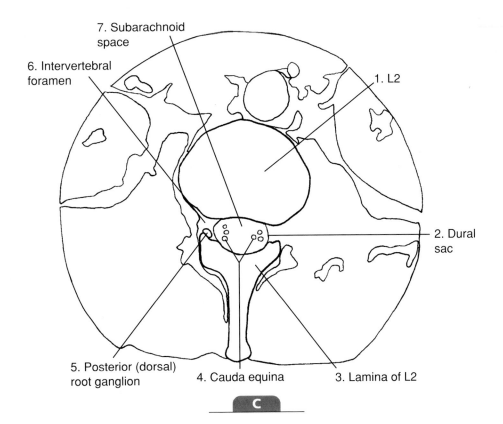

7. Subarachnoid space

6. Intervertebral foramen

1. L2

2. Dural sac

5. Posterior (dorsal) root ganglion

4. Cauda equina

3. Lamina of L2

C

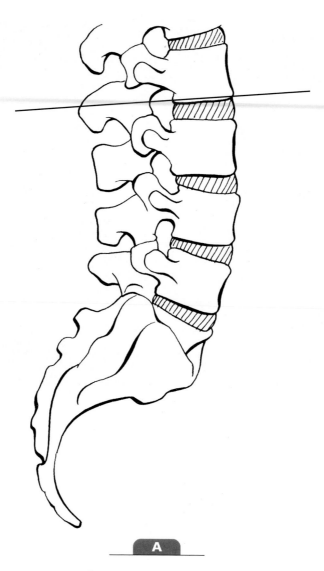

A

Figure 7-15 Axial CT image 3.

Figure 7-15 (A,B,C). As in the previous image, the intervertebral foramina in this image are between the vertebral body and the posterior vertebral arch, which includes the spinous process. Because the level of this section is through the lowest part of L2, the vertebral body is referred to as the inferior end plate, which is adjacent to the underlying intervertebral disk. Within the vertebral foramen, the dural sac is enhanced by contrast within the subarachnoid space. Within the dural sac, the radiolucent areas formed by nerve root bundles are collectively known as the cauda equina. Emerging from the right side of the dural sac, the L2 nerve roots are also enhanced by the contrast within the subarachnoid space.

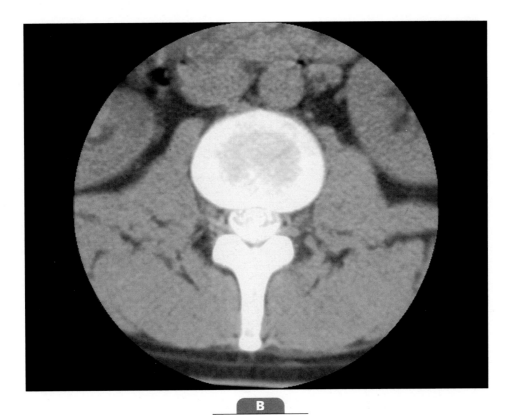

B

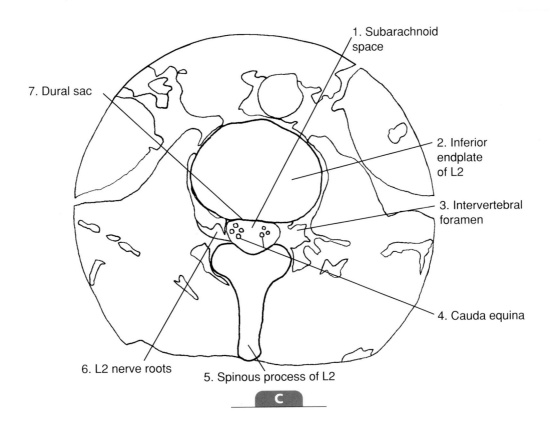

1. Subarachnoid space

7. Dural sac

2. Inferior endplate of L2

3. Intervertebral foramen

4. Cauda equina

6. L2 nerve roots

5. Spinous process of L2

C

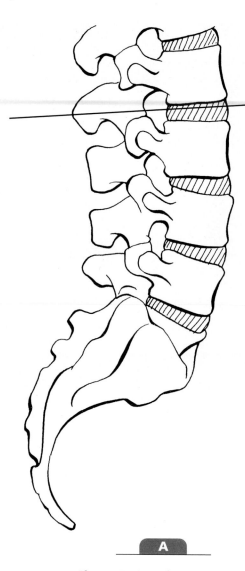

A

Figure 7-16 Axial CT image 4.

Figure 7-16 (A,B,C). Although the laminae and spinous process can still be identified on the posterior part of this image, the inferior end plate of L2 as described in the previous image has now been replaced by an intervertebral disk. Although it is difficult to find a specific boundary between the nucleus pulposus and the anulus fibrosus, the region in the center of the disk is more radiolucent than the periphery. Posterior to the intervertebral disk, the contrast-enhanced subarachnoid space is again seen within the dural sac, outlining the nerve roots representing the cauda equina. At this level, the superior articular process of L3 is found articulating with the inferior articular process of L2. To help identify the articular processes, remember that the inferior articular processes are always located "inside" compared to the superior articular processes.

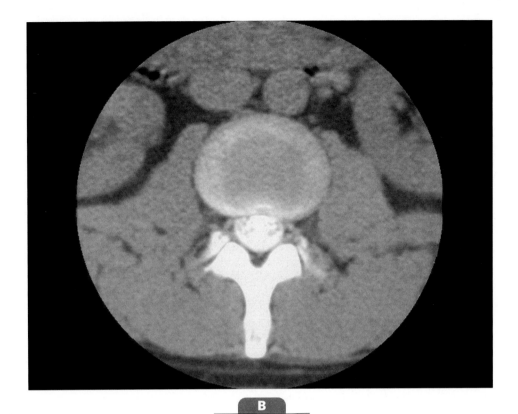

B

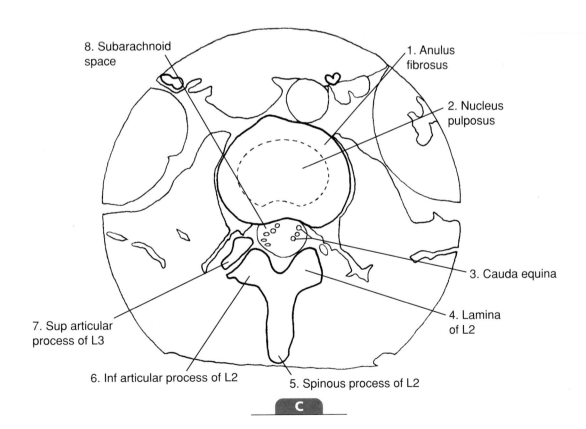

8. Subarachnoid space

1. Anulus fibrosus

2. Nucleus pulposus

3. Cauda equina

4. Lamina of L2

7. Sup articular process of L3

6. Inf articular process of L2

5. Spinous process of L2

C

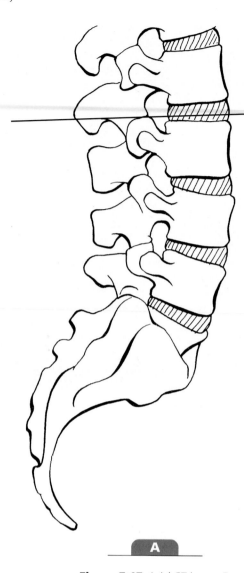

Figure 7-17 Axial CT image 5.

Figure 7-17 (A,B,C). At this level, the zygapophyseal joints are shown in cross-section on either side formed by the superior and inferior articular processes. Similar to the previous image, the spinous process of L2 can be seen separating the musculature of the back, and the intervertebral disk is demonstrated in the area previously occupied by the vertebral body. Although it is again difficult to discern a clear boundary between the regions within the intervertebral disk, the nucleus pulposus occupies the central region and is slightly more radiolucent than the surrounding anulus fibrosus. Between the intervertebral disk and the bony structures forming the posterior vertebral arch, the dural sac is enhanced by contrast within the subarachnoid space. On either side of the vertebral foramen, the intervertebral foramina are found between the posterolateral margin of the intervertebral disk and the superior articular processes of L3. Although the anatomy demonstrated within this image is normal, it clearly demonstrates how a posterolateral projection of a herniated disk could cause stenosis of the intervertebral foramen.

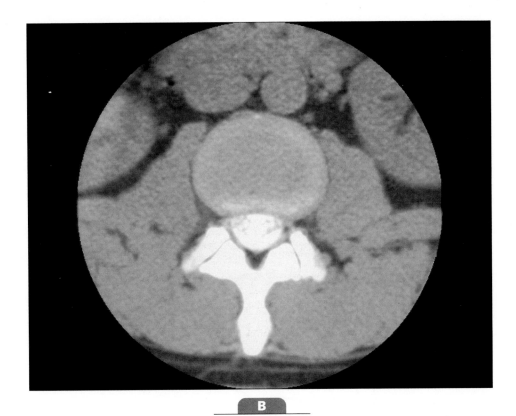

B

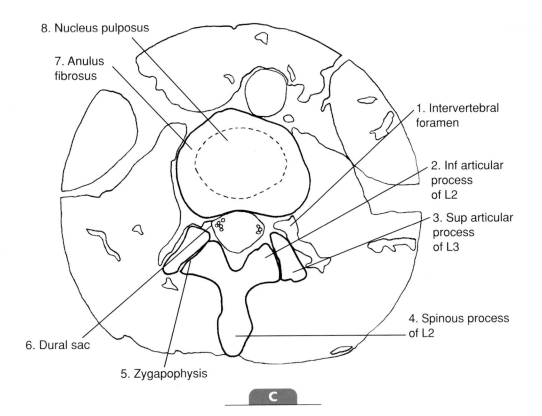

8. Nucleus pulposus

7. Anulus
fibrosus

1. Intervertebral
foramen

2. Inf articular
process
of L2

3. Sup articular
process
of L3

4. Spinous process
of L2

6. Dural sac

5. Zygapophysis

C

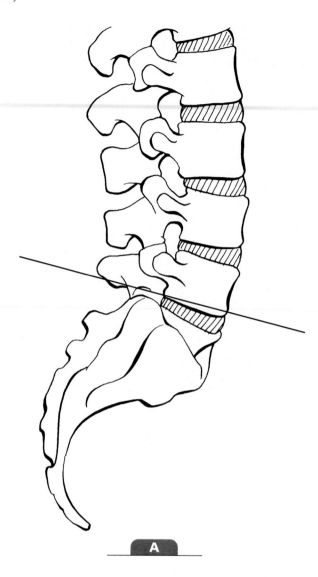

Figure 7-18 Axial CT image 6.

Figure 7-18 (A,B,C). The inferior end plate of L5 is centrally located in this image and the transverse process is shown on the left side extending toward the ilium. Posterior to the vertebral body of L5, the contents of the dural sac are enhanced by contrast within the subarachnoid space. On the right side, the sheath of dura mater is found within the intervertebral foramen surrounding the L5 nerve root. On the left side, the nerve root of S1 is beginning to separate from the contents of the dural sac. Between the vertebral body and the dural sac, a thin line of epidural space is shown that contains fat and blood vessels. Forming part of the posterior vertebral arch, the zygapophyseal joint is formed by the inferior articular process of L5 and the superior articular process of S1.

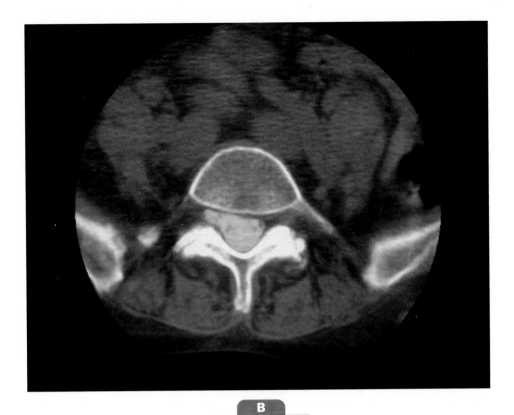

B

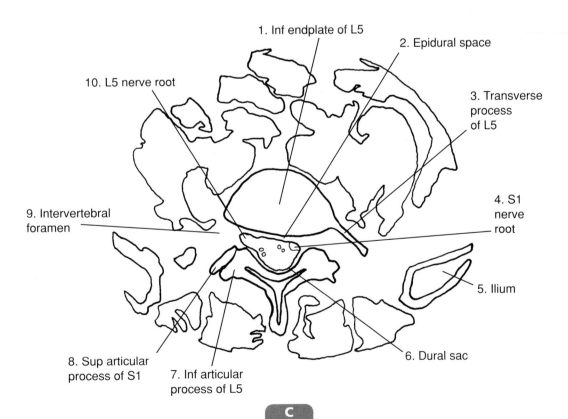

1. Inf endplate of L5

2. Epidural space

3. Transverse process of L5

10. L5 nerve root

9. Intervertebral foramen

4. S1 nerve root

5. Ilium

6. Dural sac

8. Sup articular process of S1

7. Inf articular process of L5

C

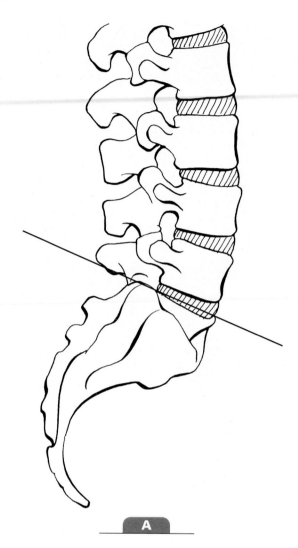

Figure 7-19 Axial CT image 7.

Figure 7-19 (A,B,C). In the central location previously occupied by the inferior end plate of L5, the intervertebral disk is shown in cross-section. The central, more radiolucent area of the disk represents the pulpy fluid known as the nucleus pulposus, which is surrounded by a concentric ring of fibrous tissue known as the anulus fibrosus. In this patient, the intervertebral disk located at L5-S1 is normal and does not cause any stenosis of the neural foramina. In the position previously occupied by the transverse process of L5, the lateral part of S1 is now shown as a triangular-shaped bone between the intervertebral disk and the iliac bones. Within the vertebral foramen, the contrast-enhanced subarachnoid space demonstrates the extent of the dura in this region. Although the nerve roots are usually more symmetrical, the S1 nerve root seen on the left side of this patient indicates the spinal nerves are coming off at a higher level on the left side. For example, the S1 nerve root is emerging from the dural sac on the left side, whereas on the right side, the S1 nerve root is not yet discernible. Forming the posterior vertebral arch, the spinous process and laminae of L5 are shown in this section to be continuous with the inferior articular processes. As described earlier, the inferior articular processes are found "inside" compared to the superior articular processes.

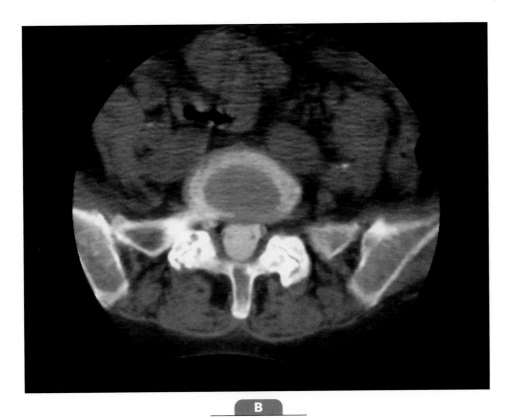

B

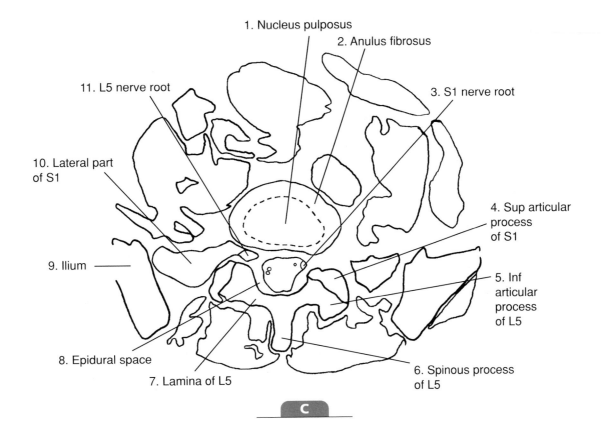

1. Nucleus pulposus

2. Anulus fibrosus

11. L5 nerve root

3. S1 nerve root

10. Lateral part
of S1

4. Sup articular
process
of S1

9. Ilium

5. Inf
articular
process
of L5

8. Epidural space

6. Spinous process
of L5

7. Lamina of L5

C

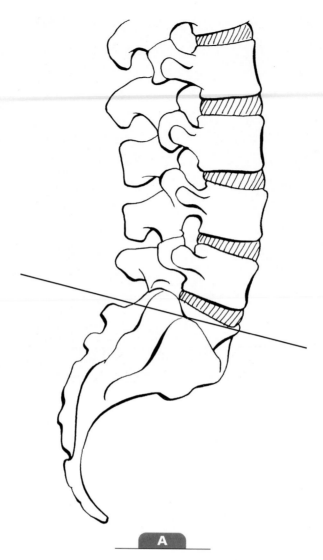

Figure 7-20 Axial CT image 8.

Figure 7-20 (A,B,C). The unique structure of the superior end plate of S1 gives the bony structure—centrally located in this image—the characteristic bat-like appearance of the sacrum. The lateral parts of the sacrum extending from the vertebral body on either side appear like wings as they extend toward the iliac bones. Posterior to the S1 segment, the oval-shaped dural sac is enhanced by contrast within the subarachnoid space and occupies a central location within the vertebral foramen. Within the dural sac, the areas of radiolucency represent the S2 through S5 nerve roots, or the lower cauda equina. Outside of the dural sac, the epidural space can be found within the vertebral foramen. Within the lateral recesses of the vertebral foramen, the S1 nerve roots can be identified on either side as they extend from the spinal cord to the sacral foramina.

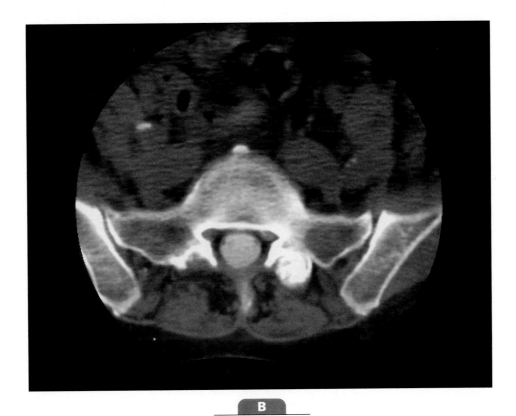

B

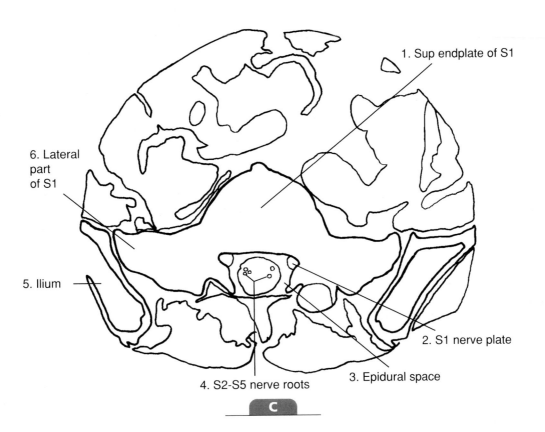

1. Sup endplate of S1

6. Lateral
part
of S1

5. Ilium

4. S2-S5 nerve roots

2. S1 nerve plate

3. Epidural space

C

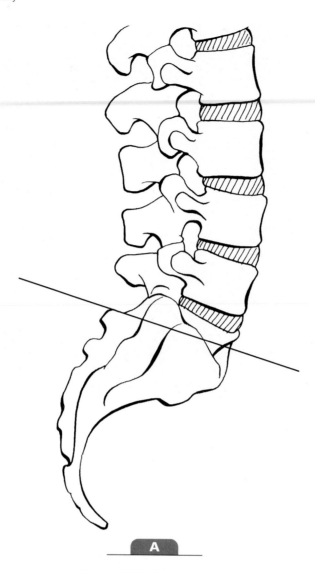

Figure 7-21 Axial CT image 9.

Figure 7-21 (A,B,C). As in the previous figure, the bat-like appearance of the sacrum in this image indicates the plane of section to be within the region of the pelvis. On either side, the lateral part of the sacrum is demonstrated articulating with the iliac bones, creating the sacroiliac joints. Although the vertebral segment of S1 typically has a round appearance, a small bony outgrowth, known as an osteophyte, is demonstrated on the anterior cortical margin. At this level, the laminae of S1 can be found on either side, forming the posterior arch around the vertebral foramen. As described in previous images, the contrast-enhanced dural sac is centrally located within the vertebral foramen and contains radiolucent areas representing the S2 through S5 nerve roots. At this level, the S2 nerve roots are within the anterolateral portion of the dural sac, and the S1 nerve roots are within the lateral recesses of the vertebral foramen.

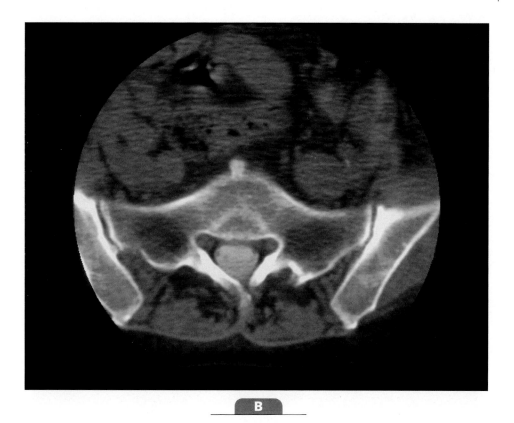

B

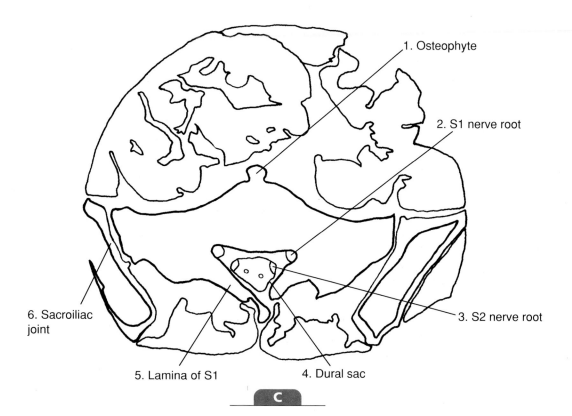

1. Osteophyte

2. S1 nerve root

3. S2 nerve root

4. Dural sac

5. Lamina of S1

6. Sacroiliac joint

C

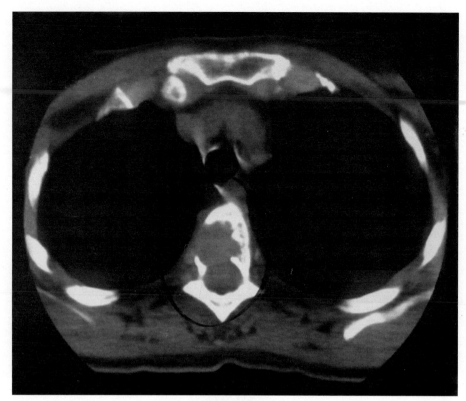

Figure 7-22

Supplement 7-1. *Figure 7-22 shows a CT scan of the chest of a 52-year-old woman. The image reveals an osteolytic lesion of the T4 vertebral body. There is a loss of the posterior cortical margin of the vertebral body; however, no epidural compression is seen. Subsequent CT scans of the abdomen and pelvis revealed multiple lytic lesions involving the skeleton consistent with metastatic disease. A biopsy revealed the osteolytic process to be a multiple myeloma, which is associated with widespread osteolytic lesions.*

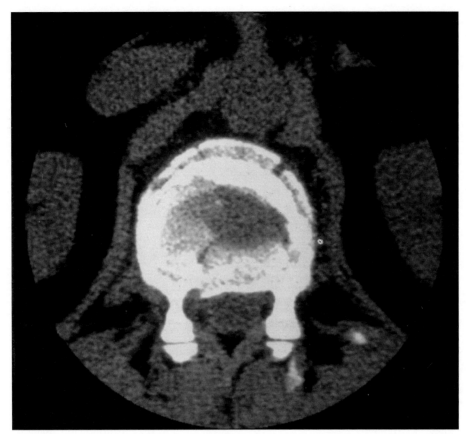

Figure 7-23

Supplement 7-2. *Figure 7-23 shows an image from a 29-year-old man who injured his back in a motor vehicle accident. The CT examination of his lumbar spine reveals a compression fracture of the L1 vertebral body. The comminuted fracture of L1 has resulted in a 5 mm displacement of the posterior wall of the vertebral body into the vertebral foramen, resulting in a slight compression of the spinal cord. As an incidental finding, this patient was also found to have six lumbar vertebrae. After surgical correction of the fracture, the patient had no signs of spinal cord injury.*

REVIEW QUESTIONS

1. There are usually_____cervical vertebrae, _____thoracic vertebrae,_____lumbar vertebrae, and_____sacral segments.

2. The_____spinal nerve is found between C1 and C2, and the_____spinal nerve is found between L5 and S1.

3. The unique feature that can be used to identify thoracic vertebrae is the_____.

4. The transverse foramina are characteristic of which of the following vertebrae?
   A. Cervical
   B. Lumbar
   C. Sacral
   D. Thoracic

5. The_____is a concentric ring of fibrous tissue forming the periphery of the intervertebral disk.

6. The intervertebral disks are responsible for approximately one-quarter of the length of the vertebral column. True or false

7. Describe the posterior longitudinal ligament.

8. The_____and_____form the posterior boundary of an intervertebral foramen.

9. The anterior border of the right L5-S1 intervertebral foramen is formed by the_____,_____, and_____.

10. The conus medullaris is usually found at which of the following vertebral levels?
    A. T1-L2
    B. L1-L3
    C. L2-L4
    D. L3-L5

11. The posterior (dorsal) nerve root carries [sensory / motor] signals.

12. In an axial section through the vertebrae, which articular process is found inside, or most medially?

13. Where does the extension of dura mater known as a dural sheath terminate?

14. The_____mater is the innermost meningeal layer.

15. The CSF within the subarachnoid space in the spine is continuous with that found within the cranium. True or false

16. In the spine, the upper and lower borders of the intervertebral foramen are formed by the
    A. Laminae
    B. Pedicles
    C. Articular processes
    D. Transverse processes

17. The_____is a loose collection of nerve roots below the level of L1.

18. The [anterior / posterior] nerve root contains a collection of nerve cell bodies known as a ganglion.

19. In axial sections, which part of the vertebral column is described as having a bat-like appearance?

20. Which of the following have the largest vertebral foramina?
    A. Cervical
    B. Thoracic
    C. Lumbar
    D. Sacral

Chapter 8

Joints

OBJECTIVES

Upon completion of this chapter, the student should be able to:

1. Define the general regions that include one or more joints.
2. List the bones forming each joint and indicate the classification and range of movements.
3. Identify and describe the unique bone structures associated with each joint.
4. Identify and describe the cartilages associated with each joint.
5. Describe the relationships of the articular surfaces within each joint.
6. Describe the major ligaments involved in stabilizing each joint.
7. Identify and describe the muscles and tendons passing around each joint.
8. Describe the origin, insertion, and action of muscles passing around each joint.
9. Describe the relationships among the structures forming each joints.
10. Correctly identify anatomical structures on patient CT and MR images of the joints.

Shoulder

ANATOMICAL OVERVIEW

The anatomy of the shoulder girdle is generally described as the junction of the upper extremity with the trunk. The shoulder girdle consists of two bones, the clavicle and the scapula, which attach to the axial skeleton via the sternoclavicular joint. On the opposite end of the shoulder girdle, the shoulder joint is formed by the glenoid fossa of the scapula, which articulates with the head of the humerus, forming an enarthrodial, or ball-and-socket, joint.

Skeletal

Humerus (*HYU-mer-ŭs*). Located in the upper arm. The largest and longest bone of the upper extremity (Fig. 8-1).

Head. The most proximal part of the humerus. It is round, forming a smooth articular (*ar-TIK-yu-lăr*) surface.

Surgical neck. A constricted part of the humerus just below the tubercles. A frequent site for fractures in the proximal end of the humerus.

Greater tubercle (*TU-ber-kl*). The small protrusion, or bump, on the lateral humerus between the head and surgical neck (Fig. 8-2). Together, the more medial lesser tubercle and the greater tubercle form a groove for the tendon of the long head of the biceps muscle.

Scapula (*SKAP-yu-lă*). Forms the posterior part of the bony shoulder. Generally described as flat and triangular (Fig. 8-1).

Acromion (*ă-KRŌ-mĒ-on*) *process*. Originates from the spine on the posterior surface of the scapula. A flattened process that extends anteriorly to articulate with the distal clavicle (*KLAV-i-kl*), forming the acromioclavicular (*ă-KRŌ-mē-ō-kla-CIK-yūlăr*) joint. Together, the acromion process and clavicle are often described as forming the roof of the shoulder joint.

Glenoid (*GLĒ-noyd*) *process*. The lateral part of the scapula. Articulates with the head of the humerus.

Glenoid fossa (*FOS-ă*). Also called the glenoid cavity. A cup-shaped depression located inside the outer edge of the glenoid process.

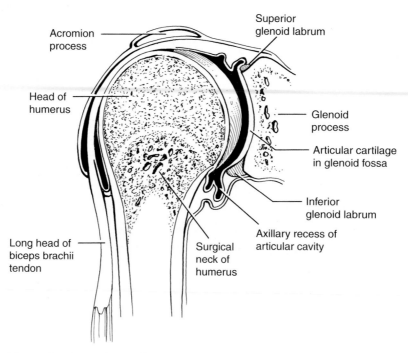

Figure 8-1 Coronal view of the shoulder.

Joint

Articular cartilage. Provides a smooth surface for the shoulder joint and covers both the glenoid cavity and the head of the humerus. Consists mostly of hyaline (*HI-ă-lin*) cartilage. Within the joint space, synovial (*sin-NO-vē-ăl*) fluid acts like oil, allowing the surfaces to slide easily on one another during movement.

Glenoid labrum (*LA-brŭm*). Surrounds the glenoid fossa. A ridge of fibrocartilage that acts to deepen the fossa and protect the bone. Because the tendon of the long head of the biceps muscle inserts on the superior glenoid process, the terminal part of the tendon is continuous with superior glenoid labrum.

Axillary (*AK-sil-ar-e*) **recess of the articular cavity.** The joint space below the inferior glenoid labrum. Lined with synovial membrane and surrounded by the connective tissue of the articular capsule. Because the shoulder joint is strengthened by muscles that run behind, above, and in front of the joint, dislocation most commonly occurs when the arm is abducted through the axillary articular capsule.

Musculature

Trapezius (*tra-PE-ze-ŭs*). Origin: ligament covering spinous processes of cervical vertebrae (*SER-vĭ-kal VER-tĕ-bre*) and thoracic vertebrae. Insertion: clavicle, medial acromion, and spine of scapula. Action: adducts and rotates scapula. NB: not shown in Figure 8-1.

Deltoid (*DEL-toyd*). Origin: upper surface of clavicle, upper surface of acromion, and spine of scapula. Insertion: deltoid tubercle of humerus. Action: abducts and rotates arm medially and laterally (Fig. 8-2).

Long head of biceps brachii (*BI-seps BRA-kē-i*). Origin: supraglenoid tuberosity (*TU-bēr-OS-i-tē*). Insertion: radial tuberosity. Action: flexes arm and forearm.

Short head of biceps brachii. Origin: coracoid (*KOR-ă-koyd*) process of scapula. Insertion: radial tuberosity. Action: supinates the hand.

Coracobrachialis (*KOR-ă-kō-brā-kē-A-lis*). Origin: coracoid process of scapula. Insertion: middle shaft of humerus. Action: flexes and adducts the arm.

Subscapularis (*sŭb-skap-yŭ-LA-ris*). Origin: subscapular fossa. Insertion: lesser tubercle of humerus and shoulder joint articular capsule. Action: rotates arm medially.

Supraspinatus (*su-pră-spi-NA-tŭs*). Origin: supraspinous fossa. Insertion: greater tubercle of humerus. Action: abducts arm (Fig. 8-3).

Infraspinatus (*in-fră-spi-NA-tŭs*). Origin: infraspinous fossa. Insertion: greater tubercle of humerus. Action: rotates arm laterally.

Teres (*TER-ez*) **major.** Origin: inferior angle of scapula. Insertion: lesser tubercle of humerus. Action: adducts, extends, and rotates arm medially.

Teres minor. Origin: axillary border of scapula. Insertion: greater tubercle of humerus. Action: rotates laterally and adducts arm.

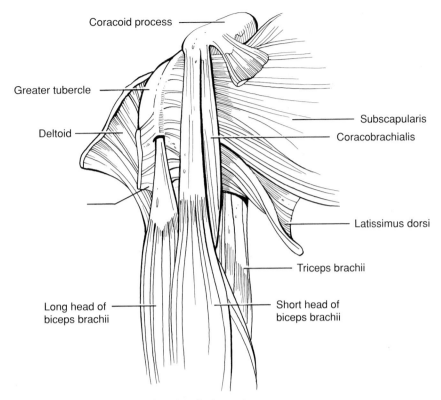

Figure 8-2 Anterior view of the brachial muscles.

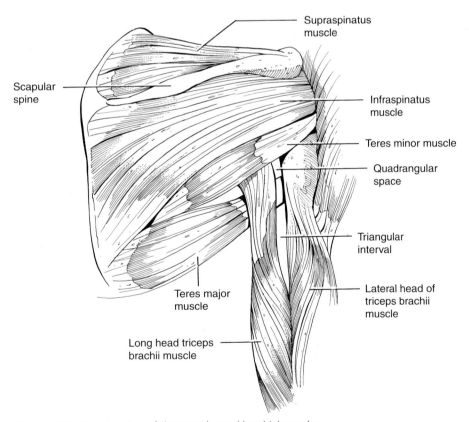

Figure 8-3 Posterior view of the scapular and brachial muscles.

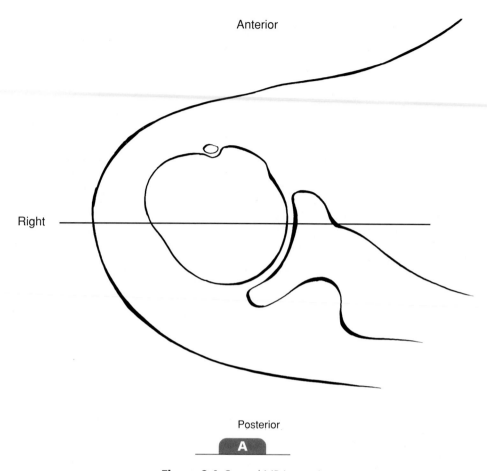

Anterior

Right

Posterior

A

Figure 8-4 Coronal MR Image 1.

CORONAL MR IMAGES

In a typical scan of the shoulder, images are generated throughout the entire region. Here, the descriptions are limited to the following four selected images described at 3.5 mm intervals from posterior to anterior through the right shoulder joint. The images were generated at the following technical factors: TR = 900, TE = 20, RF = 90°, FOV = 16 cm. Abbreviations: TR = repetition time, TE = echo-time, RF = radiofrequency, FOV = field of view.

Figure 8-4 (A,B,C). Since this image demonstrates the posterior glenohumeral joint, the bony anatomy can be used to locate the position of the section. Owing to its characteristic appearance, the humerus is shown obliquely, sectioned near the glenoid process of the scapula with the intervening glenohumeral joint. On the upper aspect of the glenoid process of the scapula, the superior glenoid labrum is labeled and represents an area of dense fibrous tissue that acts to deepen and stabilize the glenohumeral joint. Above the joint, the acromion process of the scapula is shown and is often described as forming the roof over the glenohumeral joint. Besides the bones previously described, most of the strength of the shoulder joint is provided by the surrounding musculature. Originating primarily from the spinous processes of the cervical and thoracic vertebrae, the thin flat muscle of the trapezius can be seen as it extends toward its insertion on the medial margin of the acromion process of the scapula. Below the trapezius muscle, the supraspinatus muscle is also demonstrated extending from its origin in the supraspinous fossa on the posterior aspect of the scapula to insert on the greater tubercle of the humerus. Separated by a thin line of low signal intensity, the subscapularis muscle can be identified extending from its origin on the anterior surface of the scapula to insert on the lesser tubercle of the humerus. Both the supraspinatus and subscapularis muscles form part of the rotator cuff along with the infraspinatus and teres minor, which surround the posterior articular capsule. Originating from the acromion process of the scapula and the upper surface of the clavicle, the deltoid muscle is lateral to the humerus as it extends toward its insertion on the deltoid tubercle found approximately mid-shaft on the humerus.

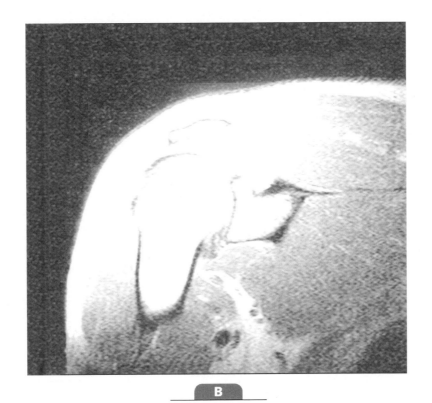

B

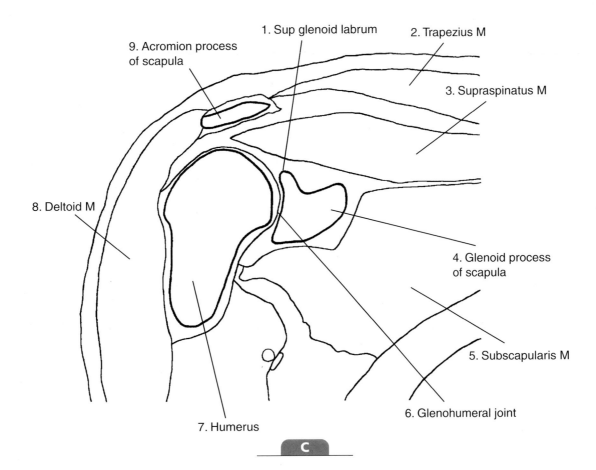

9. Acromion process
of scapula

1. Sup glenoid labrum

2. Trapezius M

3. Supraspinatus M

8. Deltoid M

4. Glenoid process
of scapula

5. Subscapularis M

6. Glenohumeral joint

7. Humerus

C

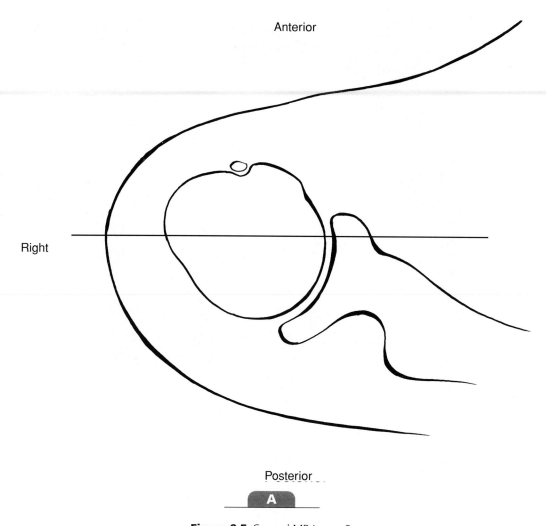

Anterior

Right

Posterior

A

Figure 8-5 Coronal MR Image 2.

Figure 8-5 (A,B,C). The acromion and glenoid processes of the scapula in this image appear much like they do in the previous image; however, the greater tubercle is clearly identified on the lateral aspect between the head and the surgical neck of the humerus. Similar to the previous image, the deltoid muscle is shown originating from the acromion process of the scapula and covers the proximal end of the humerus as it extends downward to insert on the deltoid tubercle. Medial to the deltoid muscle, the teres major muscle is shown in cross-section extending from its origin on the inferior angle of the scapula to insert on the lesser tubercle of the humerus. Next to the teres major muscle, several axillary vessels are shown in cross-section as they extend between the thoracic cage and the arm.

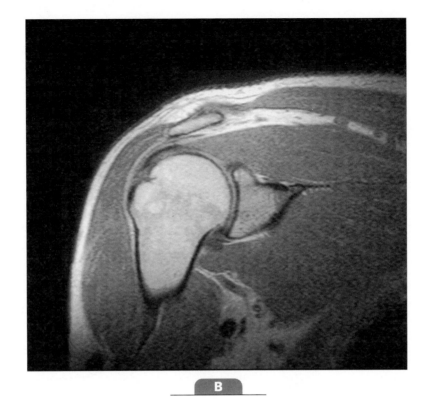

B

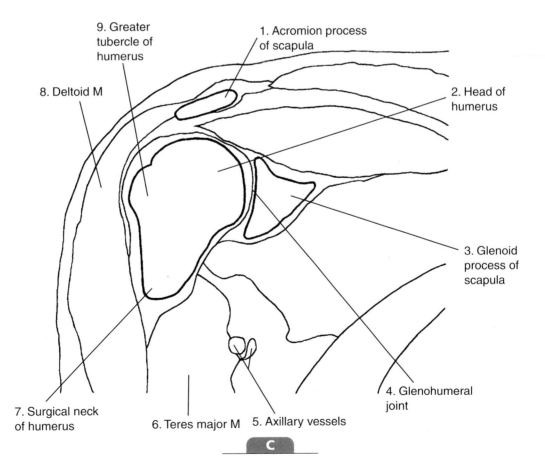

9. Greater
tubercle of
humerus

1. Acromion process
of scapula

8. Deltoid M

2. Head of
humerus

3. Glenoid
process of
scapula

4. Glenohumeral
joint

7. Surgical neck
of humerus

6. Teres major M

5. Axillary vessels

C

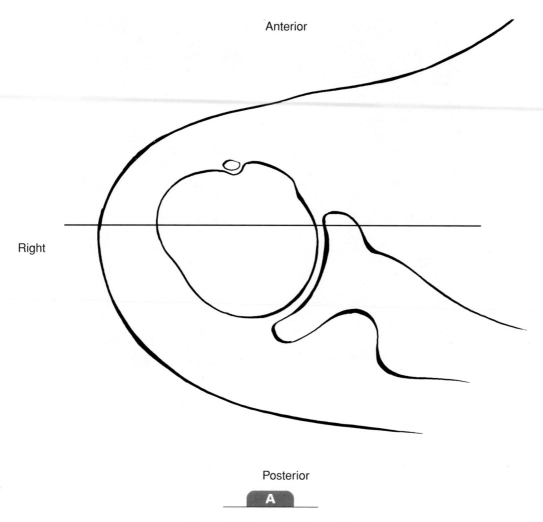

Anterior

Right

Posterior

A

Figure 8-6 Coronal MR Image 3.

Figure 8-6 (A,B,C). As in the previous images, the acromion and glenoid processes of the scapula are sectioned near the head of the humerus. Although it appears as a region of low signal intensity, the articular cartilage of the head of the humerus is labeled within the glenohumeral joint. Continuous with the glenohumeral joint, another region of low signal intensity is identified inferiorly representing the axillary recess of the articular cavity. The recess is continuous with the glenohumeral joint and decreases in size as the arm is abducted, causing an increased tension on the inferior articular capsule. Similar to the previous image, the teres major and deltoid muscles are labeled on either side of the neck of the humerus. Medially, the supraspinatus and subscapularis muscles are separated by a thin line of low signal intensity representing the body of the scapula.

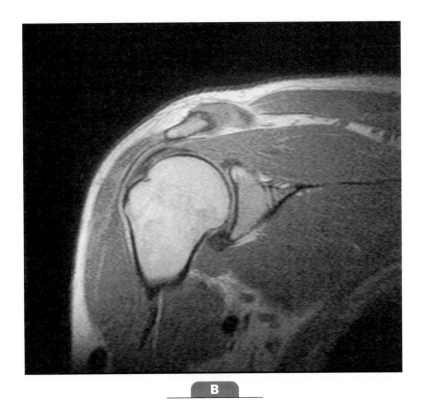

B

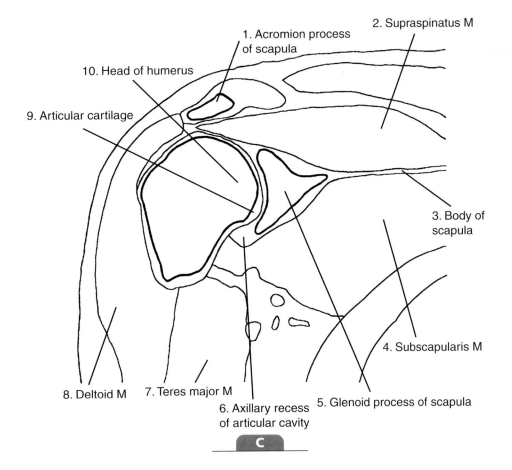

10. Head of humerus

9. Articular cartilage

1. Acromion process of scapula

2. Supraspinatus M

3. Body of scapula

4. Subscapularis M

8. Deltoid M

7. Teres major M

6. Axillary recess of articular cavity

5. Glenoid process of scapula

C

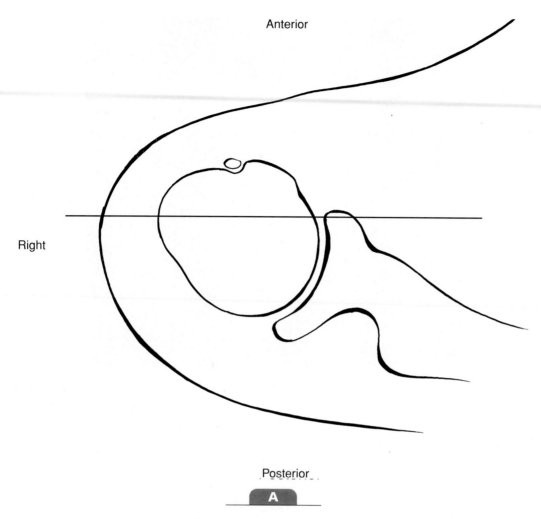

Anterior

Right

Posterior

A

Figure 8-7 Coronal MR Image 4.

Figure 8-7 (A,B,C). Because this image is anterior to the previous images, the distal end of the clavicle is now sectioned in close proximity to the acromion process of the scapula. As described earlier, the clavicle and the scapula are the bones making up the shoulder girdle and are responsible for attaching the upper extremity with the trunk of the body. The glenohumeral joint is shown between the glenoid process of the scapula and the head of the humerus. Articular cartilage not only covers the head of the humerus but is also found lining the glenoid fossa. Continuous with the articular cartilage, the glenoid labrum surrounding the edge of the glenoid fossa is sectioned, forming the upper and lower margins of the glenohumeral joint.

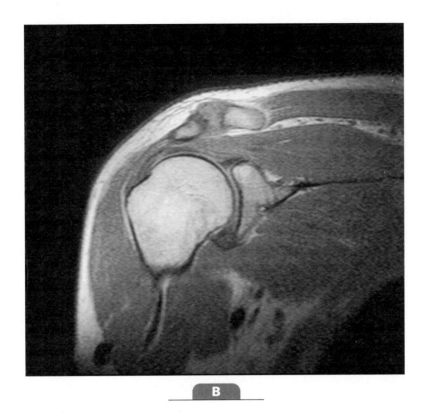

B

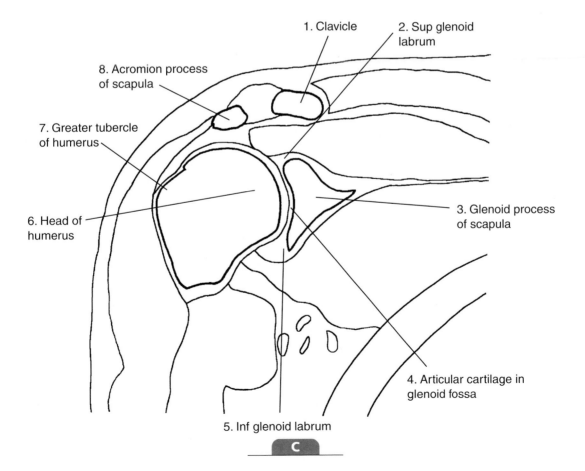

1. Clavicle

2. Sup glenoid labrum

8. Acromion process of scapula

7. Greater tubercle of humerus

6. Head of humerus

3. Glenoid process of scapula

4. Articular cartilage in glenoid fossa

5. Inf glenoid labrum

C

Elbow

ANATOMICAL OVERVIEW

The joint connecting the arm to the forearm is considered a ginglymus, or hinge-type, joint capable of flexion and extension. To form the joint, the distal humerus articulates with the proximal ends of the radius and ulna.

Skeletal

Humerus. The largest and longest bone of the upper extremity (Fig. 8-8).

Medial and lateral epicondyles (ep-i-KON-dilz). Found on the distal humerus. The medial is longer and thinner than the lateral.

Trochlea (TROK-le-e). The articulating surface on the distal humerus below the medial epicondyle. Articulates with the trochlear notch of the ulna.

Capitulum (kă-PIT-yu-lŭm). The little head or small eminence of bone on the distal humerus below the lateral epicondyle. Articulates with the fovea on the head of the radius.

Olecranon (ō-LEK-ră-non) fossa. The depression on the posterior surface of the distal humerus between the medial and lateral epicondyles.

Coronoid (KŌR-ŏ-noyd) fossa. The depression on the anterior surface of the distal humerus between the medial and lateral epicondyles.

Radius. The shorter and more lateral bone of the forearm (Fig. 8-9).

Head. The enlarged, proximal part of the radius. Appears flattened on the end that articulates with the capitulum of the humerus.

Fovea (FŌ-ve-ă). The small pit or depression on the head of the radius.

Neck. Located directly below the head. The narrow region above the radial tuberosity.

Radial tuberosity. The projection of bone on the shaft of the proximal radius. Provides attachment for the biceps muscle.

Ulna *(ÜL-nă).* The longer and more medial bone of the forearm that articulates with the distal humerus.

Olecranon process. The most proximal part of the ulna. Projects behind the distal humerus.

Coronoid process. Projection found on the proximal end of the ulna that is anterior to the distal humerus.

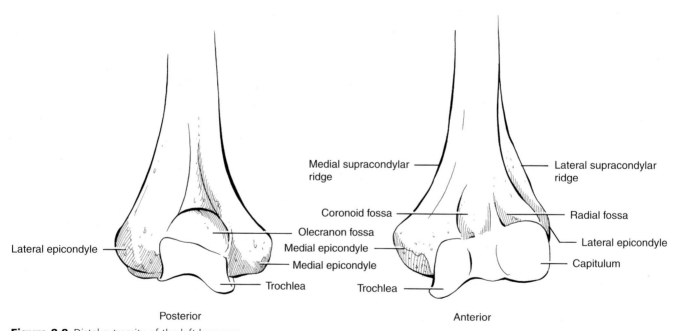

Lateral epicondyle —
Medial supracondylar ridge —
Lateral supracondylar ridge —
Coronoid fossa —
Radial fossa —
Olecranon fossa —
Medial epicondyle —
Lateral epicondyle —
Capitulum —
Trochlea —
Trochlea —

Posterior

Anterior

Figure 8-8 Distal extremity of the left humerus.

Trochlear notch. The surfaces on the olecranon and coronoid processes that articulate with the trochlea of the humerus.

Musculature

Triceps (*TRI-seps*). Origin: upper humerus and infraglenoid (*IN-fră-GLE-noyd*) tuberosity of scapula. Insertion: posterior olecranon and fascia of forearm. Action: extends forearm (Fig. 8-10).

Brachialis (*bră-ke-A-lis*). Origin: lower half anterior humerus. Insertion: coronoid process and tuberosity of ulna. Action: flexes forearm.

Brachioradialis (*BRA-ke-ō-ra-dē-A-lis*). Origin: lateral supracondylar ridge of humerus. Insertion: styloid process of radius. Action: flexes forearm.

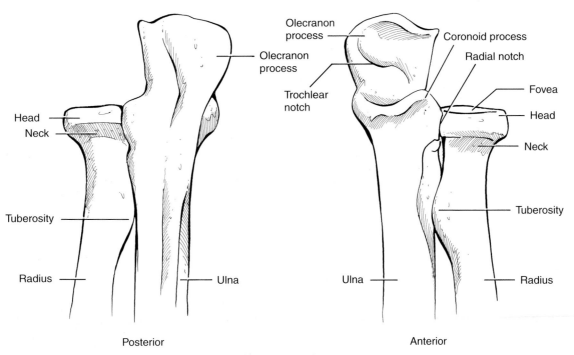

Figure 8-9 Proximal Posterior extremity of the left ulna and radius.

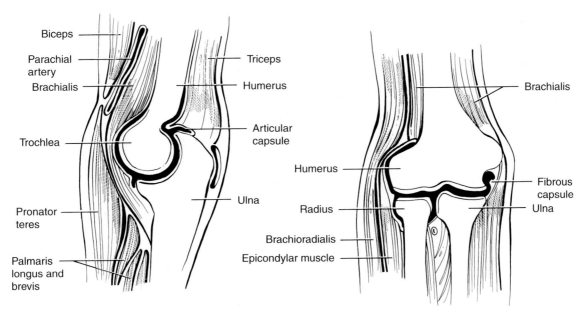

Figure 8-10 A. Sagittal section of the elbow, **B.** Coronal section of the elbow.

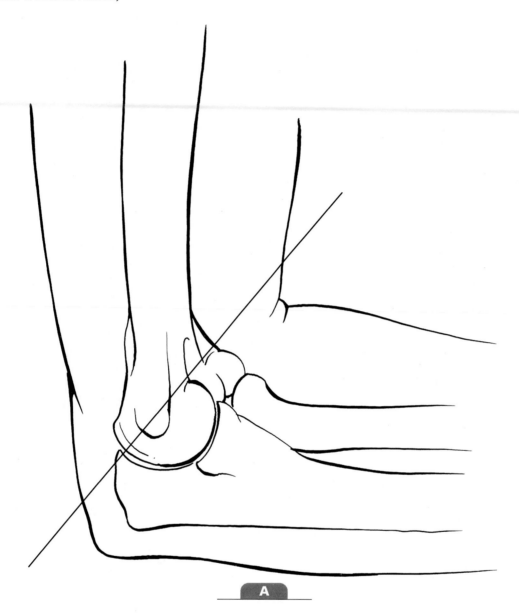

Figure 8-11 Axial MR image 1.

AXIAL MR IMAGE

The following is a selected axial MR image of the left elbow joint generated at the following technical factors: TR = 400, TE = 20, RF = 90°, FOV = 16 cm, TH = 3.5 mm. Abbreviations: TR = repetition time, TE = echotime, RF = radiofrequency, FOV = field of view, TH = slice thickness.

Figure 8-11 (A,B,C). This image demonstrates the upper elbow joint formed between the ulna and the humerus. As described earlier, the trochlear notch of the ulna is the part of the olecranon process that articulates with the trochlea of the humerus and forms the upper part of the elbow joint. On either side of the trochlea, the epicondyles of the humerus are shown in cross-section; the medial epicondyle is somewhat thinner and longer than the lateral epicondyle. On the anterior surface of the humerus, two large muscle groups can be identified as the biceps and the brachialis.

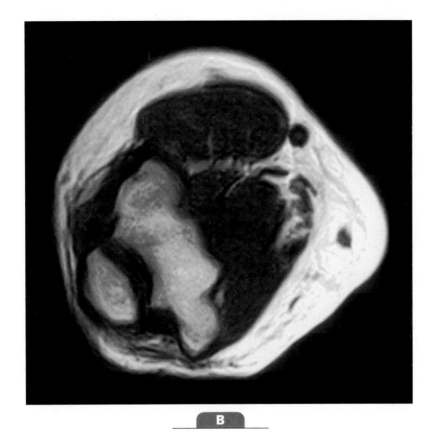

B

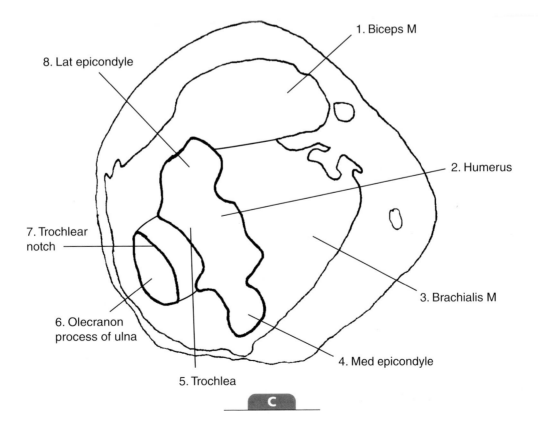

8. Lat epicondyle

1. Biceps M

2. Humerus

7. Trochlear
notch

3. Brachialis M

6. Olecranon
process of ulna

4. Med epicondyle

5. Trochlea

C

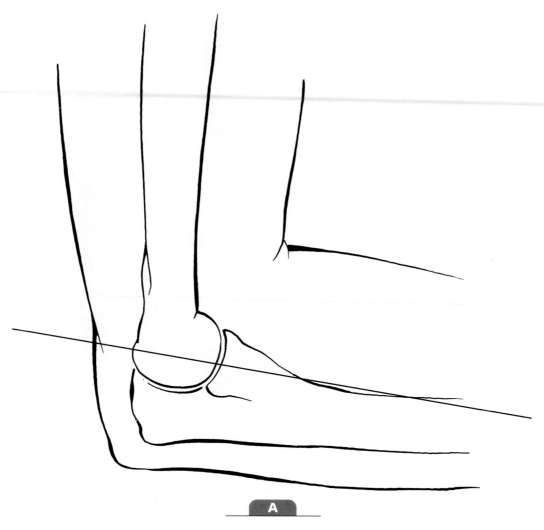

Figure 8-12 Coronal MR image 1.

CORONAL MR IMAGE

The following is a selected coronal MR image of the left elbow generated at the following technical factors: TR = 400, TE = 20, RF = 90°, FOV = 16 cm, TH = 3.5 mm. Abbreviations: TR = repetition time, TE = echotime, RF = radiofrequency, FOV = field of view, TH = slice thickness.

Figure 8-12 (A,B,C). This image demonstrates the articulation of the distal end of the humerus with both the radius and the ulna. A small part of the head of the radius is identified on the lateral side articulating with the capitulum of the humerus, found just below the lateral epicondyle. Medially, the shaft and the coronoid process of the ulna are shown aligning with the trochlea of the humerus below the medial epicondyle. On the posterior surface of the distal humerus, the olecranon fossa appears as a deep depression of low signal intensity. Above the humerus, this section shows a part of the triceps muscle on the posterior aspect of the arm. Extending downward from the upper arm, this muscle inserts on the olecranon process of the ulna and the fascia of the forearm, and acts to extend the forearm.

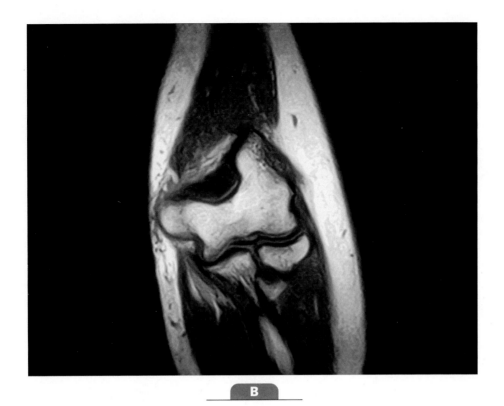

B

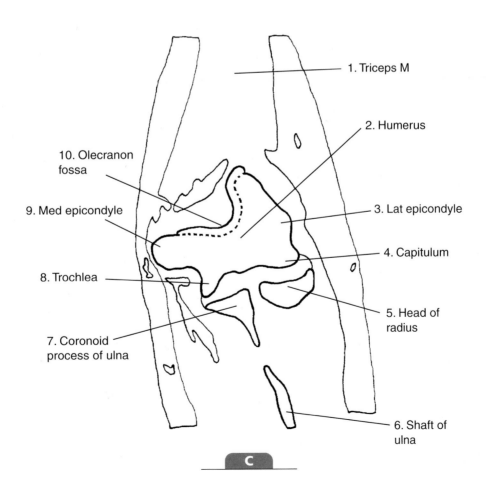

1. Triceps M

2. Humerus

10. Olecranon fossa

3. Lat epicondyle

9. Med epicondyle

4. Capitulum

8. Trochlea

5. Head of radius

7. Coronoid process of ulna

6. Shaft of ulna

C

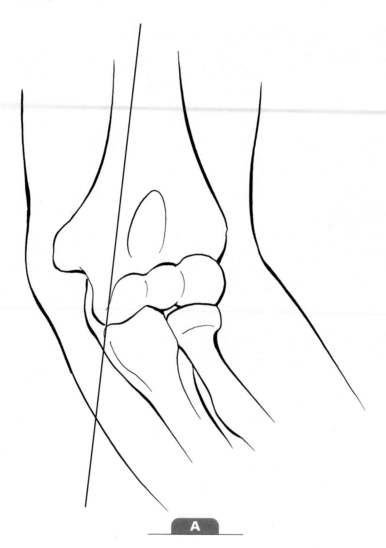

Figure 8-13 Sagittal MR image 1.

SAGITTAL MR IMAGES

The following two selected sagittal MR images of the left elbow joint were generated at 15-mm intervals from medial to lateral at the following technical factors: TR = 1100, TE = 20, RF = 90°, FOV = 16 cm, TH = 3.5 mm. Abbreviations: TR = repetition time, TE = echo-time, RF = radiofrequency, FOV = field of view, TH = slice thickness.

Figure 8-13 (A,B,C). This image shows the unique appearance of the distal end of the humerus. The shaft extends downward, narrowing as a result of the coronoid and olecranon fossae, which together cause a further narrowing of the humerus to a point at which the intervening region is nearly paper thin. Below the fossae, the humerus enlarges in a spherical manner to form the trochlea, which articulate with the proximal ulna of the forearm. Appearing as a crescent-shaped region of bone, the proximal ulna demonstrates both the coronoid and olecranon processes, which form the trochlear notch. Between the humerus and the ulna, the elbow joint space is separated from the surrounding musculature by the articu-lar capsule. In this section, the articular capsule extends from the coronoid and olecranon processes of the ulna to attach to the shaft of the humerus. The humerus separates the posterior triceps muscle from the brachialis and the biceps muscles on the anterior surface of the upper arm. The brachialis muscle, which originates from the lower half of the humerus, inserts on the coronoid process of the ulna. This position allows the brachialis muscle to flex the forearm and makes it a deeper muscle than the biceps. Shown obliquely sectioned on the anterior brachialis muscle, the brachial artery is sectioned as it extends downward along the medial border of the biceps muscle to give rise to the radial artery in the forearm.

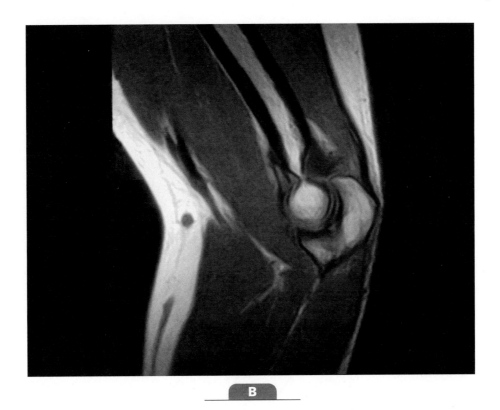

B

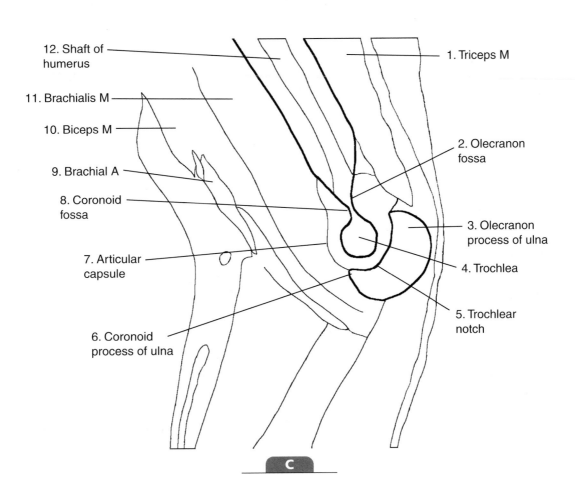

12. Shaft of humerus

11. Brachialis M

10. Biceps M

9. Brachial A

8. Coronoid fossa

7. Articular capsule

6. Coronoid process of ulna

1. Triceps M

2. Olecranon fossa

3. Olecranon process of ulna

4. Trochlea

5. Trochlear notch

C

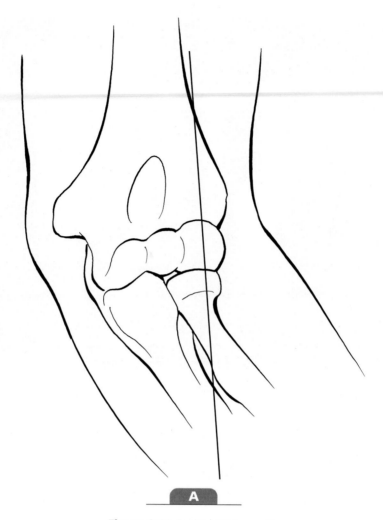

Figure 8-14 Sagittal MR image 2.

Figure 8-14 (A,B,C). This section through the lateral region of the elbow, shows the head of the radius articulating with the capitulum of the humerus. The capitulum is an enlarged region of the distal humerus that articulates with the fovea, or the depressed region on the head of the radius, to form the lateral elbow joint. On the lower part of the radius, the radial tuberosity is separated from the head by the narrowed region representing the neck of the radius. Compared to the ulna, the shaft of the radius is more anterior within the proximal forearm. Similar to the previous figure, the brachialis and biceps muscles can be identified in the upper part of the image, but the lateral location of this section also includes part of the brachioradialis muscle.

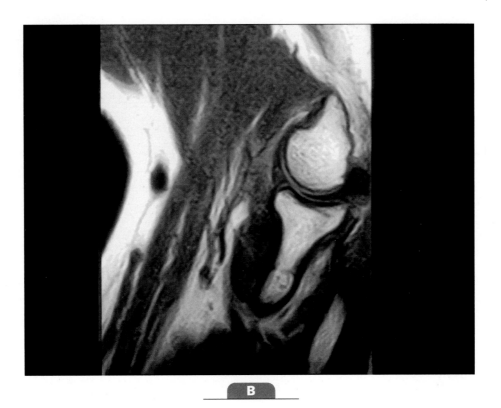

B

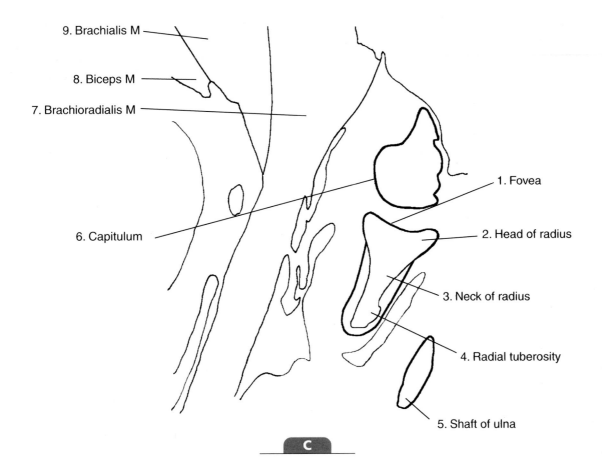

9. Brachialis M

8. Biceps M

7. Brachioradialis M

6. Capitulum

1. Fovea

2. Head of radius

3. Neck of radius

4. Radial tuberosity

5. Shaft of ulna

C

Wrist

ANATOMICAL OVERVIEW

The wrist is generally described as the part of the upper limb between the forearm and hand. Together, the carpal bones articulate to provide a wide range of movements of the hand with respect to the forearm. The wrist contains eight bones that are arranged in groups of four into proximal and distal rows (Fig. 8-15).

Skeletal

Hint: The mnemonic for remembering the order of the carpal bones, starting from the lateral side in the proximal row, is "Send *letter to Peter to tell*'m (to) *come home*."

Scaphoid (*SKAF-oyd*). Also called the navicular (*nă-VIK-yŭ-lăr*) bone. The largest and most lateral bone of the

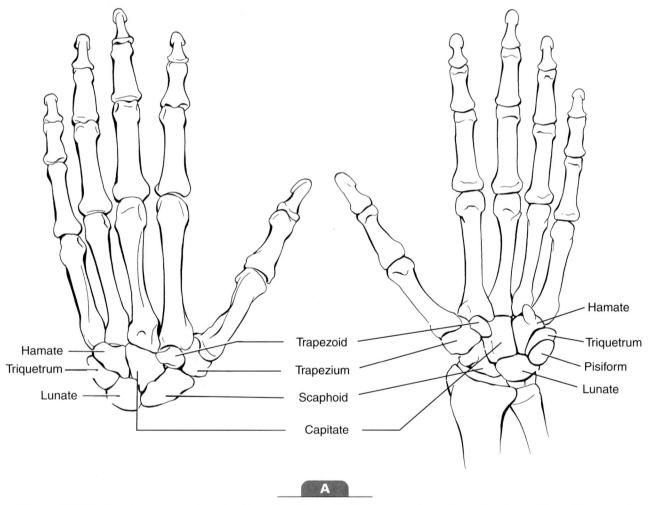

A

Figure 8-15 A. Dorsal and palmar view of wrist and hand bones. **B.** Dorsal view of muscles and tendons of the wrist and hand.
C. Palmar view of muscles and tendons of the wrist and hand.

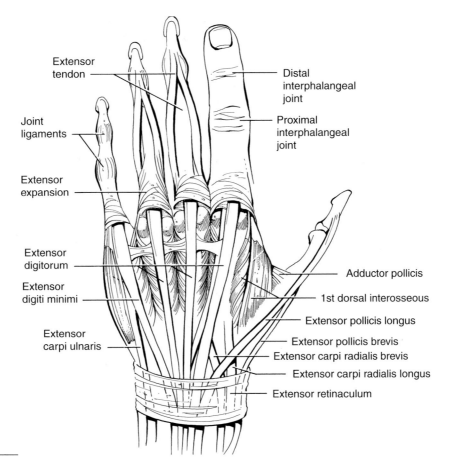

Extensor tendon

Joint ligaments

Extensor expansion

Extensor digitorum

Extensor digiti minimi

Extensor carpi ulnaris

Distal interphalangeal joint

Proximal interphalangeal joint

Adductor pollicis

1st dorsal interosseous

Extensor pollicis longus

Extensor pollicis brevis

Extensor carpi radialis brevis

Extensor carpi radialis longus

Extensor retinaculum

B

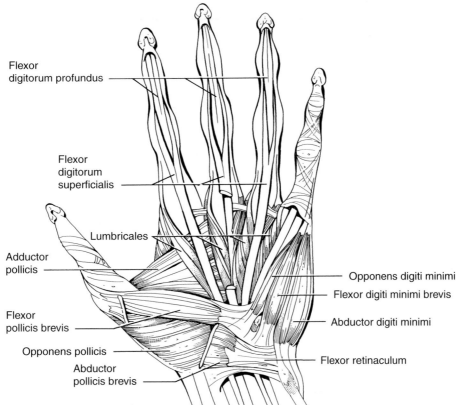

Flexor digitorum profundus

Flexor digitorum superficialis

Lumbricales

Adductor pollicis

Flexor pollicis brevis

Opponens pollicis

Abductor pollicis brevis

Opponens digiti minimi

Flexor digiti minimi brevis

Abductor digiti minimi

Flexor retinaculum

C

proximal row. Articulates with the radius. Because the radius is the only bone of the forearm that articulates with the carpal bones, the force of falls frequently results in fractures of the scaphoid bone. Approximately 75% of carpal fractures are found within this bone.

Lunate (*LU-nat*). Also called the semilunar bone. Crescent-shaped bone within the proximal row. Articulates with the radius.

Triquetrum (*tri-KWĒ-trŭm*). Also called the triangular or cuneiform bone. Pyramidal-shaped bone with an articular facet on its palmar surface for the pisiform.

Pisiform (*PIS-i-fōrm*). The most medial bone of the proximal row. Small, oval-shaped bone situated on the palmar surface of the triquetrum. Unlike the other proximal carpal bones, a muscle of the forearm, the flexor carpi ulnaris, inserts on this bone.

Trapezium (*tra-PĒ-ze-ŭm*). Also called the greater multangular bone. The most medial carpal of the distal row. Articulates with the first metacarpal (*MET-ă-KAR-păl*) and is mostly on the palmar surface of the wrist.

Trapezoid (*TRAP-ĕ-zoyd*). Also called the lesser multangular bone. Wedge-shaped bone and the smallest of the distal row of carpal bones. Articulates with the second metacarpal. On the palmar surface, it has an oblique deep groove, giving it a unique appearance in sectional images.

Capitate (*KAP-i-tat*). Also called the os magnum bone. The largest of the carpal bones and located in the center of the wrist. Articulates with the third metacarpal. Owing to its shape and location, it forms the keystone of the carpal tunnel, found on the anterior wrist.

Hamate (*HAM-at*). Also called the unciform (*ŬN-si-fōrm*) bone. The most medial carpus in the distal row. Articulates with the fourth and fifth metacarpals. Has a unique shape owing to its hook-like process on the palmar surface, the hamulus (*HAM-yu-lŭs*).

Musculature

Abductor digiti minimi (*DIJ-i-ti MIN-i-mi*). Origin: pisiform and tendon of flexor carpi ulnaris. Insertion: first phalanx (*FA-langks*) of fifth digit. Action: abducts fifth digit and flexes first phalanx.

Abductor pollicis brevis (*POL-i-sis BREV-is*). Origin: flexor retinaculum (*ret-i-NAK-yu-lŭm*), scaphoid, and trapezium. Insertion: first phalanx of the first digit. Action: abducts first digit.

Opponens (*ŏ-PŌ-nens*) **pollicis**. Origin: flexor retinaculum and trapezium. Insertion: first metacarpal. Action: abducts, flexes, and rotates the first metacarpal.

Flexor digitorum superficialis (*dij-i-TŌ-rŭm SU-per-fish-e-A-lis*). Origin: medial epicondyle of humerus, coronoid process of ulna, and mid-radius. Insertion: second phalanx of digits two through five. Action: flexes second phalanges (*f-LAN-jez*), hand, and forearm.

Flexor digitorum profundus (*prō-FŬN-dŭs*). Origin: mid-ulna and interosseous membrane. Insertion: distal phalanx of digits two through five. Action: flexes digits and flexes hand.

Extensor carpi ulnaris (*KAR-piŭl-NA-ris*). Origin: lateral epicondyle of humerus and proximal ulna. Insertion: base of the fifth metacarpal. Action: extends and abducts the hand.

Extensor digiti minimi. Origin: common extensor tendon. Insertion: first phalanx of the fifth digit. Action: extends fifth digit.

Extensor digitorum. Origin: lateral epicondyle of humerus. Insertion: bases of second and third phalanges of digits two through five. Action: extends the digits and extends the hand.

Extensor indicis (*IN-di-sez*). Origin: posterior shaft of the ulna and the interosseous membrane. Insertion: extensor digitorum tendon of the second digit. Action: extends and adducts the second digit. NB: not shown in Figure 8-15.

Extensor pollicis longus. Origin: posterior surface of ulna. Insertion: base of the last phalanx of the first digit. Action: extends first phalanx of the first digit and abducts the hand.

Extensor carpi radialis (*ra-de-A-lis*) **longus**. Origin: lateral supracondylar ridge of humerus. Insertion: base of the second metacarpal. Action: extends and abducts the hand.

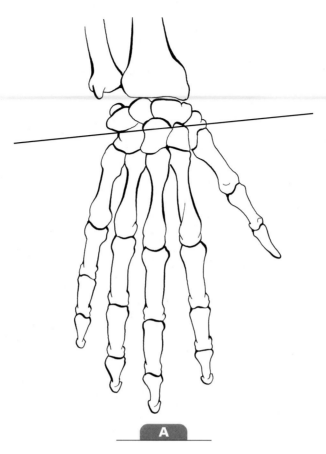

A

Figure 8-16 Axial CT image 1.

AXIAL CT IMAGES

The following two selected CT images of both wrists are described at 3 mm intervals from proximal to distal. The images were generated at the following technical factors: 120 kVp, 150 mA-s, FOV = 25 cm, TH = 3 mm. Abbreviations: kVp = kilovolt peak, mA-s = milliampere-second, FOV = field of view, TH = slice thickness.

Figure 8-16 (A,B,C). For comparison, this image includes both of the patient's wrists, which were placed side by side within the gantry. The patient's left wrist is on the right side of the image, as though the patient were facing us. In this position, the lateral parts of both wrists are located toward the middle of the image. When looking at the left wrist, the unique appearance of the hamate bone is readily distinguished owing to the presence of the hook, or hamulus, on the palmar surface. Because the plane of section is slightly higher on the left wrist, an additional carpus is shown lateral to the hamate bone. Owing to its location, the bone is the triquetrum, or the third bone of the proximal row between the hamate and the pisiform bones. Articulating with the medial side of the hamate bone, the capitate is identified and is often described as the bone within the center of the wrist. Moving medially, we note the next carpus of the distal row is the trapezoid, shown with its characteristic groove on the palmar surface. The first bone of the distal row, the trapezium, is found near the palmar surface. Together, the bones form part of a bony arch over what is known as the carpal tunnel, which contains the flexor digitorum superficialis and profundus tendons passing from the forearm into the palmar surface of the hand. In addition, the abductor digiti minimi muscle is sectioned as it extends from its origin on the pisiform bone and tendon of flexor carpi ulnaris to insert on the first phalanx of the fifth digit. On the lateral side of the wrist, the abductor pollicis brevis and opponens pollicis muscles are cross-sectioned as they originate from the flexor retinaculum and trapezium. Although reversed from the sequence described for the left wrist, all four bones of the distal row can be identified — in a slightly different plane of section — within the right wrist. Like the bones, the muscles of the right wrist are reversed in position compared to the left side. On the dorsal surface of the wrist, the tendons sectioned are collectively called the extensor tendons and include the extensor pollicis longus, extensor carpi radialis longus, extensor indices, extensor digitorum, extensor digiti minimi, and extensor carpi ulnaris.

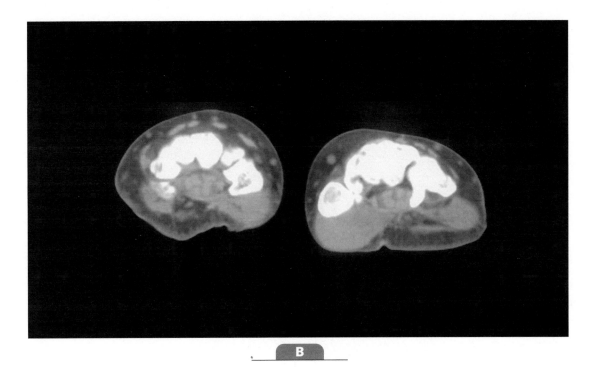

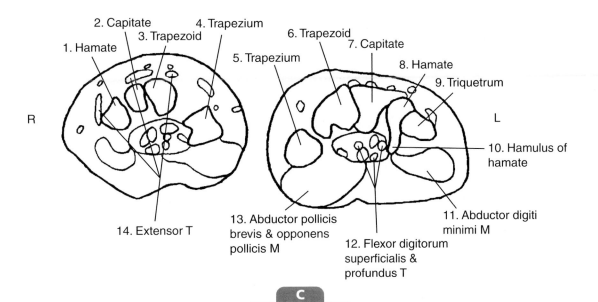

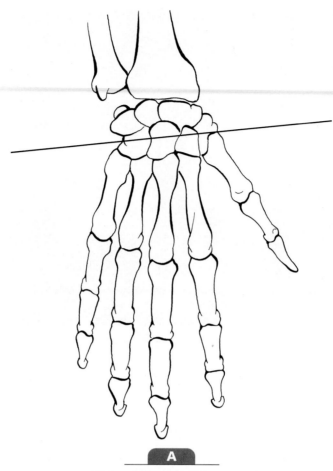

Figure 8-17 Axial CT image 2.

Figure 8-17 (A,B,C). Because this image is 3 mm distal to the previous image, the anatomy demonstrated lies closer to the metacarpals. As before, this image demonstrates both the right and left wrists. The four bones of the distal row can be identified within the right wrist. The capitate bone is in the center of the wrist separating the hamate from the trapezoid. In this position, the trapezium or most lateral bone of the distal row is demonstrated in its characteristic location toward the palmar surface. Together, these four bones form part of the bony arch over the carpal tunnel. Within the left wrist, the four bones of the distal row can also be identified in reverse sequence; the most lateral is the hamate. Although somewhat light owing to slice thickness averaging, the hamulus of the hamate bone is demonstrated on the palmar surface. Because the plane of section is slightly higher on the left wrist than on the right, the triquetrum of the proximal row is sectioned. The triquetrum separates the hamate from the small, oval-shaped pisiform bone. Much like the previous image, the flexor digitorum superficialis and profundus tendons are within the carpal tunnel and are labeled in the right wrist. The flexor tendons are separated from the abductor digiti minimi, abductor pollicis brevis, and opponens pollicis muscles by the flexor retinaculum. On the dorsal surface of the carpal bones, extensor tendons are sectioned but are not individually labeled in this image.

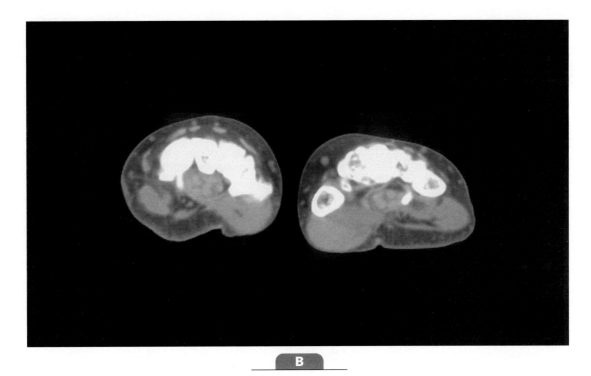

B

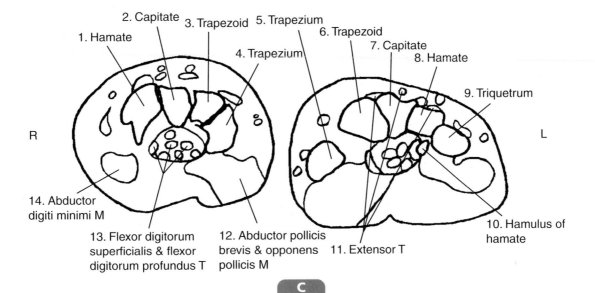

2. Capitate
3. Trapezoid
5. Trapezium
6. Trapezoid
1. Hamate
7. Capitate
4. Trapezium
8. Hamate
9. Triquetrum

R

L

14. Abductor
digiti minimi M

10. Hamulus of
hamate

13. Flexor digitorum
superficialis & flexor
digitorum profundus T

12. Abductor pollicis
brevis & opponens
pollicis M

11. Extensor T

C

Hip

ANATOMICAL OVERVIEW

Generally described as the juncture of the lower limb with the pelvic girdle, or hip bone, which is made up of the ilium, ischium, and pubis. Formed between the head of the femur and the acetabulum, the joint is considered a ball-and-socket type (enarthrosis); it is capable of a wide range of movements, including internal and external rotation.

Skeletal

Femur (*Fe-mŭr*). The longest and strongest bone in the body. Found within the thigh (Fig. 8-18).

Head. The round, proximal end of the femur that forms the ball part of the hip joint.

Greater trochanter. Projection of bone found on the lateral aspect of the proximal femur. Site of attachment for many muscles within the gluteal (*GLU-te-ăl*) region.

Fovea capitis femoris (*FŌ-ve-ă KAP-i-tis FEM-ŏ-ris*). A depression in the head of the femur where the ligamentum capitis femoris is attached. Unlike most ligaments, the ligamentum capitis femoris has little function in maintaining the structure of the joint. Instead, it acts to guide an artery through the fovea capitis to provide the major arterial blood supply to the head of the femur.

Neck. The narrowed region between the trochanters and the head of the femur that forms an angle of 120° to 125° with the shaft.

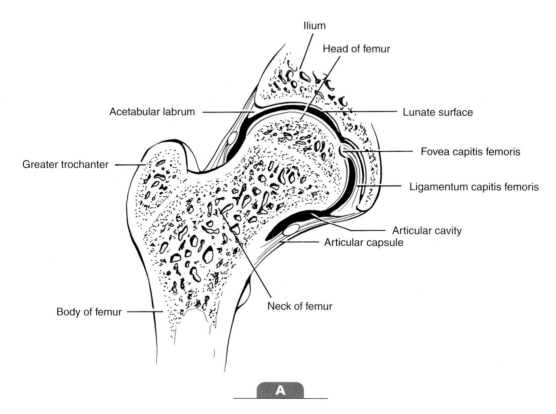

Figure 8-18 A. Coronal section of the hip. **B.** Anterior view of muscles covering the hip joint. **C.** Posterior view of muscles covering the hip joint.

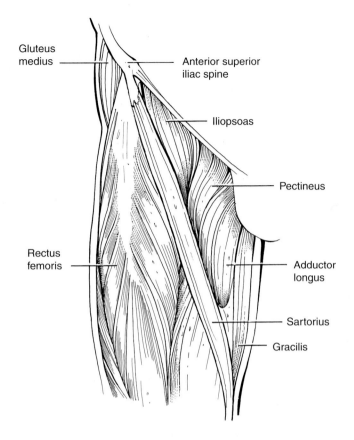

Gluteus medius

Anterior superior iliac spine

Iliopsoas

Pectineus

Rectus femoris

Adductor longus

Sartorius

Gracilis

B

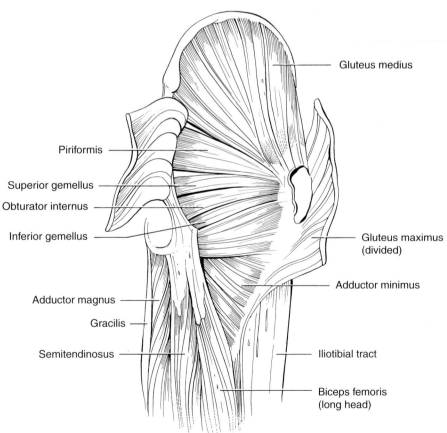

Gluteus medius

Piriformis

Superior gemellus

Obturator internus

Inferior gemellus

Gluteus maximus (divided)

Adductor minimus

Adductor magnus

Gracilis

Semitendinosus

Iliotibial tract

Biceps femoris (long head)

C

Acetabulum (*as-ĕ-TAB-yu-lŭm*). A depression on the lateral aspect of the pelvic girdle formed by the juncture of the ilium (*IL-e-ŭm*), ischium (*IS-ke-ŭm*), and pubic bones. Forms the socket of the hip joint.

Lunate surface. The crescentic-shaped articular surface within the acetabulum (Latin for "moon"). Surrounds the fossa containing the ligamentum capitis femoris.

Musculature

Iliopsoas (*IL-e-Ō-SŌ-as*). Origin: transverse processes of L1 through L5 and the upper iliac fossa. Insertion: lesser trochanter of the femur. Action: flexes the thigh and rotates the thigh laterally.

Gluteus maximus (*glu-TĒ-ŭs MAK-si-mŭs*). Origin: upper ilium and sacrotuberous ligament. Insertion: gluteal tuberosity of the femur. Action: Extends and laterally rotates the thigh.

Obturator internus (*OB-tu--rā-tŏr in-TER-nŭs*). Origin: inner obturator membrane. Insertion: greater trochanter. Action: abducts and rotates the thigh laterally.

Superior gemellus (*jĕ-MEL-ŭs*). Origin: outer ischial spine. Insertion: tendon of the obturator internus muscle. Action: abducts and laterally rotates the thigh.

Tensor fascia latae (*FASH-e-ă LA-te*). Origin: anterior iliac crest. Insertion: iliotibial tract, Action: abducts, flexes, and rotates the thigh medially. NB: not shown in Figure 8-18.

Rectus (*REK-tŭs*) **femoris.** Origin: anterior inferior iliac spine. Insertion: base of the patella. Action: flexes the thigh and extends the leg.

Sartorius (*sar-TOR-e-ŭs*). Origin: anterior superior iliac spine. Insertion: upper medial tibia. Action: flexes and rotates the thigh laterally.

Pectineus (*PEK-ti-NĒ-ŭs*). Origin: pectineal line of the pubis. Insertion: pectineal line of the femur. Action: flexes, adducts, and laterally rotates the thigh.

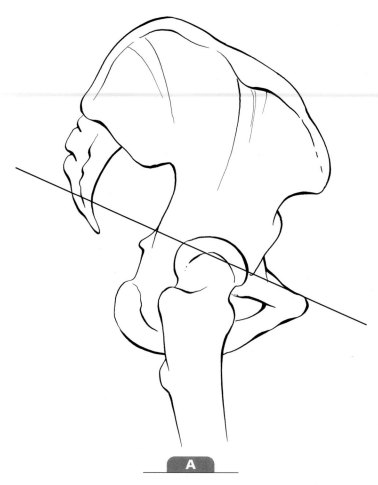

Figure 8-19 Axial CT image 1.

AXIAL CT IMAGES

The following two selected CT images of the hip joint are described at 5 mm intervals from superior to inferior. They were generated at the following technical factors: 120 kVp, 280 mA-s, FOV = 30 cm, TH = 5 mm. Abbreviations: kVP = kilovolt peak, mA-s = milliampere-second, FOV = field of view, TH = slice thickness.

Figure 8-19 (A,B,C). At this level, the coccyx is found posterior and separate from the other parts of the bony pelvis. Anteriorly, the pubic symphysis separates the two pubic bones and the pubic tubercles are shown in profile. On either side, the heads of the femurs are found within the acetabula that are formed by the bones of the pelvic girdle: pubic, ischium, and ilium. Even though the greater trochanters are shown on both sides, the left side is more inferior than the right. Within the right hip joint, the articular surface of the acetabulum, or the lunate surface, is labeled beside the acetabular fossa. Although not clearly delineated, the ligamentum capitis femoris would extend within the acetabular fossa to the fovea capitis femoris. As described earlier, the ligamentum capitis femoris has little function other than protecting and transmitting the major arterial supply to the femoral head. Covering the anterior surface of the articular capsule, the iliopsoas muscles are sectioned as they extend down to insert on the lesser trochanters. Medial to the iliopsoas muscles, the pectineus muscles are sectioned near their origin on the pubic bones and would be seen in lower sections to insert on the proximal femur. Anterolateral to the hip joints, the sartorius, rectus femoris, and tensor fascia latae muscles are sectioned as they extend downward to insert on the leg. The sartorius is more superficial than the underlying rectus femoris, and the tensor fascia latae is the most lateral of the three. On the posterior surface of the hip joint, the gluteus maximus is a large flat muscle covered with a layer of superficial fat. Deep to the gluteus maximus, the superior gemellus is sectioned, extending from its origin on the ischial spine to insert on the tendon of the obturator internus. Although the obturator internus is labeled near its origin on the inner obturator membrane, the muscle travels below the superior gemellus to insert on the greater trochanter of the femur.

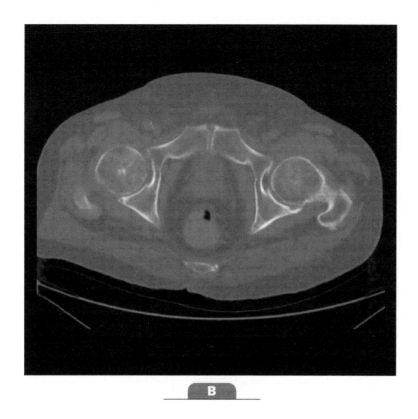

B

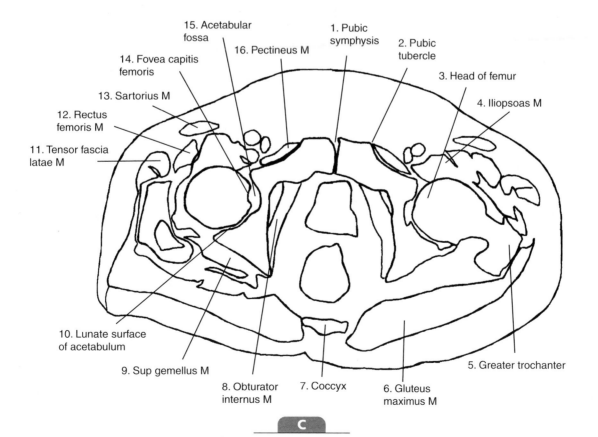

15. Acetabular fossa
16. Pectineus M
1. Pubic symphysis
2. Pubic tubercle
14. Fovea capitis femoris
3. Head of femur
13. Sartorius M
4. Iliopsoas M
12. Rectus femoris M
11. Tensor fascia latae M
10. Lunate surface of acetabulum
9. Sup gemellus M
8. Obturator internus M
7. Coccyx
6. Gluteus maximus M
5. Greater trochanter

C

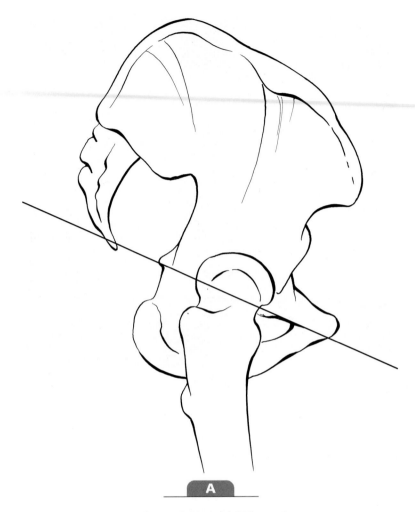

Figure 8-20 Axial CT image 2.

Figure 8-20 (A,B,C). Similar to the previous image, the coccyx is shown forming the posterior boundary of the pelvis and appearing separate from the pelvic girdle. At this lower level, the ischial and pubic bones are nearing the opening of the obturator foramen, which separates the two bones on the anterolateral aspect of the pelvis. On either side, the acetabular fossae can be identified next to the lunate surfaces of the acetabula. The heads and greater trochanters of the femurs can be identified on either side, but their appearance is slightly different, indicating the anatomy represented is slightly higher on the patient's right side. In this section, the muscles surrounding the hip joint are much the same as described in the previous section. The iliopsoas muscles are covering the anterior articular capsule, and the pectineus muscles are sectioned near their origin on the pubic bones. On the anterolateral hip, the sartorius, the rectus femoris, and tensor fascia latae are sectioned as they extend down to insert on the leg. On the posterior hip joint, the gluteus maximus is covering the superior gemellus and the obturator internus. Although the obturator internus muscle is labeled near its origin on the inner obturator membrane, the muscle extends behind the ischium and inserts on the greater trochanter of the femur. Originating from the ischial spine, the superior gemellus muscle is labeled near its insertion on the tendon of the obturator internus.

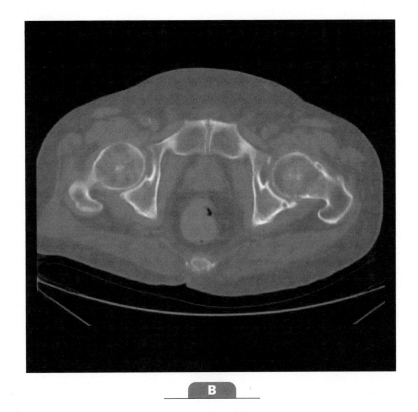

B

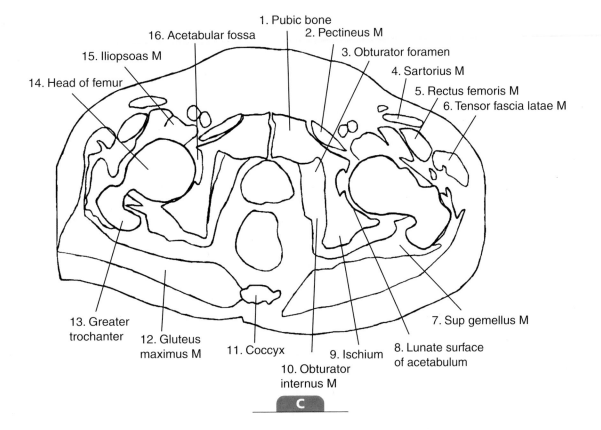

1. Pubic bone
2. Pectineus M
16. Acetabular fossa
3. Obturator foramen
15. Iliopsoas M
4. Sartorius M
14. Head of femur
5. Rectus femoris M
6. Tensor fascia latae M

13. Greater trochanter
12. Gluteus maximus M
11. Coccyx
10. Obturator internus M
9. Ischium
8. Lunate surface of acetabulum
7. Sup gemellus M

C

Knee

ANATOMICAL OVERVIEW

The knee is the largest joint in the body and is defined as the region between the thigh and the lower leg. Formed by the distal femur articulating with the tibia and the patella, the knee contains two separate joints. The joint between the femur and the tibia is considered a ginglymus, or hinge-type, joint; and the joint between the femur and the patella is arthrodial, or gliding, joint. Although the fibula does not articulate with the distal femur, ligaments between the two bones are important in stabilizing the knee joint. Much like the shoulder, ligaments are important in limiting the movements of the joint but the majority of the joint strength is provided by the surrounding musculature.

Skeletal

Femur. Its most distal part is formed by the medial and lateral condyles that are located on either side of the knee joint (Fig. 8-21). Because these rounded surfaces articulate with the tibia, they are covered with a layer of articular cartilage that helps create a smooth surface and protect the underlying bone.

Tibia (*TIB-e-ă*). Commonly called the shin bone. The second longest bone of the body. Within the lower leg, the larger and more medial bone. Its proximal end has medial and lateral condyles that articulate with those of the distal femur. Ligaments are located in the intercondyloid area (between the condylar processes). Although not shown, the

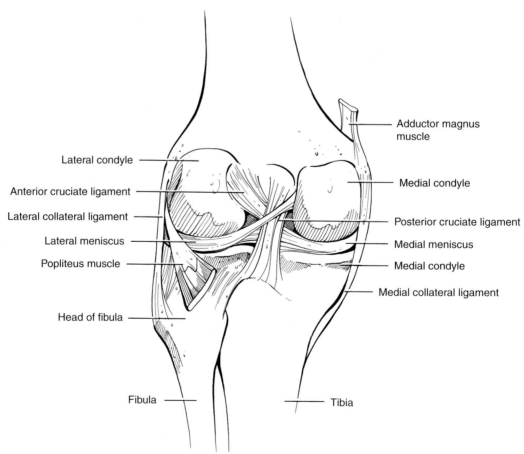

Labels (left): Lateral condyle; Anterior cruciate ligament; Lateral collateral ligament; Lateral meniscus; Popliteus muscle; Head of fibula; Fibula

Labels (right): Adductor magnus muscle; Medial condyle; Posterior cruciate ligament; Medial meniscus; Medial condyle; Medial collateral ligament; Tibia

Figure 8-21 Posterior view of the bones and ligaments of the left knee.

central intercondyloid area has intercondylar eminences where ligaments attach to the tibia.

Fibula (*FIB-yu-lă*). In the lower leg, the more slender bone found on the lateral side. Proximally, its head articulates with the lateral condyle of the tibia, forming the proximal tibiofibular joints. Distally, it articulates with the talus, forming part of the ankle joint.

Patella (*pa-TEL-ă*). Commonly called the knee cap. The largest of the sesamoid (*SES-ă-moyd*) bones. Irregularly shaped bone located in front of the knee joint (Fig. 8-22). Its rough anterior surface provides attachment for the quadriceps femoris tendon. Medial and lateral articular facets on the posterior surface join with the femur to form the femoropatellar joint.

Ligaments

Anterior cruciate (*KRŪ-shē-āt*). Round ligament extending from the anterior intercondylar fossa to the back of the lateral femoral condyle (Figs. 8-21 to 8-23). Checks exten-

sion, lateral rotation, and anterior slipping of the tibia on the femur.

Posterior cruciate. Round ligament extending from the posterior intercondylar fossa to the front of the medial femoral condyle. Checks flexion, lateral rotation, and posterior slipping of tibia on the femur.

Medial collateral. Flat ligament extending from the medial femoral condyle to the medial condyle and body of the tibia. Prevents lateral bending and checks extension, hyperflexion, and lateral rotation.

Lateral collateral. Flat ligament extending from the lateral femoral condyle to the head and styloid process of the fibula. Checks hyperextension.

Patellar. Largest ligament of the knee. Extends between the patella and the tibial tuberosity and is a continuation of the quadriceps femoris tendon below the level of the patella (Fig. 8-22). Acts to extend the lower leg.

Medial meniscus (*mě-NIS-kŭs*). Crescent-shaped ligament that attaches to the tibia in front of the anterior

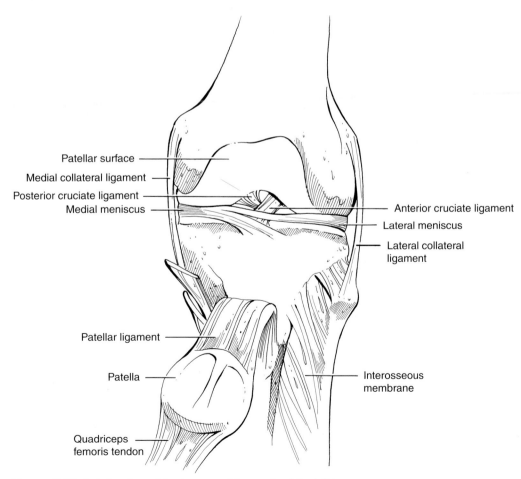

Figure 8-22 Anterior view of the bones and ligaments of the left knee.

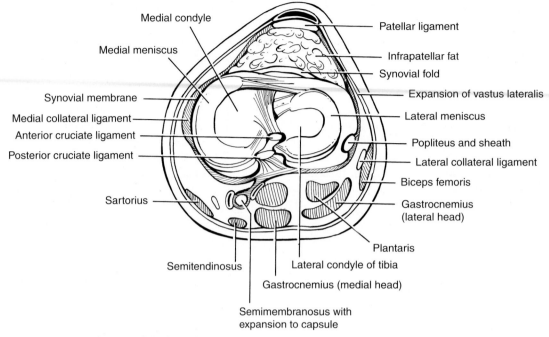

Medial condyle
Medial meniscus
Synovial membrane
Medial collateral ligament
Anterior cruciate ligament
Posterior cruciate ligament
Sartorius
Semitendinosus
Semimembranosus with expansion to capsule
Gastrocnemius (medial head)
Lateral condyle of tibia
Plantaris
Patellar ligament
Infrapatellar fat
Synovial fold
Expansion of vastus lateralis
Lateral meniscus
Popliteus and sheath
Lateral collateral ligament
Biceps femoris
Gastrocnemius (lateral head)

Figure 8-23 Axial image of the lower knee joint.

cruciate ligament and in the posterior intercondylar fossa (Fig. 8-23). Functions to deepen the medial tibial condyle.

Lateral meniscus. Nearly circular ligament that attaches to the tibia in front of the anterior cruciate ligament and behind the intercondylar eminence. Functions to deepen the lateral tibial condyle.

Musculature and Other Structures

Quadriceps (*KWAH-dri-seps*) **femoris.** Origin: inferior iliac spine and rim of acetabulum. Insertion: base of patella. Action: flexes thigh and extends lower leg.

Popliteus (*pop-li-TĒ-ŭs*). Origin: lateral condyle of femur. Insertion: posterior tibia above soleal line. Action: flexes and rotates lower leg medially.

Gastrocnemius (*gas-trok-NĒ-mē-ŭs*). Origin: medial and lateral femoral condyles. Insertion: through tendocalcaneus to posterior calcaneus. Action: flexes lower leg, plantar flexes and inverts foot

Infrapatellar fat pad. A collection of fatty tissue posterior to the patella that protects the underlying femur and tibia.

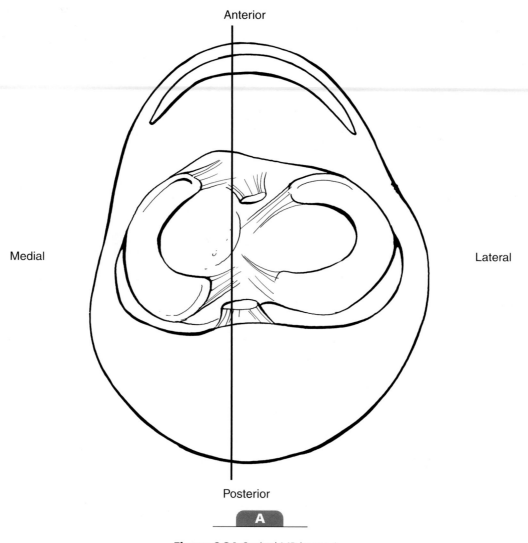

Anterior

Medial

Lateral

Posterior

A

Figure 8-24 Sagittal MR image 1.

SAGITTAL MR IMAGES

The following three selected sagittal MR images of the left knee joint were generated at 8-mm intervals from medial to lateral at the following technical factors: TR = 1100, TE = 20, RF = 90°, FOV = 16 cm, TH = 3.5 mm. Abbreviations: TR = repetition time, TE = echo-time, RF = radiofrequency, FOV = field of view, TH = slice thickness.

Figure 8-24 (A,B,C). This sagittal image demonstrates a near midsagittal section of the femur and the tibia. Because the plane of this section lies near the midline, the anterior cruciate ligament appears as a low-signal area, extending from the anterior intercondylar fossa. As the anterior cruciate ligament ascends to attach to the back of the lateral femoral condyle, it crosses the posterior cruciate ligament. As described earlier, the posterior cruciate ligament originates from the posterior intercondylar fossa and ascends to insert on the medial femoral condyle. The relationship between these two ligaments is described by the term cruciate, which means shaped like a cross. Outside the knee joint, the popliteus and gastrocnemius muscles are found posterior to the tibia, and the quadriceps femoris muscle is found on the anterior surface of the femur.

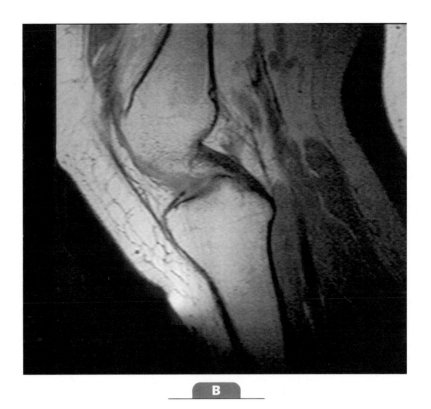

B

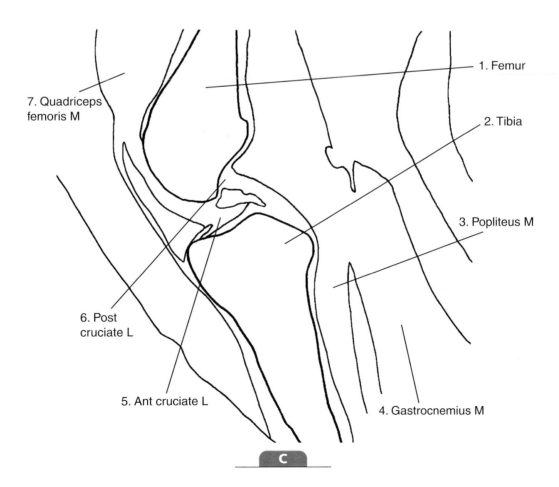

1. Femur

7. Quadriceps
femoris M

2. Tibia

3. Popliteus M

6. Post
cruciate L

5. Ant cruciate L

4. Gastrocnemius M

C

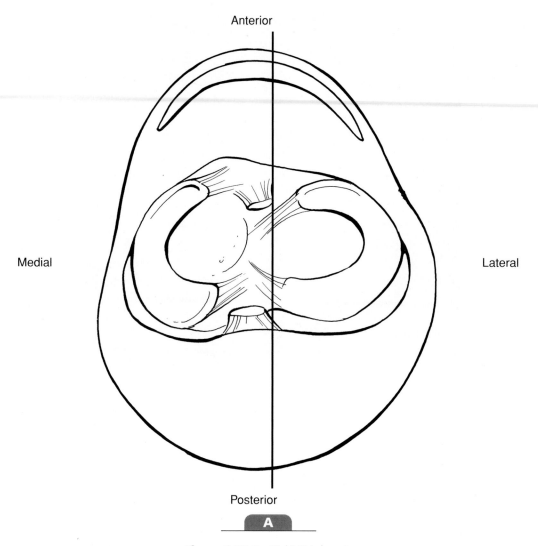

Anterior

Medial

Lateral

Posterior

A

Figure 8-25 Sagittal MR image 2.

Figure 8-25 (A,B,C). Although the femur appears much like it did in the previous image, its lower anterior part is covered with articular cartilage, indicating the beginning of the lateral femoral condyle. Anterior to the distal femur, a small section of the medial patella is demonstrated just below the space previously occupied by the quadriceps femoris muscle. The tibia looks smaller than it did in the previous figure. On the superior surface of the tibia, an inter-condylar eminence is labeled between the anterior and posterior cruciate ligaments. In this image, only the distal parts of the anterior and posterior cruciate ligaments are demonstrated near their attach-ments within the intercondylar fossae. Between the knee joint and the medial patella, an area of high signal intensity represents the area of the infrapatellar fat pad, which protects the underlying bones and joint from blows to the patella. On the posterior surface of the joint, the lateral head of the gastrocnemius muscle is found extending from its origin on the lateral femoral condyle to insert on the posterior calcaneus.

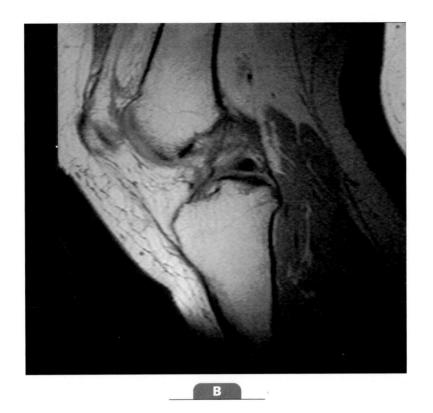

B

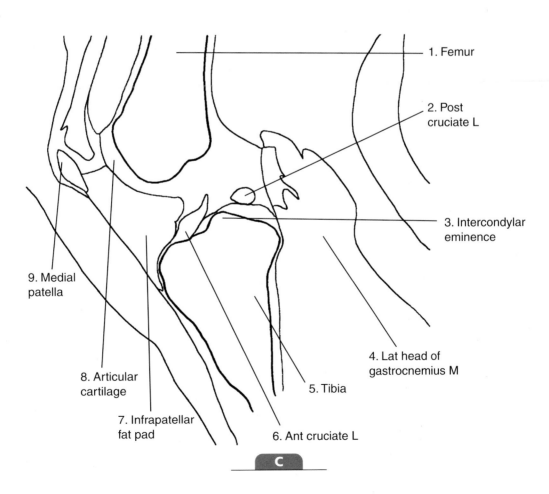

1. Femur

2. Post cruciate L

3. Intercondylar eminence

9. Medial patella

4. Lat head of gastrocnemius M

8. Articular cartilage

5. Tibia

7. Infrapatellar fat pad

6. Ant cruciate L

C

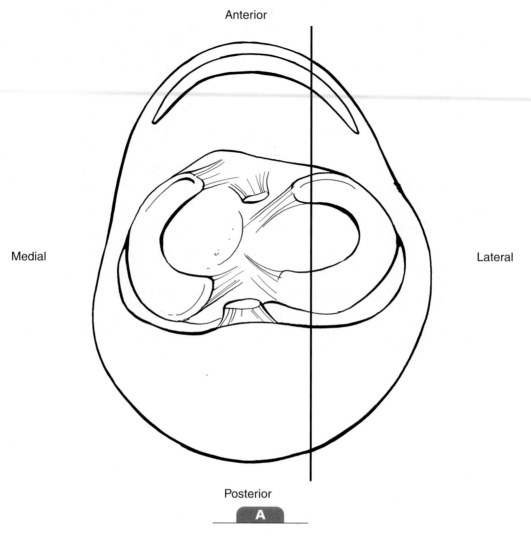

Anterior

Medial

Lateral

Posterior

A

Figure 8-26 Sagittal MR image 3.

Figure 8-26 (A,B,C). This image demonstrates the lateral femoral condyle, in full view directly behind the patella, creating the femoropatellar joint. As described earlier, the patella is embedded in the back of the quadriceps femoris tendon and is attached to the tibia via the patellar ligament. Compared to previous views, only a small part of the lateral tibia is demonstrated in this image. The proximal tibia articulates with the head of the fibula, forming the proximal tibiofibular joint. Within the knee joint, articular cartilage is shown along the periphery of the femoral condyle and the superior surface of the tibia, which are shown adjacent to one another. The anterior and posterior horns of the lateral meniscus, deepening the knee joint, are demonstrated in cross-section in regions of low signal intensity adjacent to the site of articulation between the femur and the tibia.

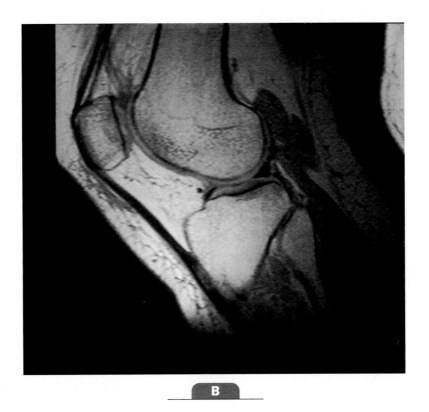

B

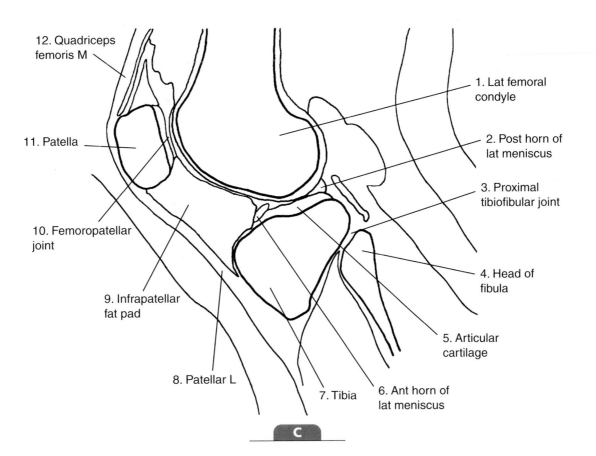

12. Quadriceps femoris M

11. Patella

10. Femoropatellar joint

9. Infrapatellar fat pad

8. Patellar L

7. Tibia

6. Ant horn of lat meniscus

5. Articular cartilage

4. Head of fibula

3. Proximal tibiofibular joint

2. Post horn of lat meniscus

1. Lat femoral condyle

C

Anterior

Medial

Lateral

Posterior

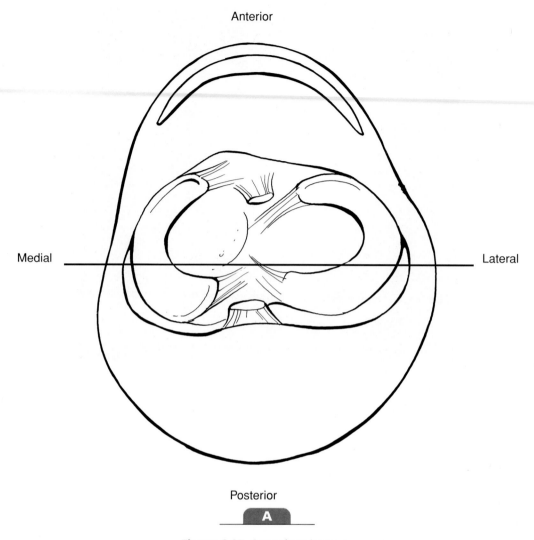

A

Figure 8-27 Coronal MR image 1.

CORONAL MR IMAGES

The following four selected coronal MR images of the left knee joint were generated at 4 mm intervals from posterior to anterior. The images were taken at the following technical factors: TR = 1100, TE = 20, RF = 90°, FOV = 16 cm, TH = 3.5 mm. Abbreviations: TR = repetition time, TE = echo-time, RF = radiofrequency, FOV = field of view, TH = slice thickness.

Figure 8-27 (A,B,C). This image demonstrates the anatomy within the posterior knee joint, including the medial and lateral femoral condyles and the proximal tibia. Between the femoral condyles and the proximal tibia, the medial and lateral menisci are in their respective locations within the posterior knee joint. Forming the medial boundary of the knee joint, the medial collateral ligament is extending from the medial femoral condyle to the proximal tibia. On the lateral side of the knee joint, the lateral collateral ligament is shown near its attachment on the lateral condyle of the femur; in more posterior sections it would be

seen to extend downward to attach to the head and styloid process of the fibula. Between the medial and lateral femoral condyles, the cruciate ligaments appear obliquely sectioned as regions of low signal intensity. The posterior cruciate ligament is shown near its distal end, or attachment in the posterior intercondylar fossa. In contrast, the proximal end of the anterior cruciate ligament is shown near the back of the lateral femoral condyle. Above the femoral condyles, the medial and lateral heads of the gastrocnemius muscles are shown originating on the distal femur.

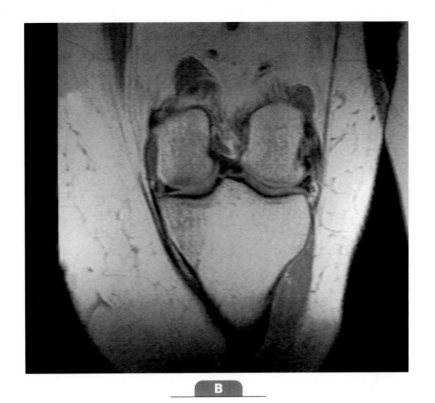

B

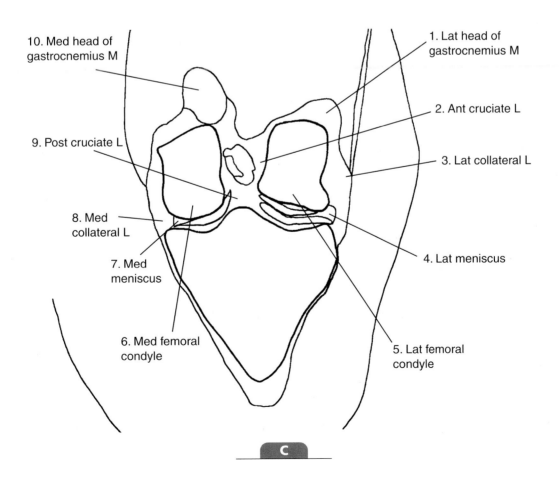

10. Med head of gastrocnemius M

9. Post cruciate L

8. Med collateral L

7. Med meniscus

6. Med femoral condyle

1. Lat head of gastrocnemius M

2. Ant cruciate L

3. Lat collateral L

4. Lat meniscus

5. Lat femoral condyle

C

Anterior

Medial

Lateral

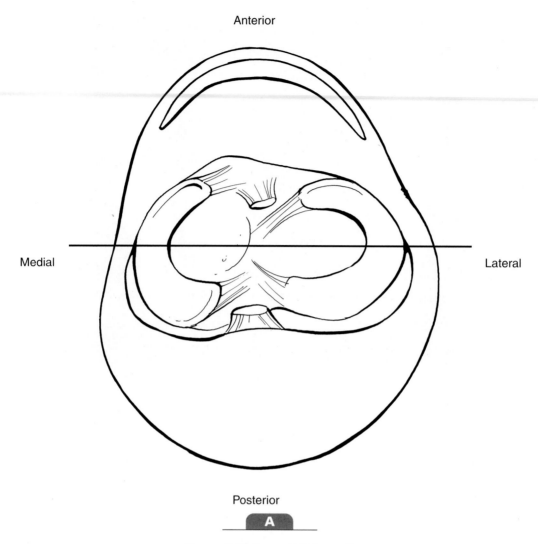

Posterior

A

Figure 8-28 Coronal MR image 2.

Figure 8-28 (A,B,C). Compared to the previous figure, the medial and lateral femoral condyles are larger, indicating we are nearing the body of the femur. Lower in the image, the proximal tibia is sectioned and clearly demonstrates the intercondylar eminence projecting upward between the femoral condyles. The medial and lateral menisci are cross-sectioned and appear as regions of low signal intensity below the femoral condyles. Extending between the medial femoral condyle and the tibia, the medial collateral ligament is shown forming the medial boundary of the knee joint. Laterally, the lateral collateral ligament is shown above the knee joint near its proximal attachment on the lateral femoral condyle. Because the lateral collateral ligament extends downward to attach to the head and styloid process of the fibula, in more posterior sections it would be shown closer to the knee joint. Found medial to the lateral collateral ligament, the popliteal tendon is originating from the lateral condyle of the femur. Between the medial and the lateral femoral condyles, the anterior and posterior cruciate ligaments appear as irregularly shaped regions of low signal intensity. The anterior cruciate ligament is sectioned near its proximal attachment on the lateral femoral condyle, and the posterior cruciate ligament is moving away from its distal attachment on the posterior intercondylar fossa.

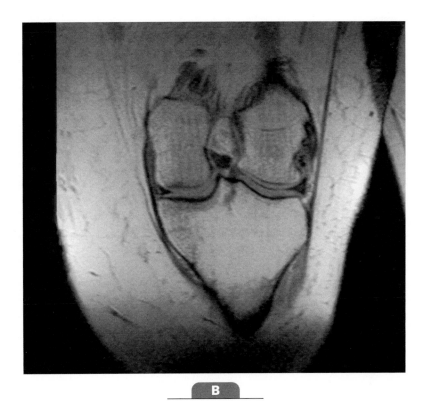

B

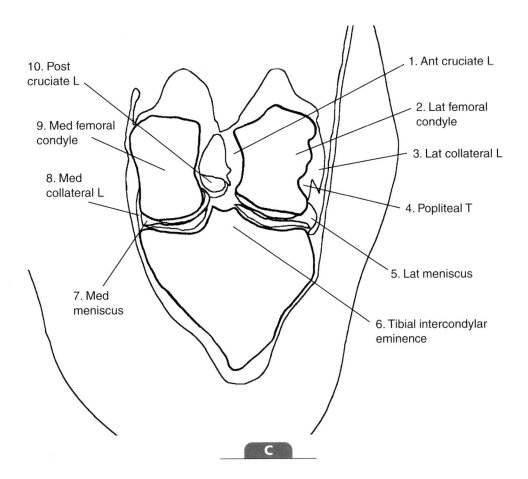

10. Post cruciate L

9. Med femoral condyle

8. Med collateral L

7. Med meniscus

1. Ant cruciate L

2. Lat femoral condyle

3. Lat collateral L

4. Popliteal T

5. Lat meniscus

6. Tibial intercondylar eminence

C

Anterior

Medial

Lateral

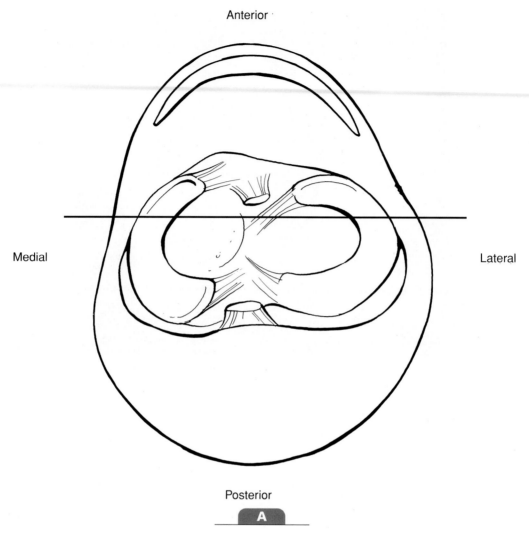

Posterior

A

Figure 8-29 Coronal MR image 3.

Figure 8-29 (A,B,C). In this image, the femoral condyles have joined with the body of the femur, and the shaft is shown extending upward. On the lower part of the image, the posterior tibia is again sectioned, demonstrating an intercondylar eminence that appears as a sharp projection upward between the medial and lateral condyles of the femur. Superior to the intercondylar eminence, the posterior cruciate ligament is sectioned medial to the anterior cruciate ligament as it extends upward to attach to the medial femoral condyle. On either side of the intercondylar eminence, the articular surfaces of the femur and the tibia are shown adjacent to each other except in regions of low signal intensity representing either the medial or lateral menisci. Forming the medial boundary of the knee joint, the medial collateral ligament is again longitudinally sectioned as it extends between the medial femoral condyle to the tibia. On the lateral surface of the knee joint, the popliteal tendon can be identified near its point of origin on the lateral femoral condyle. In this image, however, the lateral collateral ligament is indistinguishable because it separates from the articular capsule as it extends downward to attach to the head and styloid process of the fibula.

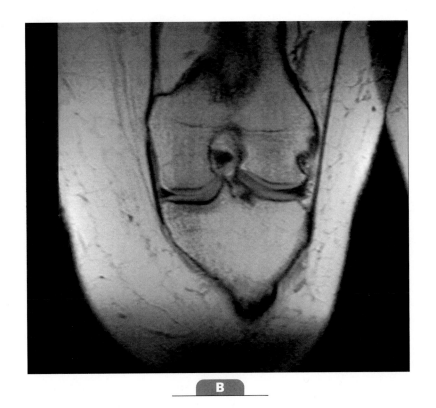

B

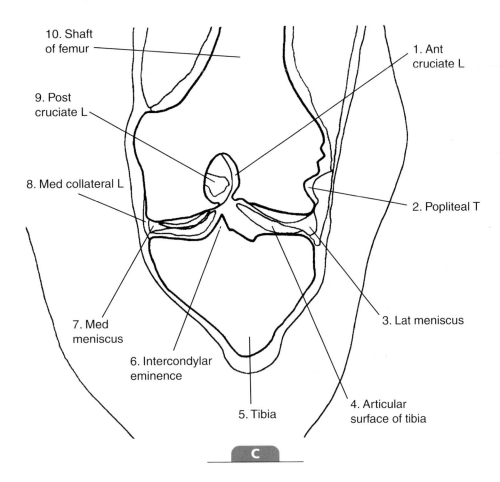

10. Shaft of femur

9. Post cruciate L

8. Med collateral L

7. Med meniscus

6. Intercondylar eminence

5. Tibia

1. Ant cruciate L

2. Popliteal T

3. Lat meniscus

4. Articular surface of tibia

C

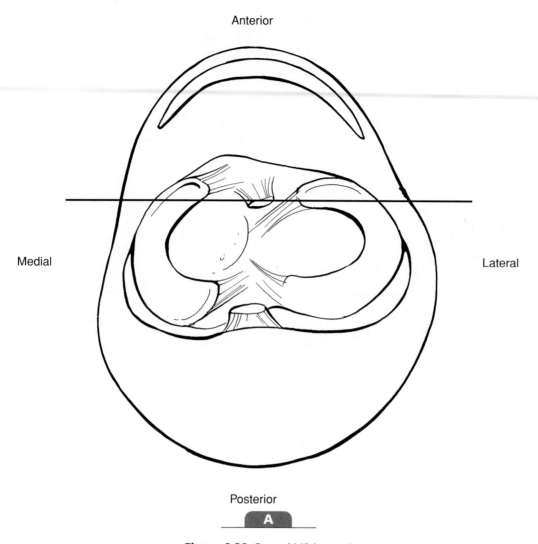

Figure 8-30 Coronal MR image 4.

Figure 8-30 (A,B,C). The medial and lateral femoral condyles are shown articulating with the proximal end of the tibia. Similar to previous images, the superior surface of the tibia is irregularly shaped owing to the intercondylar eminence projecting upward between the medial and lateral femoral condyles. Above the intercondylar eminence, the proximal end of the posterior cruciate ligament is shown near its site of attachment on the medial femoral condyle. By comparison, the distal end of the anterior cruciate ligament is shown near its origin, the anterior intercondylar fossa. On the medial side of the knee joint, a triangular region of low signal intensity represents the medial meniscus that lies adjacent to the medial collateral ligament. On the lateral side of the joint, the articular surfaces are separated by a thick lateral meniscus, indicating this plane of section traverses through the anterior part of the circular ligament.

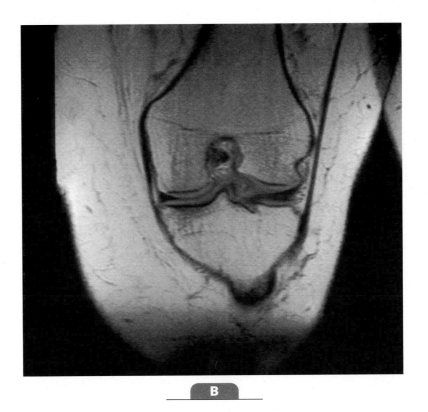

B

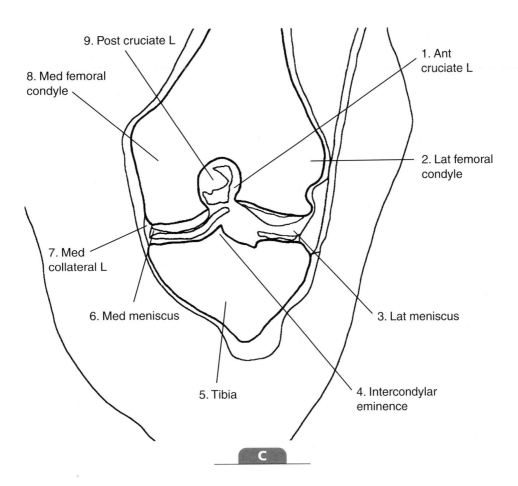

9. Post cruciate L

8. Med femoral condyle

1. Ant cruciate L

2. Lat femoral condyle

7. Med collateral L

6. Med meniscus

3. Lat meniscus

5. Tibia

4. Intercondylar eminence

C

Ankle

ANATOMICAL OVERVIEW

The ankle describes the region of articulation between the lower leg and the foot. Within this region, the ankle joint is formed by the distal tibia and fibula articulating with the talus. The ankle joint is considered a ginglymus, or hinge-type, joint that allows dorsiflexion and plantar flexion. The other movements of the foot are the result of articulations between the tarsal bones—calcaneus, talus, cuboid, navicular, and cuneiforms—which are considered arthrodial joints, because they are capable of gliding movements and have limited rotation.

Skeletal

Hint: The mnemonic for remembering the order of the tarsals is "*Come to Colorado Next 3 Christmases.*"

Calcaneus (*kal-KA-ne-ŭs*). Commonly called the heel bone; also called the os calcis. The upper part of this roughly quadrangular bone articulates with the talus and the cuboid bones (Fig. 8-31). Carries approximately 25% of the body's weight in the standing position.

Sustentaculum tali (*SŬS-ten-TAK-yū-lŭm TĀ-li*). The process on the upper medial calcaneus that acts as a shelf to

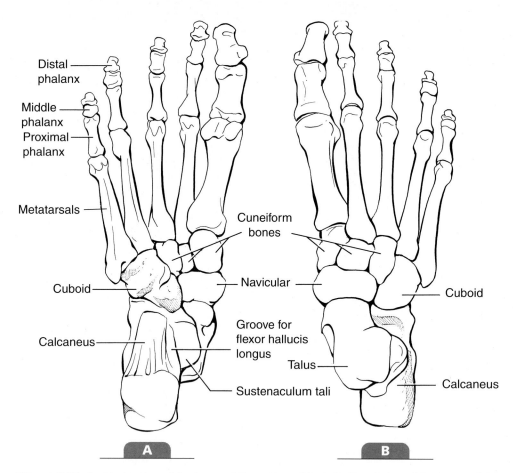

Distal phalanx
Middle phalanx
Proximal phalanx
Metatarsals
Cuboid
Calcaneus
Cuneiform bones
Navicular
Groove for flexor hallucis longus
Sustenaculum tali
Cuboid
Talus
Calcaneus

A **B**

Figure 8-31 A. Plantar view of the bones of the ankle and foot. **B.** Dorsal view of the bones of the ankle and foot.

support the head of the talus. On the lower surface, the process acts much like a pulley for the tendon of the flexor hallucis longus muscle as it passes through the medial side of the ankle.

Talus (*TĀ-lŭs*). Also called the astragalus (*as-TRAG-ă-lŭs*). The most proximal tarsal bone. Articulates with the tibia and fibula to form the ankle joint. On the distal end, it transmits approximately 50% of the body's weight to the calcaneus and navicular bones.

Cuboid (*KYŪ-boyd*). Resembles a cube and is found on the lateral side of the foot between the calcaneus and the bases of the fourth and fifth metatarsals.

Navicular (*nă-VIK-yū-lăr*). Also called the scaphoid (*SKAF-oyd*). Boat-shaped bone found between the talus and the three cuneiform bones on the medial side of the foot.

Cuneiforms (*KYŪ-nē-i-fōrmz*). Three tarsal bones located between the navicular and the bases of the first three metatarsals (Latin for "wedged shaped"). They are either numbered one to three from medial to lateral or are referred to as medial, intermediate, and lateral.

Metatarsals (*MET-ă-AR-sălz*). The five bones are numbered one to five from medial to lateral. On the proximal ends, their bases form arthrodial (gliding) joints with the cuboid and cuneiform bones. On the distal ends, their heads form ellipsoidal or condyloid joints with the proximal phalanges. In the standing position, the heads of the metatarsals of each foot bear 25% of the body's weight (10% on the first metatarsal and 3.75% each on the other metatarsals).

Musculature

Tibialis (*tib-ē-Ā-lis*) **anterior.** Origin: lateral tibial condyle and lateral tibia. Insertion: first cuneiform and base of first metatarsal. Action: dorsiflexes and inverts foot (Figs. 8-32 and 8-33).

Extensor hallucis (*HAL-lŭ-sis*) **longus.** Origin: middle anterior fibula. Insertion: distal phalanx of first digit. Action: extends first digit and everts foot.

Tibialis posterior. Origin: posterior shaft of tibia and upper shaft of fibula. Insertion: navicular, cuneiforms one, two, and three, cuboid, bases of second to fourth metatarsals. Action: adducts, plantar flexes, and inverts foot.

Flexor digitorum longus. Origin: posterior tibia below soleal line. Insertion: distal phalanges of digits two to five. Action: plantar flexes and inverts foot.

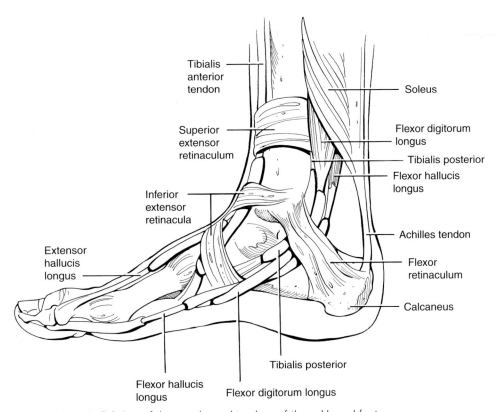

Figure 8-32 Medial view of the muscles and tendons of the ankle and foot.

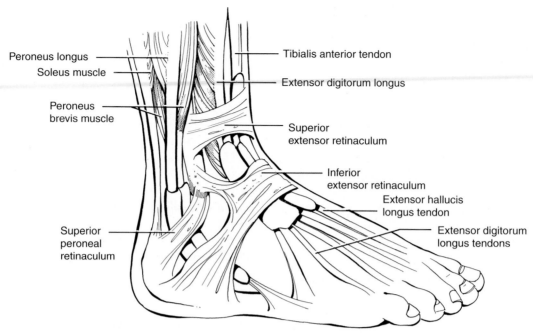

Figure 8-33 Lateral view of the muscles and tendons of the ankle and foot.

Flexor hallucis longus. Origin: lower two-thirds of posterior fibula. Insertion: distal phalanx of first digit. Action: flexes distal phalanx and inverts foot.

Extensor digitorum longus. Origin: lateral tibial condyle and anterior crest of fibula. Insertion: distal phalanges of digits two to five. Action: extends toes, dorsiflexes and everts foot.

Peroneus (*per-ō-NĒ-ŭs*) **longus and brevis.** Origin: head and shaft of fibula and lateral tibial condyle. Insertion: first cuneiform and fifth metatarsal. Action: plantar flexes and everts foot.

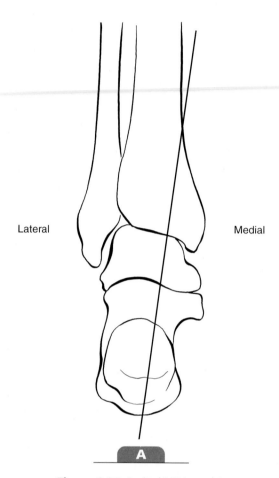

Lateral   Medial

Figure 8-34 Sagittal MR image 1.

SAGITTAL SECTION

The following are two selected sagittal MR images of the right ankle generated from medial to lateral at 100 mm intervals at the following technical factors: TR = 1100, TE = 20, RF = 90°, FOV = 16 cm, TH = 3.5 mm. Abbreviations: TR = repetition time, TE = echo-time, RF = radiofrequency, FOV = field of view, TH = slice thickness.

Figure 8-34 (A,B,C). This image demonstrates the medial side of the right ankle. With the exception of the distal tibia, all of the bones identified within this image are part of the medial arch of the foot. On the upper part of the image, the distal tibia is shown articulating with the talus, forming the ankle joint. Below the talus, interosseous ligaments extend through the subtalar joint between the talus and the calcaneus. Anterior to the talus, the boat-shaped navicular bone is cross-sectioned above the first cuneiform and the first metatarsal. On the plantar surface of the foot, it is difficult to discern the individual muscles and tendons. But on the posterior lower leg, an oblique section of the tendocalcaneus tendon is shown near its insertion on the posterior calcaneus. As described earlier for the knee, the medial and lateral heads of the gastrocnemius muscle insert through the tendocalcaneus tendon onto the posterior calcaneus and act to flex the lower leg, plantar flex, and invert the foot.

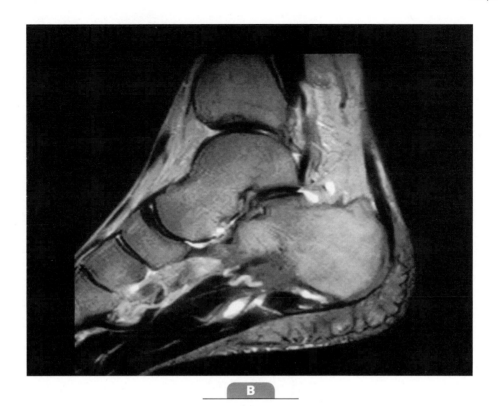

B

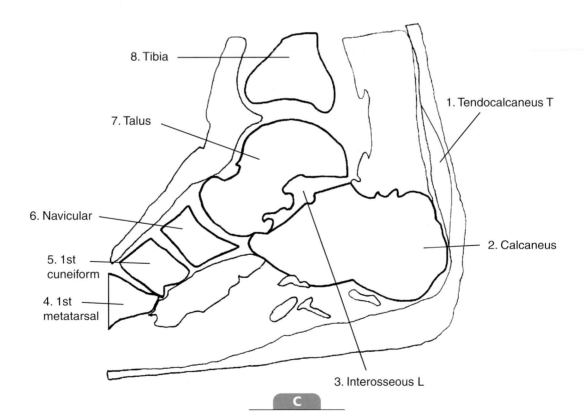

8. Tibia

7. Talus

6. Navicular

5. 1st cuneiform

4. 1st metatarsal

1. Tendocalcaneus T

2. Calcaneus

3. Interosseous L

C

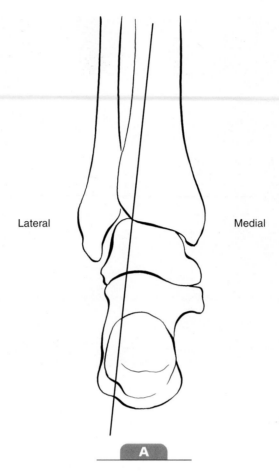

Lateral

Medial

A

Figure 8-35 Sagittal MR image 2.

Figure 8-35 (A,B,C). In contrast to the previous image, this section demonstrates much of the anatomy found within the lateral ankle. Similar to the previous image, the articulation between the distal tibia and talus form the ankle joint. Below the talus, the subtalar joint is formed between the calcaneus and the underside of the talus. Anteriorly, the talus articulates with the lateral part of the navicular and the calcaneus articulates with the cuboid, forming the calcaneocuboid joint. Because the cuneiforms are found anterior to the navicular bone, the second and third cuneiform can be identified within this image above the second and third metatarsals, respectively. As described earlier, the distal cuboid articulates with the bases of the fourth and fifth metatarsals, which are not in this section. Similar to the previous image, the tendocalcaneus tendon is found inserting on the posterior calcaneus, even though many ligaments and muscles on the plantar surface of the foot are difficult to discern.

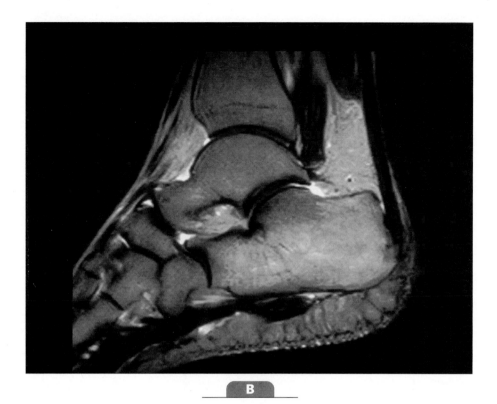

B

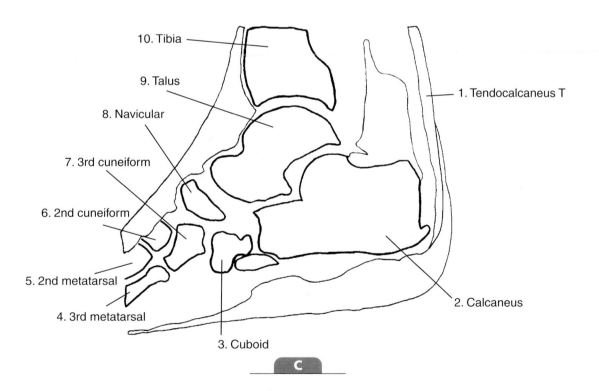

10. Tibia

9. Talus

8. Navicular

7. 3rd cuneiform

6. 2nd cuneiform

5. 2nd metatarsal

4. 3rd metatarsal

3. Cuboid

1. Tendocalcaneus T

2. Calcaneus

C

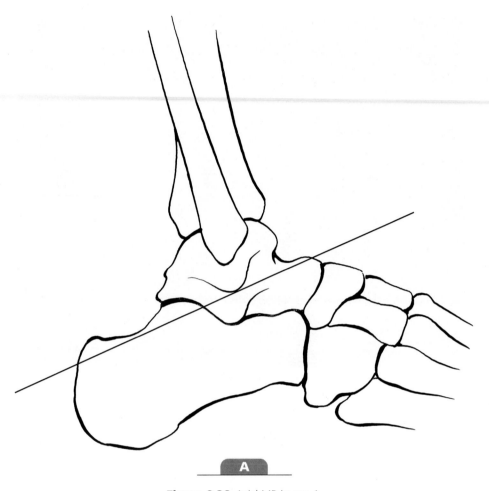

Figure 8-36 Axial MR image 1.

AXIAL MR IMAGES

The following are three selected axial MR images of the right ankle from superior to inferior generated at the following technical factors: TR = 1100, TE = 20, RF = 90°, FOV = 16 cm, TH = 3.5 mm. Abbreviations; TR = repetition time, TE = echo-time, RF = radiofrequency, FOV = field of view, TH = slice thickness.

Figure 8-36 (A,B,C). This image demonstrates the anatomy just below the ankle joint, because the two parts of the talus can be identified. The upper part of the talus, posterior to the hatched line, represents the surface that articulates with the distal tibia and fibula, forming the ankle joint. The distal part of the talus, anterior to the hatched line, articulates with the underlying tarsals. Posteriorly, the upper calcaneus appears irregularly shaped, because the sustentaculum tali is projecting medially. Appearing as low signal areas, a variety of tendons can be found surrounding these bones. Similar to the sagittal sections, the broad, flat region of low signal intensity posterior to the calcaneus represents the tendocalcaneus tendon. Medial to the sustentaculum tali, the tendon of the flexor hallucis longus muscle is shown as it extends through the medial side of the ankle from its origin on the posterior fibula to insert on the distal phalanx of the first digit. Near the anterior margin of the sustentaculum tali, the flexor digitorum longus tendon is shown as it passes along the medial side of the ankle extending from its origin on the posterior tibia to insert on the distal phalanges of the second to fifth digits. Lying near the posteromedial border of the talus, the tibialis posterior tendon is obliquely sectioned extending through the medial ankle from the muscle, which originates on the tibia and fibula, to insert on the tarsals anterior to the talus and the bases of the second to fourth metatarsals. On the anterior part of the ankle, the tibialis anterior, the extensor hallucis longus, and the extensor digitorum tendons are also sectioned as they extend downward from muscles in the lower leg to insert on the foot. On the lateral side of the ankle, the peroneus brevis and longus tendons are cross-sectioned near the anterior calcaneus.

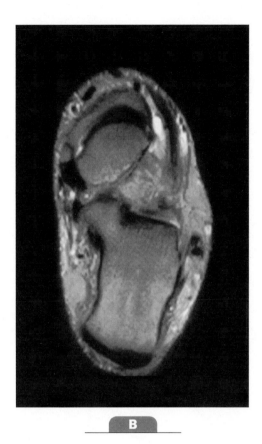

B

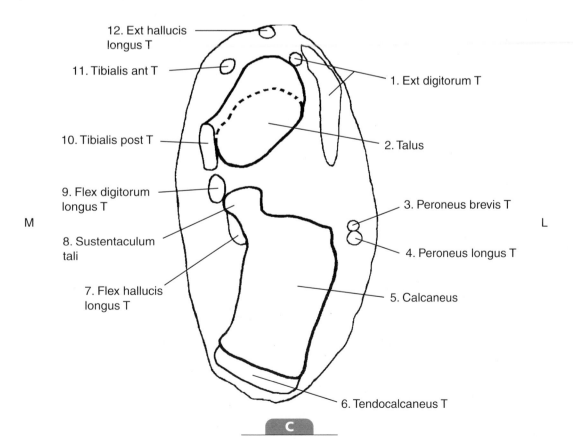

12. Ext hallucis longus T

11. Tibialis ant T

10. Tibialis post T

9. Flex digitorum longus T

8. Sustentaculum tali

7. Flex hallucis longus T

1. Ext digitorum T

2. Talus

3. Peroneus brevis T

4. Peroneus longus T

5. Calcaneus

6. Tendocalcaneus T

M

L

C

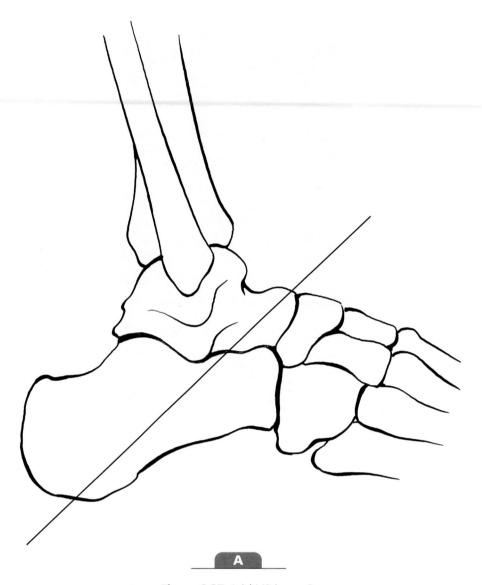

Figure 8-37 Axial MR image 2.

Figure 8-37 (A,B,C). Owing to the absence of either upper or lower articular surfaces on the talus, this image demonstrates the middle of the talus with the more posteriorly situated upper calcaneus. Similar to the previous image, the flexor hallucis longus, the flexor digitorum longus, and the tibialis posterior tendons are found on the medial side of the ankle. Anterior to the talus, the tibialis anterior tendon is sectioned extending downward to insert on the first cuneiform and the base of the first metatarsal. The most anterior tendon demonstrated is the extensor hallucis longus muscle, which originates from the anterior fibula and inserts on the distal phalanx of the first digit. Lateral to the talus, the extensor digitorum muscle tendon is sectioned as it extends downward to insert on the distal phalanges of the second to fifth digits. On the lateral side of the calcaneus, the tendons of the peroneus brevis and longus muscles are again shown in cross-section; the peroneus brevis is the more anterior. On the posterior aspect of the calcaneus, the tendocalcaneus appears as a broad, flat tendon.

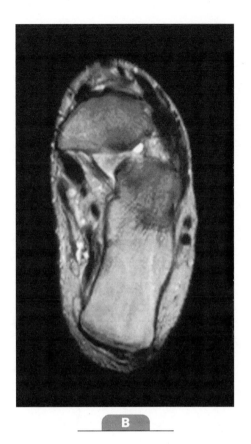

B

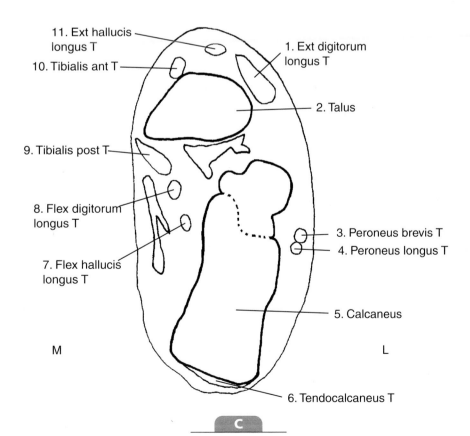

11. Ext hallucis
longus T

10. Tibialis ant T

1. Ext digitorum
longus T

2. Talus

9. Tibialis post T

8. Flex digitorum
longus T

7. Flex hallucis
longus T

3. Peroneus brevis T
4. Peroneus longus T

5. Calcaneus

M

L

6. Tendocalcaneus T

C

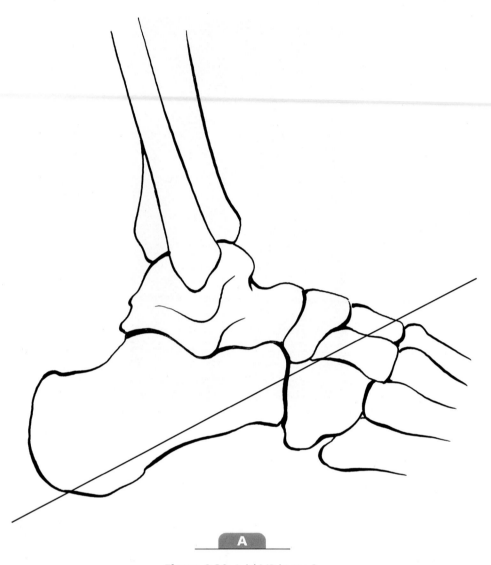

Figure 8-38 Axial MR image 3.

Figure 8-38 (A,B,C). This image is below the level of the talus and navicular and demonstrates most of the bones associated with forming the transverse arch of the foot. Posteriorly, the calcaneus is shown projecting toward the cuboid, forming the calcaneocuboid joint. Anterior and medial to the cuboid, the three wedge-shaped cuneiform bones can be identified and are labeled one, two, and three, based on their location. Similar to the sagittal images, the muscles and tendons on the plantar surface of the foot are difficult to discern; however, the peroneus brevis and longus tendons can be identified on the lateral surface of the calcaneus. As described earlier, the peroneus longus and brevis muscles originate from the upper part of the fibula and tibia and extend down around the lateral surface of the ankle to insert on the first cuneiform and fifth metatarsal.

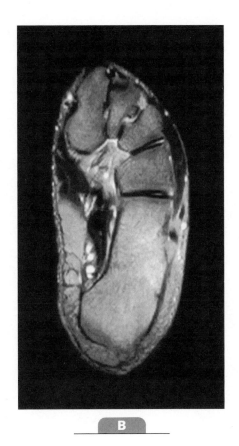

B

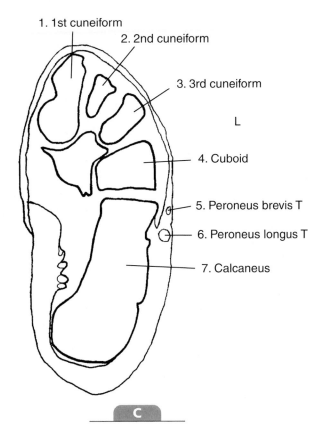

1. 1st cuneiform

2. 2nd cuneiform

3. 3rd cuneiform

M   L

4. Cuboid

5. Peroneus brevis T

6. Peroneus longus T

7. Calcaneus

C

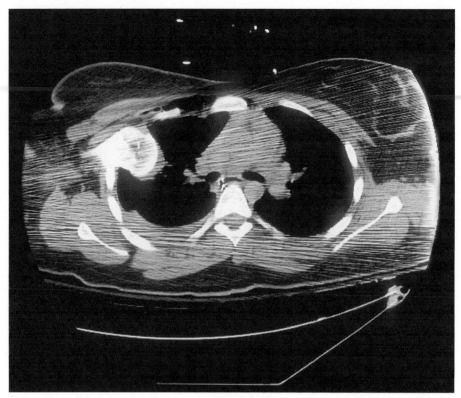

Figure 8-39

Supplement 8-1. *Figure 8-39 shows a 14-year-old girl who was in a motor vehicle accident that resulted in the dislocation of her right shoulder and upper ribs. The impact of the collision projected the right humerus through the chest wall and into the right upper lobe of the lung, causing a pneumothorax and hemothorax. The force of the trauma also caused an impaction fracture of the humeral head and an avulsion fracture of the greater tubercle. Because the right humerus could not be raised above the patient's chest for scanning, beam hardening resulted in streak artifacts that point to the shaft of the humerus. Unfortunately, the brachial plexus of nerves within the axilla were damaged by the dislocation of the humerus. After extensive surgery, the girl regained only limited use of her right arm.*

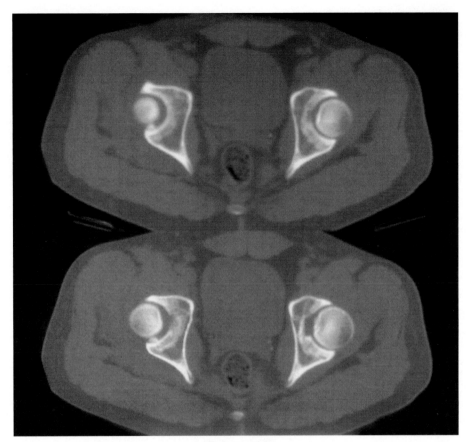

Figure 8-40

Supplement 8-2. *Figure 8-40 shows a 30-year-old man who was injured in a construction acci-dent that dislocated his right hip superolaterally and posteriorly with respect to the acetabulum. After reduction, these CT images were generated at bone window settings through the upper acetabula. On the right side, a small fragment of bone was shown between the femoral head and the posterior acetabulum. The bone fragment originated from the acetabular lip and was surgically removed. After completing physical therapy, the patient was able to resume full range of motion in his hip joint.*

REVIEW QUESTIONS

1. The ankle joint is formed between the_____, _____ and_____.
2. The ankle joint is classified as what type of joint?
   A. Ginglymus
   B. Arthrodial
   C. Enarthroses
   D. Syndesmosis
3. Describe the shoulder girdle.
4. List the bones forming the knee joint:_____, _____, and_____.
5. The hip joint is classified as what type of joint?
   A. Ginglymus
   B. Arthrodial
   C. Enarthroses
   D. Syndesmosis
6. The_____ joint is considered the largest joint in the body.
7. The_____ meniscus is described as a nearly circular ligament within the knee joint.
8. Describe the function of the glenoid labrum.
9. The capitulum is the articular surface that articulates with the ulna. True or false
10. Which of the following articulates with the base of the third metatarsal?
    A. Cuboid
    B. Navicular
    C. Second cuneiform
    D. Third cuneiform
11. Describe the attachments of the lateral collateral ligament.
12. List the muscles making up the rotator cuff found within the shoulder.
13. The coronoid fossa is located on the [anterior / posterior] side of the humerus.
14. The cuboid is found on the [medial / lateral] side of the ankle.
15. The trochlea of the humerus articulates with the
    A. Glenoid fossa
    B. Clavicle
    C. Radius
    D. Ulna
16. On an axial image of the ankle, which tendon is *not* found on the medial surface of the leg?
    A. Peroneus longus
    B. Tibialis posterior
    C. Flexor hallucis longus
    D. Flexor digitorum longus
17. List in order from lateral to medial the proximal row of carpal bones.
18. Approximately 75% of carpal fractures are found within the_____.
19. The anterior cruciate extends from the_____ intercondylar fossa to the back of the_____ femoral condyle.
20. The hamulus is found on which carpal bone?
    A. Scaphoid
    B. Hamate
    C. Capitate
    D. Lunate

Answers to Review Questions

Chapter 2

1. The azygos vein is located inside the right posterior thoracic cage adjacent to the right side of the vertebral bodies. It drains the posterior thorax and upper abdomen into the superior vena cava.
2. C
3. Lamina
4. True
5. A
6. C
7. A
8. A
9. Left
10. B
11. Left
12. Parietal pleura / visceral pleura
13. Upper
14. B
15. The vein that drains the left axillary vein of the upper limb and shoulder girdle into the left brachiocephalic vein. Compared to adjacent structures, the vein lies just anterior and adjacent to the left subclavian artery.
16. B
17. A
18. Hilum
19. 2 / 2 / 7 / 2 / 4 / 1
20. Left atrium

Chapter 3

1. Diaphragm / greater or false pelvis
2. Right renal vein
3. The spleen lies against the diaphragm on the upper left side of the abdomen within the thoracic cage. Its size and shape vary considerably, partially depending on the adjacent structures. The anterior surface is next to the stomach, the posterior surface is next to the left kidney, the superior surface is next to the diaphragm, and the inferior surface is next to the left splenic flexure of the colon.
4. C
5. Hepatic duct, portal vein, and proper hepatic artery

6. B
7. Caudate
8. It is found immediately posterior to the stomach and the pancreas.
9. Celiac trunk, superior mesenteric, renal, inferior mesenteric, and common iliac
10. A
11. D
12. Vein
13. The major part of digestion occurs in the small intestine, which extends from the termination of the stomach to the large intestine. The small intestine ranges from 5 to 8 m in length and is made up of three segments: the duodenum, the jejunum, and the ileum.
14. Gallbladder
15. Fundus, body, and pyloric
16. Visceral peritoneum / parietal peritoneum
17. Right
18. Inferior mesenteric / splenic
19. The mesentery is a double layer of peritoneum that encloses the intestine and attaches it to the abdominal wall. Owing to constant moving and changes in shape, much of the intestine is described as having no fixed position but is only loosely organized by the mesentery. The mesentery also contains the arteries and veins of the intestines and is a site for fat storage within the body.
20. C

Chapter 4

1. Internal iliac artery
2. D
3. Ilium / pubis / ischium
4. False
5. B
6. C
7. D
8. A
9. Above
10. A
11. Posterior
12. C

13. D
14. D
15. Fundus: the dome-shaped roof of the uterus found above the oviduct. Body: the largest part of the uterus; centrally located and tapered in shape. Cervix: the most inferior constricted region of the uterus opening into the vagina.
16. D
17. D
18. Vertebral foramina
19. Fornix
20. The first image must be above the iliac crest, and the last image must be below the ischium.

Chapter 5

1. Base of the skull
2. Vomer and ethmoid
3. Ovale
4. This pair of bones forms the posterior part of the hard palate. Because the bones are L-shaped, they also form part of the lateral walls and floor of the nasal cavity.
5. B
6. Also referred to as the inner lobe of the brain, the insula lies at the bottom of the Sylvian fissure and is covered by the frontal, parietal, and temporal lobes.
7. Dura mater / arachnoid mater / pia mater
8. C
9. Located on either side, the fornix is an arched tract of fibers that join together posteriorly under the splenium of the corpus callosum. Together, these arches form the roof of the third ventricle.
10. A
11. A
12. Deep within the temporal lobe, this curved sheet of gray matter extends upward into the floor of the lateral ventricle. Considered part of the limbic system, the hippocampal formation is involved in the emotional aspects of behavior.
13. Superior cistern
14. D
15. Magnum
16. Arising from the internal carotid artery near the hypothalamus, the artery extends laterally as it travels upward through the Sylvian fissure.
17. A
18. Sphenoid
19. A
20. D

Chapter 6

1. Base of the skull / bony thoracic cage
2. Axis
3. D

4. Third
5. C
6. Laryngeal vestibule / glottic space / infraglottic space
7. It is located between the posterior tongue and the epiglottis, on either side of the median glossoepiglottic fold.
8. True
9. C3 / C4
10. C
11. It is a space within the larynx bounded by the vestibular folds and the vocal folds, also called the ventricle.
12. C
13. False
14. Thyroid cartilage / anterior
15. Valleculae
16. Arytenoid / cricoid
17. A
18. Nasopharynx / oropharynx / laryngeal pharynx
19. Thyroid
20. Subclavian

Chapter 7

1. 7 / 12 / 5 / 5
2. C2 / L5
3. Costal facets on the vertebral body and transverse processes
4. A
5. Anulus fibrosus
6. True
7. It is a layer of dense connective tissue tightly attached to the posterior surfaces of vertebrae and intervertebral disks, extending from C2 to the sacrum
8. Inferior articular process / superior articular process
9. L5 vertebral body / L5-S1 intervertebral disk / S1 vertebral segment
10. B
11. Motor
12. Inferior articular process
13. Within the intervertebral foramen at the origin of the spinal nerve
14. Pia
15. True
16. B
17. Cauda equina
18. Posterior
19. Sacrum
20. A

Chapter 8

1. Talus / tibia / fibula
2. A
3. The shoulder girdle consists of two bones—the clavicle and the scapula—that attach to the axial skeleton via

the sternoclavicular joint. On the opposite end of the shoulder girdle, the shoulder joint is formed by the glenoid fossa of the scapula, which articulates with the head of the humerus to form a enarthrodial, or ball-and-socket, joint.

4. Femur / tibia / patella
5. C
6. Knee
7. Lateral
8. This ridge of fibrocartilage acts to deepen the glenoid fossa and protect the bone.
9. False
10. D
11. It extends from the lateral femoral condyle to the head and styloid process of the fibula.
12. Supraspinatus, subscapularis, infraspinatus, and teres minor
13. Anterior
14. Lateral
15. D
16. A
17. Scaphoid, lunate, triquetral, and pisiform
18. Scaphoid
19. Anterior / lateral
20. B

Glossary

A

Abduct. To move away from midline; opposite of adduct.

Adduct. To move toward the midline of the body; opposite of abduct.

Afferent. Carrying toward a center.

Alveolus. A small, hollow area or cavity; bony socket of a tooth; pouch in lung air sac.

Ampulla. A sac-like dilation of a duct or tube.

Annulus. A ring-shaped opening or structure.

Antrum. A nearly closed cavity or chamber; often within a bone.

Artery. A blood vessel that carries blood away from the heart.

Articular. Refers to an articulation or a joint.

Articulation. A joint or connection between bones.

Atrophy. A wasting away of tissue; results in a decrease in tissue size.

Axial. A section perpendicular to the median.

Axillary. Pertaining to the armpit.

Axon. The process of a neuron that carries the impulse away from the cell body.

Azygos. Certain vessels or nerves not in pairs.

B

Benign. An abnormal slow growth of tissue that remains discrete in an area.

Bifurcate. To divide or separate into two parts.

Body. The broadest or longest mass of a structure.

Brachial. Pertaining to the arm.

Bursa. A sac or pouch of synovial fluid located between friction points, especially in the region of the joints.

C

Cancer. A malignant, invasive growth of abnormal tissue that has the capability to spread throughout the body.

Cardiac. Pertaining to the heart.

Cartilage. A tough fibrous connective tissue.

Central nervous system. The brain and the spinal cord.

Chronic. Persisting for a long time.

Concave. Having a curved, depressed surface.

Condyle. A rounded projection at the end of a bone that articulates with another bone.

Convex. Having a curved protruding surface.

Coronal. A longitudinal section that runs at right angles to sagittal planes dividing the body into anterior and posterior parts.

Cortex. The outer surface layer of an organ.

Costal. Pertaining to the ribs.

Cranial. Pertaining to the skull.

Crest. A bony ridge or border.

Cruciate. Overlapping or cross-shaped structures.

Cyst. A sac with a distinct wall containing fluid or other material.

D

Dendrite. The process of a neuron that conducts the impulse toward the cell body.

Diaphragm. Any partition that separates one area from another.

Diarthrosis. A freely movable joint.

Dislocation. Displacement of a bone from a joint space.

Distal. Farthest from the center or the midpoint.

Dorsal. Pertaining to the back or posterior.

Duct. A canal or passageway.

E

Edema. An abnormal accumulation of fluid within the body causing swelling.

Efferent. Carrying away from an area or an organ.

Epicondyle. An elevation near a condyle.

Extremity. A limb, such as the arm or the leg.

F

Fascia. A connective tissue wrapping around muscular structures and other tissues.

Fissure. A groove or cleft.

Flexor. A muscle that decreases the angle between bones.

Foramen. A hole or opening in a bone or between body cavities.

Fossa. A shallow depression often forming an articular surface.

Fovea. A small pit or depression for attachment rather than articulation.

Fundus. The base of an organ.

G

Ganglion. A group of nerve cell bodies usually located outside the central nervous system.

Genu. Any structure that resembles a flexed knee.

Gland. An organ specialized to secrete or excrete substances within the body.

Glenoid. Having the form of a shallow cavity or articular depression or socket of a joint.

Gyrus. A convolution on the outer cerebral cortex.

H

Hematoma. A blood clot located outside a blood vessel.

Hypertrophy. An increase in the size of a tissue or organ beyond normal growth.

I

Inguinal. Pertaining to the groin region near the thigh.

Innervation. The supply or distribution of nerve stimuli to a part.

Insertion. The place of attachment for a muscle on the movable end.

Invert. To turn inward.

J

Joint. The junction of two or more bones forming an articulation.

Jugular. Belonging to the neck.

L

Labia. A lip-like structure.

Lacrimal. Pertaining to tears.

Lamina. A plate or thin layer.

Ligament. A concentration of fibrous tissue connecting bones or parts.

Lobe. A curved or rounded structure or projection.

Lumen. The space inside a tube.

Lymph. The watery fluid in lymph vessels.

M

Malignant. Pertains to diseases that are likely to spread.

Meatus. The external opening of a canal.

Medial. Toward the midline of the body.

Mesentery. The double layer of peritoneum that attaches the intestine to the posterior abdominal wall.

Mucous membranes. The membranes that line the digestive, respiratory, reproductive, and urinary tracts.

Muscle. Organ capable of contraction and producing movement.

Myelin. The white substance forming a sheath around the axon of some nerve cells.

N

Nasal. Relating to the nose.

Neoplasm. Any new and abnormal growth of tissue.

Nerve. A group of nerve cell fibers found outside the central nervous system.

Neuron. The basic unit of the nervous system made up of the nerve cell body plus its processes.

Nucleus. A collection or concentration of nerve cell bodies within the central nervous system.

O

Omentum. Folds of peritoneum connecting the abdominal viscera with the stomach.

Optic. Pertaining to the eye.

Organ. A part of the body composed of two or more tissues to perform a specialized function.

Origin. The end of attachment of a muscle that remains fixed during contraction.

P

Palate. The roof of the mouth.

Palmar. The anterior surface of the hands.

Palpation. Examination by touch.

Parenchyma. The functional or glandular components of an organ.

Peripheral nervous system. A system of nerves connecting the outer parts of the body with the central nervous system.

Plexus. A network of nerves, blood vessels, or lymphatics.

Proximal. Toward the attached end of a limb or the center.

Pulmonary. Pertaining to the lungs.

R

Ramus. A branch of a bone, vessel, or nerve.

Renal. Pertaining to the kidney.

S

Spine. A short, pointed projection of bone.

Stroma. The supportive elements of an organ including connective tissue, nerves, and vessels.

Sulcus. A furrow or linear groove that is not as deep as a fissure.

Supine. The body lying horizontally with the face upward.

Suture. Immovable joints that bind bones together.

Symphysis. A slightly movable joint between the right and left sides of the pelvis, which join in the midline.

Systemic. Pertaining to the whole body.

T

Tendon. A dense band of fibrous tissue that join a muscle to a bone.

Tissue. A group of similar cells that form a distinct structure.

Trauma. An injury or wound usually produced by external forces acting on the body.

Trochanter. A large blunt process.

Trochlea. A spool-shaped or pulley-like articular surface.

Tubercle. A small rounded process or bump.

Tuberosity. A large conspicuous bump, larger than a tubercle.

Tumor. An abnormal growth of cells.

V

Vas. A duct or vessel that conveys a liquid.

Vein. A vessel carrying blood away from the tissue toward the heart.

Ventral. Toward the anterior or the front.

Ventricle. A small cavity or pouch; found in the heart and brain.

Vesicle. A liquid filled pouch or sac.

Vestibule. A chamber or space resembling an entrance to some other body cavity or space.

Viscera. The internal organs.

Bibliography

A

Afifi AK, Bergman RA. Basic neuroscience. Baltimore: Urban & Schwarzenberg, 1980.

Agur AMR, Lee MJ. Grant's atlas of anatomy. 9th ed. Baltimore: Williams & Wilkins, 1993.

Akesson EJ, Loeb JA, Wilson-Pauwels L. Thomson's core textbook of anatomy. 2nd ed. Philadelphia: Lippincott, 1990.

Anderson D, Keith J, Novak P, Elliot M. Dorland's illustrated medical dictionary. 28th ed. Philadelphia: Saunders, 1994.

Anderson JE. Grant's atlas of anatomy. 8th ed. Baltimore: Williams & Wilkins, 1983.

B

Ballinger PW. Merill's atlas of radiographic positions and radiologic procedures. 7th ed. 3 vols. St. Louis: Mosby, 1991.

Barrett CP, Anderson, LD, Holder LE, Poliakoff SJ. Primer of sectional anatomy with MRI and CT correlation. 2nd ed. Baltimore: Williams & Wilkins, 1994.

Basmajian JV, Slonecker CE. Grant's method of anatomy. 11th ed. Baltimore: Williams & Wilkins, 1989.

Bates B. A guide to physical examination. 3rd ed. Philadelphia: Lippincott, 1983.

Berquist TH. Pocket atlas of MRI body anatomy. 2nd ed. Philadelphia: Lippincott & Raven, 1995.

Bo W, Wolfman N, Krueger W, Meschan I. Basic atlas of sectional anatomy with correlated imaging. 2nd ed. Philadelphia: Saunders, 1990.

Bontrager KL. Textbook of radiographic positioning and related anatomy. 3rd ed. St. Louis: Mosby Year Book, 1993.

C

Cahill DR, Orland MJ. Atlas of human cross-sectional anatomy. Philadelphia: Lea & Febiger, 1984.

Christoforidis JA. Atlas of axial, sagittal, and coronal anatomy with CT and MRI. Philadelphia: Saunders, 1988.

Clemente CD, ed. Gray's anatomy of the human body. 30th ed. Philadelphia: Lea & Febiger, 1985.

Crafts RC. A textbook of human anatomy. 3rd ed. New York: Churchill Livingstone, 1985.

E

Eisenberg RL. Clinical imaging: an atlas of differential diagnosis. 2nd ed. Gaithersburg, MD: Aspen, 1992.

Eisenberg R, Dennis C. Comprehensive radiographic pathology. St. Louis: Mosby, 1990.

Ellis H, Logan BM, Dixon A. Human cross-sectional anatomy atlas of body sections and CT images. Oxford, UK: Butterworth-Heinemann, 1991.

F

Frick H, Kummer B, Putz R. Wolf-Heidegger's atlas of human anatomy. 4th ed. Farmington, CT: Karger, 1990.

G

Gardner E, Gray DJ, O'Rahilly R. Anatomy: a regional study of human structure. 4th ed. Philadelphia: Saunders, 1975.

Grossman CG, Gonzalez CF, Palacio E. Computed brain and orbital tomography. Technique and interpretation. New York: Wiley, 1976.

H

Hamilton WJ, ed. Textbook of human anatomy. 2nd ed. St. Louis: Mosby, 1976.

Hollinshead WH, Rosse C. Textbook of anatomy. 4th ed. New York: Harper & Row, 1985.

House EL, Rosse C. A systemic approach to neuroanatomy. 3rd ed. New York: McGraw-Hill, 1979.

I

International Anatomical Nomenclature Committee. Nomina anatomica. 6th ed. Baltimore: Waverly, 1989.

K

Kelley LL, Petersen CM. Sectional anatomy. St. Louis: Mosby, 1997.

L

Lane A, Sharfaei H. Modern sectional anatomy. Philadelphia: Saunders, 1992.

Langman J, Woerdeman MW. Atlas of medical anatomy. Philadelphia: Saunders, 1982.

Laudicina PF. Applied pathology for radiographers. Philadelphia: Saunders, 1989.

Lee JKT, Sagel SS, Stanley RJ. Computed body tomography with MRI correlation. 2nd ed. New York: Raven, 1989.

M

Mace DM, Kowalczyk N. Radiographic pathology for technologists. 2nd ed. St. Louis: Mosby Year Book, 1994.

McGrath P, Mills P. Atlas of sectional anatomy. Farmington, CT: Karger, 1985.

McMinn RMH, Hutchings RT. Color atlas of human anatomy. 2nd ed. Chicago: Year Book Medical, 1988.

Meschan I. An atlas of anatomy basic to radiology. Philadelphia: Lea & Febiger, 1975.

Moore KL. Clinically oriented anatomy. 3rd ed. Baltimore: Williams & Wilkins, 1992.

N

Nolte J. The human brain. 3rd ed. St. Louis: Mosby, 1992.

Norkin C, LeVange P. Joint structure and function: a comprehensive analysis. Philadelphia: FA Davis, 1983.

Novellin RA, Squire LF. Living anatomy, a working atlas using computed tomography, magnetic resonance and angiography images. Philadelphia: Hanley & Belfus, 1987.

P

Pansky B. Review of gross anatomy. 5th ed. New York: Macmillan, 1984.

R

Robbins SL, Kumar V. Basic pathology. 4th ed. Philadelphia: Saunders, 1987.

Rodgers AW. Textbook of anatomy. New York: Churchill Livingstone, 1992.

Romanes GJ, ed. Cunningham's manuals of practical anatomy. 15th ed. 3 vols. London: Oxford University Press, 1986.

S

Seeram ERT. Computed tomography technology. Philadelphia: Saunders, 1982.

Slaby FJ, McCune SK, Summers RW. Gross anatomy in the practice of medicine. Philadelphia: Lea & Febiger, 1994.

Smith JW, Murphy TR, Blair JSG, Lowe KG. Regional anatomy illustrated. New York: Chuchill Livingstone, 1983.

Snell RS. Clinical anatomy for medical students. 4th ed. Boston: Little, Brown, 1992.

Soderberg GL. Kinesiology, application to pathological motion. Baltimore: Williams & Wilkins, 1986.

T

Tortora GR, Anagnostakos NP. Principles of anatomy and physiology. 4th ed. New York: Harper & Row, 1984.

Twietmeyer A, McCracken T. Regional guide to human anatomy. Philadelphia: Lea & Febiger, 1988.

W

Wagner M, Lawson TL. Segmental anatomy. New York: Macmillan, 1982.

Wegener OH. Whole body computed tomography. 2nd ed. Boston: Blackwell Scientific, 1992.

Weir J, Abrahams PH, eds. An imaging atlas of human anatomy. St. Louis: Mosby Year Book, 1992.

Wicke L. Atlas of radiologic anatomy. 5th ed. Philadelphia: Lea & Febiger, 1994.

Williams PL, Warwick R, eds. Gray's anatomy. 36th ed. Philadelphia: Saunders, 1980.

Woodburne RT. Essentials of human anatomy. 9th ed. New York: Oxford University Press, 1994.

Index

Pages in *italics* indicate illustrations.

577